Paediatrics

A CLINICAL GUIDE FOR NURSE PRACTITIONERS

For Jonathan and Caitlin Carr, you two are my everything

For Butterworth-Heinemann:

Commissioning Editor: Susan Young
Project Development Manager: Catherine Jackson
Project Manager: Derek Robertson
Design Direction: George Ajayi

Paediatrics

A CLINICAL GUIDE FOR NURSE PRACTITIONERS

Edited by

Katie Barnes RGN, RSCN, BSc (Hons), MSc, MPH, CPNP
Certified Paediatric Nurse Practitioner

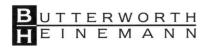
BUTTERWORTH
HEINEMANN

An imprint of Elsevier Science Limited
EDINBURGH LONDON NEW YORK OXFORD PHILADELPHIA ST LOUIS SYDNEY TORONTO 2003

BUTTERWORTH-HEINEMANN
An imprint of Elsevier Science Limited

First published 2003

ISBN 07506 49577

British Library Cataloguing in Publication Data
A catalogue record for this book is available from the British Library

Library of Congress Cataloging in Publication Data
A catalog record for this book is available from the Library of Congress

Note
Medical knowledge is constantly changing. As new information becomes available,
changes in treatment, procedures, equipment and the use of drugs become necessary.
The editor, contributors and the publishers have taken care to ensure that the
information given in this text is accurate and up to date. However, readers are strongly
advised to confirm that the information, especially with regard to drug usage, diagnosis
and illness management, complies with the latest legislation and standards of practice.

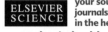 your source for books,
journals and multimedia
in the health sciences
www.elsevierhealth.com

The
publisher's
policy is to use
**paper manufactured
from sustainable forests**

Printed in China

Contents

Contents

Contributors

Editor

Katie Barnes MSc MPH BSc(Hons) CPNP
Katie Barnes is a Certified Paediatric
Nurse Practitioner (CPNP) who emigrated
from America in 1997. Originally from
Cape Cod, she received her undergraduate
nurse training in Boston at Northeastern
University in 1986 and subsequently
moved to New York City where she
completed a Master of Science degree in
Paediatric Primary Care at Columbia
University in 1989. After achieving her
National Board Certification as a PNP,
she was named as a Fellow in the National
Association of Paediatric Nurse
Practitioners and began working with
disenfranchised children on mobile
medical units in the New York homeless
and foster care systems. Katie followed
this with a PNP position in paediatric
haematology at Columbia-Presbyterian
Medical Centre until she travelled to the
jungles of Guatemala to work with Mayan
children in rural villages. She returned
from Central America to conduct a
community-based, randomised controlled
trial for the New York City Department
of Health and Columbia University
School of Public Health where she also
completed a Master of Public Health in
1996. Upon arriving in England, she
worked as a lecturer in child health and a
paediatric nurse practitioner (PNP) until
she moved to Liverpool in 2002 (where
she continues her practice and consulting
work). During her 6 years in England,
Katie has been very fortunate to
collaborate in the education, training
and policy development of advanced
paediatric nursing practice; she lectures,
consults and presents widely on a variety
of educational, clinical and advanced
practice policy issues.

Medical Consultant

Peter Wilson MBChB, MRCPCH
Peter received his medical degree in
1993 from the University of Cape Town,
South Africa. After working in primary
care paediatrics for 2 years he arrived in
the UK where he has worked in
paediatrics ever since. He became
a member of the Royal College of
Paediatrics and Child Health in 1997
and is currently in his final year as
a Specialist Registrar in paediatric and
cardiac intensive care at Great Ormond
Street Hospital. His special interests are
sepsis and the critically ill child.

Pharmacy Consultant

Sara Higginson BPharm, MRPharmS
Sara qualified as a pharmacist from
Bradford University in 1992 and
subsequently accepted a post at Ipswich
Hospital in Suffolk. In 1994 she received
her London Diploma in Pharmacy
Practice from the London School of
Pharmacy. Sara chose to pursue paediatric
and neonatal pharmacy in 1997.

Contributors

Andrea G Abbott DBO(T) BSc(Hons) SRO
Clinical Tutor/Orthoptist,
Maidstone Ophthalmic Hospital,
Maidstone
    10.7 Amplyopia and strabismus

Dolsie Allen MSc RN CFNP
Former Senior Lecturer,
Nurse Practitioner Programme,
Saint Martin's College, Lancaster
    14.3 Vulvo-vaginitis in the
       prepubescent girls
    14.5 Sexually transmitted infections

Gilly Andrews RGN ENBAO8 ENB8103
Clinical Nurse Specialist in
Family Planning,
King's College Hospital
NHS Trust, London
    14.4 Adolescent contraception

Katie Barnes MSc MPH BSc(Hons) CPNP
Consultant, National Nursing
Leadership Programme, Manchester;
Certified Paediatric Nurse Practitioner,
Old Swan NHS Walk-in Centre,
Liverpool; Visiting Lecturer,
Paediatric Nurse Practitioner
Programme, City University,
Saint Bartholomew School of Nursing
and Midwifery, London;
Guest Lecturer, Paediatric Nurse
Practitioner Programme, Saint Martin's
College, Lancaster
    1. A developmental approach to the
       history and physical
    2. Anatomical and physiological
       differences in paediatrics
    3. Care of the adolescent
    4. General principles in the assessment
       and management of the ill child
    5. Pharmacology in paediatrics
    12.1 Acute abdominal pain
    15.1 Acute fever

Kelly A Barnes DMD
Endodontic Resident, Department of
Endodontics, Boston University School of
Dental Medicine, Boston, USA
    10.4 Common oral lesions
    10.5 Common oral trauma

Breidge Boyle MSc BSc RGN RSCN
Advanced Nurse Practitioner
(Neonatal), Great Ormond Street
Hospital, London
Appendix 2 Age-appropriate B/P and
vital signs

Gill Brook CBE RSCN RGN
Clinial Nurse Specialist, Liver Disease,
Birmingham Children's Hospital NHS
Trust, Birmingham
    12.4 Jaundice

Sara Burr BN(Hons) RN ENBN18 FETC Dip TropNurs
Independent Dermatology Nurse
King's Lynn
    9.6 Cellulitis
    9.9 Impetigo

Julie Carr RGN
Paeditric Dermatology Specialist
Nurse, Sheffield Children's Hospital,
Sheffield
    9.2 Acne

Angela Casey BEd RGN RSCN DipNurs
Endocrine Nurse Practitioner,
Birmingham Children's Hospital,
Birmingham
    12.7 Delayed sexual development

Deborah Chadwick BSc(Hons) RGN RSCN ENB148 ENB415
Lecturer, Pre-registration Nursing – Child
Branch, School of Health Studies, Edge
Hill College, Ormskirk
    13.5 Head injury

Anita Flynn MSc DipHE RSCN RGN SEN
Lecturer, Child Nursing, School of
Health Studies, Edge Hill College,
Liverpool
    13.3 Pain assessment and
    management

Suzanne Garbarino-Danson BSc(Hons) DipHE RN(Child) NP(Paediatrics)
Paediatric Nurse Practitioner,
Children's Ward,
Cumberland Infirmary, Carlisle
    15.8 Meningitis

Steve Gill RGN RSCN
Paediatric Dermatology Nurse
Specialist, Birmingham Children's
Hospital, Birmingham
    9.10 Infantile sebhorrhaeic dermatitis

Michele Harrop BA(Hons) Dip(Asthma and Allergy) RSCN RGN
Paediatric Respiratory Nurse Specialist,
Whiston Hospital, Prescott
    11.1 Asthma and wheezing

Pamela A Hayes RGN RSCN
Endocrine Nurse Practitioner,
Birmingham Children's Hospital,
Birmingham
    12.8 Premature sexual
    development

Anna Hunter MSc BSc CertEd NPDip OND RGN
Senior Lecturer and Nurse Practitioner
    10.1 Congenital blocked
    nasolacrimal duct

Sara Higginson BPharm MRPharmS
Pharmacist, The Ipswich Hospital NHS
Trust, Ipswich
    5. Pharmacology in paediatrics
    13.3 Pain assessment and
    management

Judy Honig EdD CPNP
Associate Dean, Student Services;
Assistant Professor of Clinical Nursing,
School of Nursing, Columbia University,
New York
    10.3 The red eye

Monica Hopkins BNurse MSc PGDipEd PGAdvPrac RSCN RGN RHV
Advanced Nurse Pactitioner, Royal
Liverpool Children's NHS Trust,
Liverpool
    15.4 Pyrexia of unknown origin

Lynn J Hunt BSc Nurse Practitioner Diploma
Soho NHS Walk-in-Centre, London
    7. Paediatric telephone advice and
    management
    Melanie Hutton
    13.2 Lacerations

Katherine Jenner BA(Hons) RSCN RGN RNT
formerly Senior Lecturer, Nursing and
Child Health, Suffolk College, Ipswich
    Appendix 1 Overview of child
    development

Ritamarie John MSN EdD(c)
PNP Program Director, Assistant
Professor of Clinical Nursing,
Columbia University School of Nursing,
New York, USA
    11.5 Syncope
    11.6 Chest pain

Ruth Johnson BSc(Hons)
Paediatric Diabetic Liaison Nurse,
West Cumberland Hospital,
Whitehaven, Cumbria
    13.1 Limp and hip pain

Paulajean Kelly BA(Hons) MSc RGN RSCN PGCE
Former Lecturer/Practitioner,
Paediatric Ambulatory Care Unit,
Homerton University Hospital NHS
Trust/City University London;
Lecturer in Child Health,
Kings College London, London
    9.5 Burns

Debby Laws BSc
Senior Lecturer in Nursing, Suffolk
College, Ipswich
    Appendix 4 Child protection
    resources

Sandra Lawton RN OND RNDip(Child) ENB393
Nurse Consultant, Dermatology Queen's
Medical Centre, Nottingham
    9.13 Psoriasis

Maureen Lilley BSc(Hons)
Ambulatory Day Care, Yorkhill NHS
Trust, Glasgow
    9.7 Food allergies

Jane Linward SRN RSCN
Clinical Nurse Specialist, Birthmark Unit,
Great Ormond Street Hospital,
London
    9.4 Birthmarks

Adele McEvilly RGN RSCN
Paediatric Diabetes Specialist
    12.6 Diabetes mellitus

Nan D McIntosh BSc(Hons) Nurse Practitioner Diploma RSCN RGN
Haematology Nurse Practitioner
Schiehallion Unit, Yorkhill NHS Trust,
Glasgow
    15.9 Bruising in the healthy child

Janet Marsden MSc BSc RGN OND MCMI
Senior Lecturer Department of Health
Care Studies, Manchester Metropolitan
University, Manchester
    10.2 Eye trauma
    10.3 The red eye

Joan M Marshall BSc(Hons)
Nurse Practitioner, Short-Stay Ward,
Yorkhill NHS Trust, Glasgow
    11.4 Stridor and croup

Jan Mitcheson MSc BA(Hons) PGCE RGN RHV
Senior Lecturer, Suffolk College, Ipswich
    9.12 Pediculosis humanus capitus
    (head lice)

Emma Murphy DipHE RN(Child)
Former Auxulogist/Growth Nurse,
Department of Paediatric Endocrinology,
Birmingham Children's Hospital,
Birmingham
    12.9 Short stature

Diane Norton MSc BSc(Hons) PGDE RSCN RM SRN
Lecturer in Children's Nursing,
St Bartholomew's School of Nursing
and Midwifery, City University,
London
    8. Transcultural nursing
    considerations
    12.5 Threadworms

Thomas R Ollerhead BDS LDSRCS DMD
Diplomate to the American Board
of Endodontics;
Clinical Director of Postgraduate
Endodontics,
Boston University School of Dental
Medicine, Boston, USA
    10.4 Common oral lesions
    10.5 Common oral trauma

Sally Panter-Brick BSc
Paediatric Nurse Practitioner,
Cumberland Hospital, Carlisle
   12.3 Acute Gastro-enteritis
Jill Peters BSc(Hons) RGN Nurse Practitioner
Diploma
Dermatology Nurse Practitioner,
Ipswich Primary Care Trust and Ipswich
Hospital Trust, Ipswich
   9.1 'My child has a rash'
Susan Peter MSc
Paediatric Advanced Nurse Practitioner,
Perth, Western Australia
   11.2 Bronchiolitis
Lee M Ranstrom BSN MS CPNP
Captain, USAF, Langley Air Force Base,
USA
   10.6 Acute otitis media
   13.5 Head injury
Rebecca C Robert BSc(Hons) MSc
PhD CFNP
Certified Family Nurse Practitioner,
Junior Investigator,
Instituto de Investigación Nutricional,
Lima, Peru
   10.2 Eye trauma
Mary Evelyn Robinson BSc(Hons)
MSc CPNP
Major, United States Air Force;
Certified Paediatric Nurse Practitioner
   14.1 Urinary tract infection
Jean Robinson BSc RGN RSCN
Clinical Nurse Specialist, Dermatology
Children's Services, St Bartholomew's
Hospital, London
   9.3 Atopic eczema
Diane Scott MSc BSc(Hons)
Nurse Consultant, Child Health
Directorate Burnley General Hospital,
Burnley
   15.7 Parvovirus B19 infection
   (Fifth disease/erythema infectiousum)
Karen Selwood MSc BSc(Hons)
Advanced Nurse Practitioner, Royal
Liverpool Children's Hospital NHS Trust,
Liverpool.
   15.3 Lymphadenopathy
Debra Sharu MSc BA(Hons) PGDip RGN
RSCN
Senior Lecturer, Royal College of
Nursing Development Centre,
South Bank University, London

   15.2 Glandular fever (Epstein-Barr
infection)
   15.6 Varicella
Fiona Smart MA BEd(Hons) RGN RSCN
DipN RNT
Nurse Practitioner/Emergency
Practitioner, St Martin's College,
Carlisle
   1. A developmental approach to the
history and physical
Linda Smith BSc(Hons) DipHE
East Suffolk Community Children's
Nursing Team Leader, Central Suffolk
Primary Care Trust
   12.2 Constipation and encopresis
   14.2 Enuresis
Annabel L Smoker MA Bsc(Hons)
PGDipEA RGN
Lecturer, School of Nursing and
Midwifery, University of Southampton,
Southampton
   9.8 Fungal skin infections
Karen Spowart MSc RSCN
Former Paediatric Dermatology Nurse
Specialist, Queen Elizabeth Hospital for
Childen, London;
Paediatric Diabetes Nurse Specialist,
Chelsea and Westminster NHS Trust,
London
   9.15 Viral skin infections (warts and
molluscum contagiosum)
Jayne Taylor PhD BSc(Hons) DipN(Lond)
RGN RHV Cert Ed RNT
Previously Dean of Health and Head of
Nursing and Midwifery, Suffolk College,
Ipswich
   3. Care of the adolescent
Sarah Todd
   2. Anatomical and physiological
differences in paediatrics
Rosemary Turnbull BSc(Hons) RSCN
Paediatric Dermatology Specialist
Nurse, Chelsea & Westminster Hospital,
London
   9.11 Nappy rash
   9.14 Scabies
John Walter BSc(Hons) RN CPNP
Certified Paediatric Nurse Practitioner;
Former Adjunct Faculty,
University of Arizona,
College of Nursing, Tucson,
Arizona USA;

Former Adjunct Faculty, Arizona State
University, College of Nursing,
Tempe, Arizona USA
   6. Internet resources for the NP
Cheryl Ward BSc
Community Children's Nurse, Central
Suffolk Primary Care Trust, Ipswich
   12.2 Constipation and encopresis
   14.2 Enuresis
Sigrid Watt MSc DipNEd RSCN SRN
RCNT RNT
Paediatric Nurse Practitioner Programme
Leader, City University, London;
St. Bartholomew School of Nursing and
Midwifery, London
   8. Transcultural nursing
considerations
   15.5 Roseola
Elinor White BSc(Hons) SRN RSCN
Paediatric Nurse Practitioner, West
Cumberland Hospital, Cumbria
   11.3 Penumonia
   13.4 Febrile seizures
Jo Williams MSc DPSN RGN RSCN
Advanced Nurse Practitioner, ENT,
Diana Princess of Wales Children's
Hospital, Birmingham
   10.6 Acute otitis media
Peter Wilson MBChB MRCPCH
Paediatric Intensive Care Fellow, Great
Ormond Street Hospital, London
   12.10 Ingestions and poisonings
   14.6 Painful male genitalia

Editorial consultant
Sue J Vernon BA(Hons) RGN RSCN
Doctoral Student; Honorary Senior
Research Associate,
University of Newcastle, Department of
Clinical Medicine Science (Paediatrics);
Senior Nurse, Paediatric UTI Service
Royal Victoria Infirmary, Newcastle

Preface

The academic preparation and role development of the nurse practitioner in the UK has largely focused on adult patients. This is in contrast to the clinical setting where the percentage of paediatric consultations in busy ambulatory sites (e.g. primary care, accident and emergency, walk-in centres, etc.) may approach 30–40%. A large proportion of nurse practitioners (NPs) that care for children do not have extensive paediatric experience, nor a children's nursing qualification. In formalised NP programmes, typically there is very little paediatric content. Even for paediatric advanced practitioners working in specialist areas (e.g. paediatric oncology, dermatology, paediatric acute care, etc.) knowledge of common paediatric conditions outside the scope of their individual specialties may be lacking. *Paediatrics: A Clinical Guide for Nurse Practitioners* is an attempt to address these gaps and the paucity of reference material with regard to paediatric advanced nursing practice. As such, the main objectives of the book are: (1) to offer nurse practitioners (both developing and experienced providers) a *pragmatic* and *clinically focused*, UK-based text that outlines important components to be considered when assessing and managing health problems among infants, children and adolescents; (2) to provide nurse practitioners with information that has *immediate* relevance to their advanced practice in paediatrics; and (3) to furnish nurse practitioners with a paediatric advanced nursing text that is *not* setting dependent (i.e. not specific to primary or acute care but instead can be utilised in numerous settings). While the future may see

paediatric nurse practitioners (PNPs) as the standard of advanced nursing care for infants, children and adolescents, NPs currently in the clinical front line are likely to benefit from a paediatric clinical reference text. It is from this rationale that *Paediatrics: A Clinical Guide for Nurse Practitioners* was derived.

Part One (*Clinical Issues in Paediatrics*) contains practical information pertaining to a variety of subjects that are intrinsic to paediatric advanced nursing practice. Part Two (*Common Paediatric Problems*) outlines the clinical assessment, diagnosis and management of numerous paediatric ambulatory conditions that are often encountered, assessed and/or managed by NPs. The chapters in Part Two are arranged in a 'systems' format, with the individual conditions (or presenting complaints) comprising the sub-content of each chapter. Individual sections in the book attempt to address their specific content in a consistent format. This objective is easily achieved in Part Two as each topic begins with some basic background information about the subject and then proceeds to discuss the pathophysiology, historical information, important physical examination findings, list of differential diagnoses, initial management, follow-up and indications for referral. This format is not so readily applied to the topics in Part One, where the subject matter does not lend itself so easily to this format (e.g. *Internet Resources for the Nurse Practitioner*). However, it is my hope that the practitioner reaching for this text in the middle of a busy clinic session, for the most part, knows what to expect and where to find the relevant information. Each section concludes with a list of

'Paediatric Pearls' (i.e. important points garnered from years of clinical practice) and a comprehensive bibliography. Appendices 1–3 include reference material, largely pertaining to childhood growth and development, such as age appropriate vital signs and child growth charts. Appendix 4 lists numerous child protection resources for the NP. As there is a wealth of information related to child protection currently in the literature and also because of the complexity of the issues, the decision was made to address child protection in a reference-only approach rather than outlining its assessment, diagnosis and management (as in the other sections). This decision was not intended to minimise the importance of child protection in advanced paediatric practice, but rather it was an attempt to provide the NP with a broad range of information related to child protection that could subsequently be applied on an individual basis (concurrently with local resources and procedures).

While the book is not the definitive guide to paediatrics, it is an *initial* attempt to assist both the acute care NP (that may be queried by a mother about her child's eczema) and the primary care NP (that may find a healthy 13 year old in the consulting room asking why she has not started puberty) with the information required for initial assessment, diagnosis and management of a range of paediatric ambulatory conditions. *It is my sincerest hope that it is useful to you in your everyday practice.* I welcome your feedback and your expertise, especially as it relates to the book's format, content and/or conditions that are not covered (e.g. paediatric mental health issues, broader range of injuries, illnesses, etc.). As such, please do not hesitate to contact me with your comments; I can be reached through Elsevier Sciences, Health Sciences Division or directly at KBarnes574@aol.com.

Lastly, this book would never have arrived at publication without the contributions (both direct and indirect) of a number of people that stayed buckled up through many a bumpy ride. Their participation was essential and they deserve mention here: David and Joan Barnes, gave me roots, wings, perseverance and a commitment to excellence; Kelly and David Barnes were at the ready if I needed them and usually made me smile; Joan and Ian Carr came to the rescue on numerous occasions, while Judy Honig, Lenny Shapiro, Becky Robert, Mary Doyle and Jim and Karen White have been long-standing sources of support and friendship (irrespective of the many miles between us). Mary Seager, the Butterworth-Heinemann staff and the 'new team' at Elsevier Science have been a pleasure to work with; Fred Walker always came up with the thoughtful comment; Douglas and Zilah Atfield and Christine Foster have never been far away (thankfully); and Karen Morgan and Rod and Barbara Gathercole provided much needed gentleness and 'good ears'. All of the contributors possessed monumental patience and great humour while Sara Higginson and Peter Wilson have been outstanding collaborators. Petula and India Cook (and company) were lifesavers while R. Goswamy (and team) helped to create dreams to be held. Finally, I owe a tremendous debt of gratitude to the hundreds of children and families that allowed me to work with them over many years (and in many places); despite my mistakes you have taught me how to care, not to judge and often reminded me of the importance of listening. *To all of you I extend a huge, heart-felt and resounding thank-you!*

In peace,
Katie Barnes

CLINICAL ISSUES IN PAEDIATRICS

CHAPTER **1**

A Developmental Approach to the History and Physical Examination in Paediatrics

Katie Barnes and Fiona Smart

INTRODUCTION

- Children are not miniature adults and as such, the nurse practitioner (NP) caring for children will require an appreciation of age and development-related issues that impact the care of children. This includes an understanding of the anatomical and physiological differences across the age groups (see Ch. 2) and a working knowledge of child development (see Appendix 1). This section will outline the developmental springboard from which the paediatric history and physical examination are launched. Note that Chapter 3 (Care of the Adolescent) discusses this unique group in greater detail.
- *Flexibility* is an important prerequisite to paediatric consultations; observe the child's response and let this guide your interactions.
- Considerations of *safety* are likewise imperative when working with children. Think about the proximity of electrical outlets, equipment in the examination area (otoscopes, ophthalmoscopes) and other hazards that are easily reached by inquisitive fingers (electrical cords, lamps, needles). *Never leave a child unattended on the examination table.*
- Be *organised* (without forgetting about flexibility). Equipment should be accessible and in working order; things can easily slip into chaos, especially with toddlers or families with numerous children in the consultation room at the same time.
- Table 1.1 summarises important developmental considerations.

INFANTS (BIRTH TO 12 MONTHS)

- Attachment and trust are the key developmental issues of infancy and the infant–carer dyad is pivotal. Therefore, it is important that the NP respects this relationship and involves the parent(s) in all aspects of the physical examination. In addition, stranger and separation anxiety play an increasingly important role when assessing children older than 7 months. Stranger anxiety tends to peak at 9 months, whereas distress related to a separation from caregivers may continue to influence social interactions into the toddler period. Note however, that there are wide variations with both of these behaviours.
- A birth history (gestational age at birth, birth weight, prenatal care, intrauterine exposures, problems during labour, delivery or the neonatal period) is particularly relevant in this age group as an assessment of potential vulnerability may be necessary (e.g. traumatic birth and risk for developmental delays). In addition, the parent's observations regarding the infant's growth, development and illness-related behaviours are required in order to assess the infant within a broader context. Lastly, information about the family's ability to cope with a sick infant is requisite for the negotiation of a realistic plan of care.
- The physical examination of a young infant (less than 5 months of age) is relatively straightforward and can usually proceed in a cephalocaudal manner. The examination of older infants will likely require flexibility in the examination sequence. However, if presented with a sleeping infant, the NP should take advantage of the opportunity to assess the heart, lungs and possibly the abdomen. It is important to provide a warm, protective environment for the infant, as she will not be happy if the examination room is cold and she is undressed and exposed. Young infants can be examined on the table, whereas older infants (especially those that can sit) may be happier on the parent's lap. It is often helpful to position yourself opposite the parent (putting knees together) to form a 'human examination table.' Note that if the older infant does need to be placed on the examination table, be sure to keep the parent in full view and keep the infant in a sitting position (she will not like lying down). Smile at the infant—she'll smile back. Likewise, be sure to use a gentle touch and tone of voice. Cooperation can be assisted by the use of distracters such as rattles, snapping fingers or tongue depressors.

Table 1.1   A Developmental Approach to the History and Physical Examination in Paediatrics

Developmental Considerations

Infants (birth to 12 months)	Toddlers (1–2 years)	Pre-schoolers (3–5 years)	School-agers (6–11 years)	Adolescents (12–18 years)
• Most dramatic and rapid period of growth and development • Attachment and trust are key issues • Stranger anxiety appears >6 months • Separation anxiety starts to affect social interactions at approx. 9 months • Safety is an issue as gross and fine motor development progress rapidly	• Separation and stranger anxiety continue to influence social interactions • Autonomy, egocentrism and negativism are major developmental issues • Parent is a 'home-base' for explorations • Fears bodily harm • Verbal communication skills limited • Safety continues to be an important issue	• Developing sense of initiative is important • Able to 'help', participate and cooperate • Knows most body parts and some internal parts • Fears bodily harm • Verbal communication skills more advanced • Cognition characterised by egocentricity, literal interpretations and magical thinking	• Sense of industry important; articulate and active participant in care • Increased self-control • Understands simple scientific explanations (cause and effect); thinking still concrete	• Increasing independence • Time of tremendous growth and change • Orientation to the future • Separates easily from parents • Peer group important • Knows basic anatomy and physiology • Has own opinions/ideas • Active and articulate participant in care

Age-related History

Infants	Toddlers	Pre-schoolers	School-agers	Adolescents
• Birth history • Carer's observations of infant growth and development • Parental observations of illness behaviours • Family coping with illness	• Birth history • Reaction to increasing independence • Family coping with toddler issues: struggles, tantrums, negativity and discipline • Caretaker's perception of growth/development • Family stress levels and perceptions of illness	• Family coping • Child's understanding of illness • Parental expectations of illness	• Child's understanding and role in illness and its management • School performance, enjoyment and presence of any problems at school • Hobbies • Family coping	• HEADSS history • Parent/adolescent relationship • See Chapter 3

A Developmental Approach to the Physical Examination

• Three rules in the examination of children and adolescents: *flexibility* (adjust your technique according to the child's response); *safety* (do not leave the child unattended on the examination table, careful with outlets and equipment); and *organisation* (things can easily slip into chaos)
• Allow the child's age and developmental level to guide your history and physical examination
• Atmosphere and environment are important (e.g. warm room, appropriate decoration, use of toys, consider special needs of adolescents, unhurried social environment, try and limit the number of people in the room)
• Incorporate health education and growth and development anticipatory guidance into the examination
• Move from the easy/simple → more distressing; use positive reinforcement and 'prizes'
• Use demonstration and play to your advantage (play equipment or 'spares', paper doll technique, crayons, blocks)
• Expect an age-appropriate level of cooperation; explain what will be involved in the physical examination and tell the child what she needs to do (e.g. hold still, open your mouth)

Infants	Toddlers	Pre-schoolers	School-agers	Adolescents
• Keep parent in view • Before 6 months examination on table; after 6 months examination in parent's lap • Undress fully in warm room • Careful with nappy removal • Distract with bright objects/rattles • Soft manner; avoid loud noises and abrupt movements • Have bottle, dummy or breast handy • Vary examination sequence with activity level (if asleep/quiet auscultate heart, lungs, abdomen first) • Usually able to proceed in cephalocaudal sequence • Distressing procedures last (ears and temperature)	• Most difficult group to examine • Approach gradually and minimise initial physical contact • Leave with parent (sitting or standing if possible) • Allow to inspect equipment (demonstration usually not helpful) • Start examination distally through play (toes, fingers) • Praise, praise, praise • Parent removes clothes • Save ears, mouth and anything lying down for last • Use restraint (with parent) only if necessary	• Allow close proximity to parent • Usually cooperative; able to proceed head to toe • Request self-undressing (bit by bit exposure—modesty important) • Expect cooperation • Allow for choice when possible • If uncooperative, start distally with play • Allow brief inspection of equipment with brief demonstration and explanation • Use games/stories for cooperation • Paper doll technique very effective • Praise, reward and positive reinforcement	• Usually cooperative • Child should undress self; privacy important; provide drape/gown if possible • Explain function of equipment; use of 'spares' helpful • Examination can be important teaching exercise • Head–toe sequence • Praise and feedback regarding normalcy is important	• Give the option of parental presence • Undress in private; provide gown • Expose one area at a time • Physical examination can be an important teaching exercise • Head–toe sequence • Feedback regarding normalcy is important • Anticipatory guidance regarding sexual development (use Tanner staging) • Matter-of-fact approach to examination (and history) • Encourage appropriate decision-making skills

Avoid loud noises, jerky movements and blocking the infant's view of the parent. Save distressing manoeuvres for last.

TODDLERS (12 MONTHS TO 2 YEARS)

- Developmental issues impacting the physical examination of toddlers are a function of their growing independence, characteristic negativity (as an expression of emerging autonomy), egocentricity and fear of bodily harm. In addition, separation and stranger anxiety continue to make social interaction challenging. The parent will be a 'home base' for exploration as the toddler alternates between investigation and parental reassurance. Communication is restricted by a limited vocabulary and, as verbal skills are insufficient for expression, the toddler will physically act out fear, upset and anxiety.
- Important historical information to obtain in the assessment of toddlers includes much of the same information included with infants (e.g. birth history, growth and development history and illness behaviours). However, some additional information is necessary in order to best negotiate a plan of care: parental reaction(s) to the toddler's increasing independence; the extent of tantrums/struggles and handling of discipline; difficulties with the toddler's degree of negativity; and family stress levels (e.g. a family that is struggling with developmentally appropriate tantrums and negativity may find the added stress of illness-related irritability very difficult).
- Toddlers are the most difficult age group to examine. Start with a gradual approach, initially avoiding eye contact with the toddler while smiling and speaking happily with the carer. Setting out distracters, such as blocks or other toys (remember infection control principles) during the history (while still avoiding direct eye contact with the toddler) allows the child to become more familiar with you before the examination is attempted. Consider what the most important

parts of the physical examination are and set these as a priority. Avoid becoming involved in a power struggle by having the parent undress the child. Begin the examination distally, and work towards the centre of the body. Keeping the toddler's fingers busy through playing with the blocks, may lessen the likelihood of the stethoscope being pulled out of your ears. Leave the examination of mouth, ears and any system which requires the toddler to lie down until last. Use restraint (with the parent's permission and assistance) only if absolutely essential. Praise is important, as are calm and reassuring tones.

PRE-SCHOOLERS (3–5 YEARS)

- Interactions with the pre-schooler are far easier than with toddlers. Fear of bodily harm remains an issue, but most pre-schoolers are outgoing and unafraid as long as contact with the parent is maintained and they are told what is going to happen. Communication skills are far more advanced and the pre-schooler will know most body parts (including some internal ones). Games can be used to very good effect, including storytelling, colouring and the 'paper doll technique' (i.e. the child's outline is traced onto the examination table paper for explanations and building rapport). The pre-schooler's developing sense of initiative can likewise be used positively; praise the child for being so 'brave', 'grown-up' and 'helpful'. The pre-schooler can follow simple instructions (e.g. dressing, undressing, putting toys away) and again these behaviours should be praised and/or rewarded (child-friendly stickers are a big treat). Note however, that cognition may be characterised by egocentricity, literal interpretations and magical thinking; communication should be direct, clear and unambiguous (e.g. *checking* your temperature rather than *taking* your temperature).
- Additional history specific to the pre-schooler includes family coping with the illness and the child's

understanding of what made her unwell. Discuss parental expectations of the illness as part of the history in order to obtain an idea of whether these are appropriate for the child's age and illness course.
- The physical examination of the pre-school child can be quite fun. It is likely that the pre-schooler will be quite comfortable on the examination table (but be sure to keep mother close at hand) and that the physical examination can proceed in a head to toe direction (although sometimes it is best to save mouth and ears for last). Privacy is an issue, so it is probably best to undress one part at a time (the child can do this); if the child is very hesitant, start with the shoes (or proceed as with the toddler). Allow the child to play with and inspect the equipment (it is very handy to have a 'spare' play stethoscope). It is important to explain to the child what will be involved when the heart, lungs, abdomen, etc., are examined; demonstrations on a nearby doll (or the tracing of the child) can be invaluable. Allow the child choice when possible: *'Which should we listen to first, your heart or your lungs?'*. Praise and positive reinforcement throughout the examination will not only have pay-offs for the immediate consultation, but also will set the tone for future interactions. The pre-school period is when the foundations of the patient–NP relationship can take shape. As such, the expectation is that the child is an active and positive participant in her own health (and health care) which is an important concept in the development of healthy lifestyle choices.

SCHOOL-AGER (6–11 YEARS)

- These children are usually willing participants and curious about what is involved in their physical examination and care management. They are articulate and possess much greater self-control (as compared to the younger age groups). Their sense of accomplishment and mastery is important and they will understand simple scientific explanations (i.e. cause and effect). However, their thinking remains concrete (although there is wide variation in older children) and validation should be sought as to whether the child understands what has been discussed: i.e. *'Can you explain back to me what you need to do to take care of your cold?'*.

- It is important to elicit from both the parent and the child what they believe is responsible for the illness and how they have been managing it at home. Enquire about school performance, school enjoyment, hobbies and presence of any problems at school.
- The physical examination of the school-age child should be able to proceed as for an adult. Be aware that modesty is an issue; good technique includes exposing only the area that needs to be examined. The child will likely wish to dress/undress themselves (provide privacy); use of an examination gown or drape is beneficial. Explain to the child what is being done throughout the examination. Use the normal physical examination findings as a way to discuss positive health behaviours and the structure/function of the body.

ADOLESCENTS (12–18 YEARS)

- This is a period of tremendous growth and change for the adolescent: physically, emotionally and cognitively. Adolescence is a time of increasing independence and a strong attachment to the peer group. The older adolescent will have a future orientation (i.e. plans for further education, training, etc.), whereas the younger adolescent will be starting to question authority. The adolescent is sure to have her own opinion of health and illness and as such, management and follow-up will need to be negotiated. Privacy is important and the option of an interview with or without the parent present should be explored (especially with older adolescents).
- Specific historical information relevant to the adolescent is discussed in Chapter 3.

- The physical examination of the adolescent is similar to that of an adult. It is important to use it as an opportunity for health education and anticipatory guidance; be sure to reinforce normal findings. The adolescent is likely to be very self-conscious and extra consideration should be given to privacy: e.g. allow the adolescent to undress in private, expose a single area at a time and provide drapes and gown. Explain to the adolescent the importance of establishing the sexual maturity rating (Tanner staging) and use this as a springboard to a discussion of sexual development and health. Remember that size and physical maturity are not good predictors of chronological age; always treat an adolescent according to her age (see Ch. 3).

PAEDIATRIC PEARLS

- Flexibility, organisation and safety are essential prerequisites in paediatric practice.
- Atmosphere and environment are important; keep the consulting room warm, bright, cheery and age-appropriate.
- The child's age and developmental level should lead your history and physical examination; different ages often require different approaches. However, there is wide variation in behaviours and responses *across* and *within* age-groups; allow the child's actions to guide you. Remember that size and physical maturity are not good predictors of chronological age (especially with adolescents).
- Use the history and physical examination as an opportunity for health education, growth and development teaching and discussion of healthy lifestyle choices.
- Move from the easy/simple to the more distressing (i.e. leave the ear and throat examination in toddlers until last).
- Use demonstration and play to your advantage with younger patients.
- Expect an age-appropriate level of cooperation; explain what you are going to do and what the child should

do in clear, unambiguous terms. Praise children for cooperative behaviour and note that small 'prizes' (i.e. stickers) can be good motivators and reinforcers.

BIBLIOGRAPHY

Algranati PS. The pediatric patient: an approach to history and physical examination. Baltimore: Williams & Wilkins; 1992.

Algranati PS. Effect of developmental status on the approach to physical examination. Pediatr Clin North Am 1998; 45(1):1–23.

Allen HD, Golinko RJ, Williams RG. Heart murmurs in children: when is a workup needed? Patient Care 1994; 15 April:123–151.

Burns C, Barber N, Brady M, Dunn A. Pediatric primary care: a handbook for nurse practitioners, 2nd edn. New York: WB Saunders; 2000.

Burton DA, Cabalka AK. Cardiac evaluation of infants. Pediatr Clin North Am 1994; 41(5):991–1015.

Church JL, Baer KJ. Examination of the adolescent: a practical guide. J Pediatr Health Care 1987; 1(2):65–72.

Craig CL, Goldberg MJ. Foot and leg deformities. Pediatr Rev 1993; 14(10):395–400.

Engel J. Pediatric assessment, 3rd edn. New York: Mosby; 1997.

Gill D, O'Brien N. Paediatric clinical examination, 3rd edn. London: Churchill Livingstone; 1998.

Jarvis C. Physical examination and health assessment, 2nd edn. Philadelphia: WB Saunders; 1996.

Killam PE. Orthopedic assessment of young children: developmental variations. Nurse Pract 1989; 14(7):27–36.

Kleiman AH. ABC's of pediatric ophthalmology. J Ophthalmic Nurs Technol 1986; 5(3):86–90.

Ledford JK. Successful management of the pediatric examination. J Ophthalmic Nurs Technol 1987; 6(3):96–99.

Litt IF. Pubertal and psychosocial implications for pediatricians. Pediatr Rev 1995; 16(7):243–246.

McCann J, Voris J, Simon M, et al. Comparison of genital examination techniques in prepubertal girls. Pediatrics 1990; 85(2):182–187.

Moody Y. Pediatric cardiovascular assessment and referral in the primary care setting. Nurs Pract 1997; 22(1):120–134.

Neinstein LS. Adolescent health care: a practical guide, 3rd edn. Baltimore: Williams & Wilkins; 1996.

Bibliography

Rudolph MC, Levene MI. Paediatrics and child health. Oxford: Blackwell Science; 1999.

Rudy C. Developmental dysplasia of the hip: what's new in the 1990's. J Pediatr Health Care 1996; 10(2):85.

Thomas DO. Assessing children—it's different. RN 1996; 59(4):38–44.

Unti SM. The critical first year of life: history, physical examination and general developmental assessment. Pediatr Clin North Am 1994; 41(5):859–873.

Vessey JA. Developmental approaches to examining young children. Pediatr Nurs 1995; 21(1):53–56.

Wong DL. The paper doll technique. Pediatr Nurs 1981; 7:39–40.

Wong DL, Wilson D. Whaley and Wong's nursing care of infants and children, 6th edn. St. Louis: Mosby; 1999.

CHAPTER 2

Anatomical and Physiological Differences in Paediatrics

Sarah Todd and Katie Barnes

INTRODUCTION

- There are many differences in the anatomy and physiology among infants, children and adolescents.
- Whereas changes in physical appearance, motor abilities and cognition are obvious indicators of maturation, parallel development of internal organs, body systems and physiological pathways is simultaneously occurring.
- These developmental changes follow a characteristic pattern that includes periods of growth acceleration and deceleration (which may vary with the specific system(s) involved). It should be noted that while the *rate* of developmental and/or maturational changes can vary from child to child, the *sequence* of development (for the most part) is the same for all children.
- The anatomical and physiological differences outlined in this chapter are intended to provide an overview rather than a comprehensive discussion of paediatric anatomy and physiology. For a more in-depth discussion, the reader is referred to the Bibliography Section at the end of the chapter.

INFANTS AND TODDLERS (BIRTH TO 2 YEARS)

- The first 12 months of life are the most rapid period of growth and development (intrauterine period excepted). In addition, there are

significant differences in body proportions, metabolic rates and body fluid composition as compared to older children and adults. Individual body systems (e.g. neurological, cardiovascular and genitourinary) likewise have a developmental component with implications for function and/or capacity. While the growth rate slows during the second year of life, growth parameters—i.e. height, weight and head circumference—are important indicators of well-being. An infant or toddler that is *not* growing is a cause for concern and as such, a slowing and/or change in a child's growth rate should prompt further assessment. The increased proportion of water in body fluids, increased insensible losses (related to higher metabolic rates) and a decreased ability to concentrate urine place infants and toddlers at greater risk of dehydration and/or electrolyte disturbances during an episode of acute vomiting and diarrhoea.
- A summary of the changes among infants and toddlers is given in Table 2.1.

PRE-SCHOOL AND SCHOOL-AGE CHILDREN (3–11 YEARS)

- Throughout the pre-school and school-age years there is maturation and stabilisation of all body systems. It is a period of relatively steady growth that should follow the trajectory

established during infancy and toddlerhood. Body proportions are more adult-like, with both the protuberant abdomen and lordosis of toddlerhood commonly disappearing by 4 years of age. The typical appearance of children in this age group is slender, leggy, agile and posturally erect. Gradual increases in bone and muscle growth result in a doubling of strength and physical capabilities by 11 years of age. However, muscles remain functionally immature until adolescence and are more readily damaged by excessive activity and/or overexertion. In addition, bone mineralisation is likewise incomplete and children of this age group are less resistant to pressure and muscle pull. As such, guidance regarding age-appropriate physical activity may be necessary when young footballers or cricketers present with overuse syndromes. Likewise, attention should be given to carrying heavy loads (i.e. full book bags); backpacks should have equal weight distribution, with both straps used simultaneously.
- There is wide variation in physical growth and development towards the end of the school-age period. These discrepancies are due to disparities in physical maturation that occur across gender (girls maturing earlier than boys) and within gender (early developers as opposed to 'late-bloomers'). These differences become increasingly apparent as the child approaches the latter half of the

Table 2.1 Anatomical and Physiological Differences among Infants and Toddlers

System	Anatomical/physiological difference
General	• Most rapid period of growth (i.e. weight, height, head circumference) during the first 12 months • Increased proportion of water in the composition of body fluids (65–75% at birth) • The head and trunk constitute a greater proportion of total body surface area (TBSA) with associated clinical implications (e.g. burn management). The head and trunk of infants constitute 45% of TBSA, while they account for 40% of TBSA among toddlers • Increased metabolic rates, as a function of the larger body surface area (BSA) in relation to active tissue mass. This results in an increased production of metabolic wastes and slightly higher insensible losses • Immature hypothalamus contributes to poor temperature control among newborns
Ear, nose and throat and mouth	• External auditory canal relatively short and straight • Eustachian tube is short and broad and in close proximity to the middle ear • Maxillary and ethmoid sinuses are small; usually not aerated for approximately 6 months • Sphenoid and frontal sinuses underdeveloped • By 2½ years of age, 20 deciduous teeth have usually erupted
Pulmonary	• The respiratory tract is shorter and as such, the trachea, bronchi and lower respiratory structures are in very close proximity. Transmission of infectious agents is much more efficient • Respiratory efforts in infants are largely abdominal • Poor immunoglobulin A (IgA) production in pulmonary mucosa combined with a narrower tracheal lumen and lower respiratory structures causes the infant to be more prone to respiratory difficulties from oedema, mucus or foreign body aspiration • Less alveolar surface for gaseous exchange • Differences in the angle of access to the trachea among various age groups; implications for airway clearance and/or support during resuscitation • Upper airway sounds are much more easily transmitted to the chest of young children, making auscultation of the lower respiratory tract challenging
Cardiovascular	• Heart is higher and more horizontal in the chest cavity • Resting heart rate is markedly greater than adult norms • Sinus arrhythmia is normal finding (e.g. heart rate increases during inspiration, decreases with expiration)
Gastrointestinal	• The abdomen tends to be prominent with poor muscle tone. Shape of stomach remains round until approximately 2 years of age • In infancy, the ascending and descending portions of the colon are short compared with the transverse colon • There is a deficiency of the starch-splitting enzyme amylase during early infancy. This prevents optimal handling of polysaccharides. Lipase activity is low, while trypsin activity is adequate from birth • Stomach capacity is small but increases rapidly with age, while gastric-emptying time is faster during infancy. Both have implications for frequency and amount of feeds • During infancy, the proportionately longer gastrointestinal tract is a source of greater fluid loss (especially during episodes of acute diarrhoea)
Neurological	• By the end of the first year of life, the brain has reached approximately two-thirds of its adult size. During the second year brain growth decelerates; however, by 24 months of age, the brain is approximately four-fifths of its adult size • There is a significant increase in the number and complexity of dendrite connections, the number and size of neurones and glial cells, and rapid myelinisation of nerve pathways occurring • This period of cellular proliferation is dependent on good nutritional status as nervous system myelinisation is dependent on an adequate intake of fats (i.e. children under age 2 require 30% more fat for neural development and as such, reduced fat milk should not be included in their diet.)
Genitourinary	• Glomerular filtration rate (GFR) and urine output are decreased in the neonatal period. By the end of the second week of life, these parameters have increased rapidly • Ability to concentrate, dilute or acidify urine is limited and urea clearance is low • By 12 months of age, the GFR approaches adult levels • Control of the anal/urethral sphincters is acquired gradually as spinal cord myelinisation is completed (18 months to 2 years)
Immune system	• IgG in newborn period is almost entirely maternal IgG • IgG levels reach a nadir at about 3 months of age. A rise occurs as the infant begins to produce his own immunoglobulins (40% of adult level by 12 months). Adult levels are reached by the end of the second year • Significant amounts of IgM are produced after birth; adult level produced by 9 months • Infants < 3 months are at greater risk of Gram-negative bacterial infection • Ability to synthesise IgA, IgD and IgE much less developed • Lymph system develops rapidly after birth • Antibodies of major blood group system (ABO) usually appear by 2 months
Haemopoietic	• Fetal haemoglobin comprises 80% total haemoglobin at birth; falls to 5% by 4 months of age • Leucocyte count high and may reach its highest at about 7 months • Lymphocyte count is highest during the first year of life

school-age period and if extreme (or unique) can contribute to significant stress for the children and their families. Anticipatory guidance related to height and weight relationships, rapid or slow growth, and development (or delay) of secondary sexual characteristics is important (see Ch. 12). In addition, physical maturity is often not well correlated to cognitive, social and emotional maturity. While an 8-year-old child may look like a 12-year-old adolescent (as well as the reverse) it is imperative to match behavioural expectations to

Table 2.2 Anatomical and Physiological Differences in Pre-school and School-age Children	
System	Anatomical/physiological difference
Head	• Face tends to grow proportionally • Jaw widens to prepare for eruption of permanent teeth • First permanent teeth often erupt during seventh year of life • Frontal sinus develops by seventh year of life • Enlargement of nasal accessory sinuses
Cardiopulmonary	• Heart and respiratory rates decrease with a rise in blood pressure. Heart rate shows an inverse relationship to body size • Heart reaches adult position in thoracic cavity by 7 years of age • Under 7 years of age, respiratory movement is principally abdominal or diaphragmatic. Among older children, particularly girls, movement is chiefly thoracic • Episodes of respiratory infections are often frequent during pre-school and school-age years
Gastrointestinal	• Fewer stomach upsets compared with younger ages • Stomach elongates until approximately 7 years and then assumes shape and anatomical position of the adult stomach • Improved maintenance of blood sugar levels and increased stomach capacity have implications for the timing of meals (i.e. decreased need for prompt and frequent feedings) • Caloric needs less than during infancy/toddlerhood and less than they will be in adolescence
Musculoskeletal (MSK)	• Great increase in bone and muscle growth • Muscles remain functionally immature. More readily damaged by overuse • Spine becomes straighter • Bones continue to ossify, but mineralisation incomplete (until puberty)
Genitourinary	• Onset of pubertal changes and sexual development may start at the end of the school-age years • Bladder capacity greatly increased (however this varies widely); it is, however (generally) greater in girls than boys
Immune system	• By 10–12 years of age, lymphatic tissues are at the peak of their development and generally exceed their adult size; regression of tissue (to adult size) occurs during adolescence • Matured immune system is able to localise and respond to acute infection; response to infection more like that of an adult

the child's emotional, social and cognitive level.

• An overview of the anatomical and physiological changes of this age group are outlined in Table 2.2.

ADOLESCENTS (12–18 YEARS)

• Adolescence is a period of profound physiological change that includes final maturation of all body systems. The most striking of these changes are the increases in height, weight, body proportions and secondary sexual development that give the adolescent a very adult-like appearance. The development of secondary sexual characteristics and changes in physical growth are collectively referred to as puberty. While there is wide variation in the timing of pubertal changes, the sequence in which these changes occur is the same for all children. The adolescent's greater physical endurance and strength are due to an increase in the size and strength of the heart, increased blood volume and increased systolic blood pressure. Likewise, the lungs increase in length and diameter with resultant increases in respiratory volume, vital capacity and respiratory functional efficiency. Other internal organs such as the kidneys, liver and stomach increase in size and capacity, reaching a peak at about 14 years of age. There is maturation of the musculoskeletal system, haemopoietic system (with corresponding attainment of adult blood values) and an increase in the proliferation of neurological support cells and growth of the myelin sheath in the nervous system. This allows for faster neural processing, with corresponding improvements in coordination and more advanced cognitive capabilities. Lastly, there is maturation of the reproductive system with the onset of menarche in girls (although this may occur during the school-age years) and the ability for seminal emissions in boys.

• Anatomical and physiological changes of adolescents are summarised in Table 2.3. Note that while adolescence has been outlined as a single stage, there are differences between early, middle and late adolescence (see Further Reading).

PAEDIATRIC PEARLS

• A child that is not growing is a cause for concern; further investigation is required.

• While the *rate* at which developmental and/or maturational changes occur can vary from child to child, the *sequence* of development (for the most part) is the same for all children.

• The close proximity of the upper and lower respiratory structures among infants and young children can make assessment of the lower respiratory tract challenging in the presence of significant upper airway congestion. Listening (with the stethoscope) at the nose of a congested child before moving to the chest may familiarise the NP with the sounds coming from the upper respiratory tract and thus enable a distinction between upper airway 'noise' and lower respiratory adventitious sounds. In addition, switching to the bell of the stethoscope while auscultating the chest can contribute to a degree of 'noise' filtering.

• The location of the heart higher up and more horizontal in the chest cavity of infants and young children has implications for the apical impulse, which is laterally displaced from the mid-clavicular line in this age group.

• Use age-appropriate vital sign values and account for increases related to fever or distress. Likewise, it is important to obtain age-appropriate normal values in the interpretation of any haematological parameters in children.

• A sinus arrhythmia (heart rate increasing on inspiration, decreasing on expiration) is a normal finding in paediatrics.

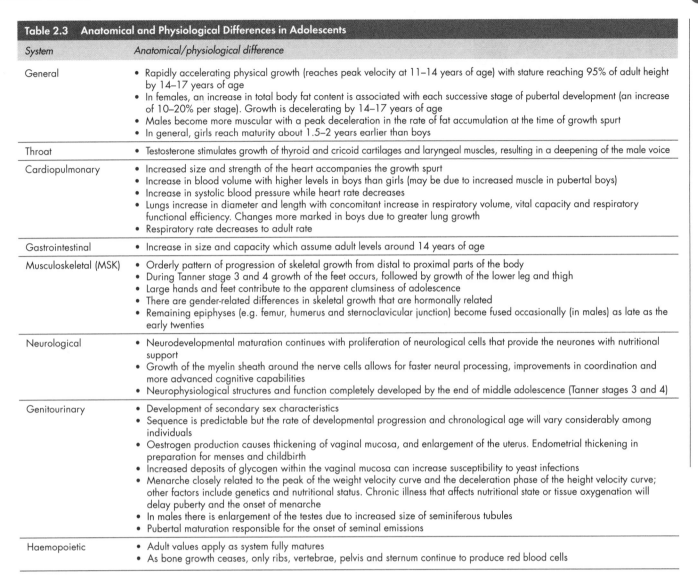

Table 2.3 Anatomical and Physiological Differences in Adolescents

System	Anatomical/physiological difference
General	• Rapidly accelerating physical growth (reaches peak velocity at 11–14 years of age) with stature reaching 95% of adult height by 14–17 years of age • In females, an increase in total body fat content is associated with each successive stage of pubertal development (an increase of 10–20% per stage). Growth is decelerating by 14–17 years of age • Males become more muscular with a peak deceleration in the rate of fat accumulation at the time of growth spurt • In general, girls reach maturity about 1.5–2 years earlier than boys
Throat	• Testosterone stimulates growth of thyroid and cricoid cartilages and laryngeal muscles, resulting in a deepening of the male voice
Cardiopulmonary	• Increased size and strength of the heart accompanies the growth spurt • Increase in blood volume with higher levels in boys than girls (may be due to increased muscle in pubertal boys) • Increase in systolic blood pressure while heart rate decreases • Lungs increase in diameter and length with concomitant increase in respiratory volume, vital capacity and respiratory functional efficiency. Changes more marked in boys due to greater lung growth • Respiratory rate decreases to adult rate
Gastrointestinal	• Increase in size and capacity which assume adult levels around 14 years of age
Musculoskeletal (MSK)	• Orderly pattern of progression of skeletal growth from distal to proximal parts of the body • During Tanner stage 3 and 4 growth of the feet occurs, followed by growth of the lower leg and thigh • Large hands and feet contribute to the apparent clumsiness of adolescence • There are gender-related differences in skeletal growth that are hormonally related • Remaining epiphyses (e.g. femur, humerus and sternoclavicular junction) become fused occasionally (in males) as late as the early twenties
Neurological	• Neurodevelopmental maturation continues with proliferation of neurological cells that provide the neurones with nutritional support • Growth of the myelin sheath around the nerve cells allows for faster neural processing, improvements in coordination and more advanced cognitive capabilities • Neurophysiological structures and function completely developed by the end of middle adolescence (Tanner stages 3 and 4)
Genitourinary	• Development of secondary sex characteristics • Sequence is predictable but the rate of developmental progression and chronological age will vary considerably among individuals • Oestrogen production causes thickening of vaginal mucosa, and enlargement of the uterus. Endometrial thickening in preparation for menses and childbirth • Increased deposits of glycogen within the vaginal mucosa can increase susceptibility to yeast infections • Menarche closely related to the peak of the weight velocity curve and the deceleration phase of the height velocity curve; other factors include genetics and nutritional status. Chronic illness that affects nutritional state or tissue oxygenation will delay puberty and the onset of menarche • In males there is enlargement of the testes due to increased size of seminiferous tubules • Pubertal maturation responsible for the onset of seminal emissions
Haemopoietic	• Adult values apply as system fully matures • As bone growth ceases, only ribs, vertebrae, pelvis and sternum continue to produce red blood cells

• Appearances can be deceiving; always match expectations of the child to their emotional, social and cognitive levels. Ask a child's age; never assume it based on physical development.

BIBLIOGRAPHY

Behrman R, Vaughan W. Nelson's textbook of pediatrics, 16th edn. St. Louis: WB Saunders; 1999.

MacGregor J. Introduction to the anatomy and physiology of children. London: Routledge; 2000.

Wong D. Nursing care of infants and children, 6th edn. St. Louis: Mosby; 1999.

CHAPTER 3

Care of the Adolescent

Jayne Taylor and Katie Barnes

INTRODUCTION

- Defining adolescence is in itself problematic and there is no consensus view about when adolescence starts and when it finishes. The nurse practitioner (NP) should be familiar with the legal parameters of adolescence, such as the law around alcohol consumption and consenting sexual intercourse. Otherwise, the NP needs to be aware that adolescence is a complex period of change in the physical, intrapsychic and social domains and that each individual will experience it in a unique way.
- Adolescence is generally a time of good health and adolescents tend not to access health care services as much as younger children or adults. They can therefore be seen as a neglected population and services specifically for them are largely underdeveloped. However, adolescence is a time when many young people will start to engage in risky behaviours that can have, or lead to, longer-term consequences: e.g. experimentation with drugs, alcohol and tobacco; the start of sexual activity; and dietary and exercise habits.
- Emotional and social development is also important during this period, as young people seek to find their own unique place in society. Many young people are, during this time, emotionally impressionable. The developmental tasks of the adolescent can be defined as detailed in Box 3.1.
- Adolescent visits to the health centre, clinic or surgery provide a unique opportunity for one-to-one health education, risk assessment, lifestyle counselling and health interventions.

Box 3.1   Developmental tasks of adolescence
• Adjusting to, and accepting, physical changes that occur as part of normal developmental processes
• Moving towards a level of independence that is acceptable within the individual's cultural grouping
• Developing social skills that are appropriate within adult society and the world of work
• Achieving balance in work and/or study and leisure activities
• Finding an identity that is not in conflict with personal values and beliefs and that has a 'good fit' feel about it
• Developing desired educational and vocational skills and abilities

As such, goals of the adolescent interview are to determine the nature of any health problems and assess risk; to develop and maintain therapeutic relationships; to educate and motivate the adolescent around positive lifestyle choices; and to provide ongoing monitoring of any identified problems.
- Confidentiality is an important and complex issue for the NP. The adolescent's right to expect confidentiality hinges legally on his or her ability to form a confidential relationship with the practitioner. By implication this means that if the adolescent cannot form such a relationship then the practitioner has what amounts to a duty to disclose information learned to those with parental responsibility, or in the case of for example, child abuse, to the local authority. If the adolescent is capable of forming a confidential relationship then the general rule is that they should be treated as one would treat an adult in respect of confidentiality.
- The adolescent's right to consent to, or refuse, treatment is also complex. An adolescent above the age of 16 may give consent to treatment as can those under the age of 16 if, in the opinion of the practitioner, he or she is capable of understanding the nature and potential consequences of a procedure or treatment regime. In the latter case the adolescent would be deemed to be '*Gillick competent*'. Refusal to consent to treatment is technically the other end of the same continuum, but in law it is not treated this way as the law has no application in respect of refusal to consent. If an adolescent who is deemed to have '*Gillick competence*' refuses treatment, those with parental responsibility cannot overrule the decision of the child and in such cases the court has to decide what the best interests of the adolescent are.
- The Department of Health has issued guidelines with regard to informed consent and working with children. The document is available on line at http://www.doh.gov.uk/consent.

HISTORY

- Key communication skills for working with adolescents include facility with bidirectional communication; accurate, non-verbal expression (and recognition) of emotions; a communication style that is sensitive to the adolescent's feelings; attentive listening and a non-judgemental, direct questioning style with regard to psychosocial issues.

- The episodic history as outlined in Chapter 4 does not include an assessment of important psychosocial issues of adolescence. Each encounter with an adolescent provides the sensitive and astute clinician with a chance to establish a rapport and lay the foundation of a therapeutic relationship. Because adolescents as a population do not routinely access preventive services, it is important to provide assessment (and potential intervention) of risk-taking behaviours as part of every episodic interview.

- H–E–A–D–S–S is a useful mnemonic that incorporates the relevant psychosocial issues of adolescence in a history-taking format that proceeds from the least-threatening to the more sensitive factor. Risk assessment as part of the adolescent interview is vital so that interventions can be targeted and appropriate:
  - H = home environment: where living, who else living at home, relationships at home, etc.
  - E = education (or employment): how school is going, plans for the future, strengths, marks, etc.
  - A = activities: hobbies, fun things done with friends, what happens with free time, etc.
  - D = drug use: useful to preface with acknowledgement that many young people experiment with drugs, alcohol or smoking and then proceed to enquire about the adolescent's (and their friends) use. *Many young people experiment with drugs, alcohol and cigarettes. Have you or your friends tried them? What have you tried?'*
  - S = sexuality: as this is a sensitive subject, prefacing the interview with acknowledgement that adolescence is a time when there is growing interest in sexual relationships can let the adolescent know that sexuality is a legitimate topic. Likewise, reassure the adolescent that he can ask any questions or voice any concerns he may have (especially as some adolescents do not have anyone knowledgeable to talk to about sex). It is also crucial to put the sensitive nature of a sexual history into the context of a

general health assessment. More specifically, let the adolescent know that since sexual activity can affect his health (now and in the future) sexual health is part of overall well-being; for example, it is just as important as dental health. As such, treating problems early (or better yet, preventing them in the first place) is important. It is vital to assess the adolescent's risk of sexually transmitted infection (STI), STI knowledge and behaviours, contraception knowledge/practices, and to rule out the possibility of sexual abuse or pressure for sexual intimacy.
  - S = suicide/depression: screening for potential suicide and depression risk includes enquiries regarding sleep disorders, appetite or behaviour changes, feelings of 'boredom', emotional outbursts or impulsive behaviour, history of withdrawal/isolation, feelings of hopelessness/helplessness, past suicide attempts or depression, history of suicide or depression in the family, history of recurrent serious 'accidents', psychosomatic symptomatology, suicidal ideation, decreased affect during interview, and preoccupation with death (clothing, music, art, etc.).

PHYSICAL EXAMINATION

- The physical examination provides an excellent opportunity for health education. During the assessment of various body systems such as the heart, lungs and skin adolescents can be reassured with regard to normal variants, expected changes associated with puberty and/or specific concerns. However, given the adolescent's likely reluctance to undress and acute self-consciousness, efforts aimed to put patients at ease during the physical examination (respect for privacy, minimal exposure of various body parts, etc.) should be doubled.
- Check (and plot) height and weight.
- Assessment of sexual maturity (e.g. Tanner staging) should be made (see Ch. 12).

- Note that adolescents may consider the physical examination as an 'optional' part of a consultation: e.g. an adolescent female seeking care in order to obtain contraceptive services and during the history disclosing that she is also engaging in risky behaviours/unprotected sexual intercourse. An internal examination (with STI cultures) is not usually a requisite for contraception. However, current rates of STIs (especially chlamydia) have increased dramatically in the adolescent population with far-reaching implications for later sexual and reproductive health. This should be explained to the adolescent as part of the decision-making process with regard to an internal pelvic examination.
- If an internal examination is going to be performed, the utmost care and sensitivity should be taken, as an unpleasant experience may deter the adolescent from seeking care in the future. Careful explanations and anticipatory guidance throughout the examination is imperative. Use of a specially designed, patient-held mirror allows the adolescent to observe the examination while in progress and can be very useful.

MANAGEMENT

- It is important that the adolescent 'buys into' the management plan. More specifically, the adolescent needs to understand (and be happy with) treatment, follow-up and symptoms that indicate a need to return for more care. In short, most health care delivered to adolescent populations is negotiated care. It is often helpful to obtain verbal agreement to the plan before the end of the consultation: *'Is _____ going to be manageable for you?' 'Are you all right with the plan we've developed for this problem?'.*
- Behavioural interventions need to be achievable for the adolescent. Advising adolescents to perform unrealistic self-care activities will likely result in poor concordance with the management plan and a reticence on the part of the adolescent to access care in future (as it wasn't helpful the last time).

- Patient education needs to be appropriate to the adolescent's level of development and specific to his/her issues. In developing a teaching or follow-up plan for the adolescent patient, a strong foundation of growth and development is mandatory. There are big differences in development between early, middle and late adolescents.

FOLLOW-UP

- Adolescents often have access problems with regard to health services and follow-up. It is important that extreme sensitivity is exercised with any follow-up contact. If follow-up is likely to be required, ask the adolescent what they would like to do and, as such, negotiate the management of all follow-up care.

PAEDIATRIC PEARLS

- All communications with adolescents need to be direct, truthful and thoughtful. Relationships with adolescents take time to build but are easily damaged if they are not treated with respect.
- Adolescents can smell hypocrisy from a mile away: never pretend to be something you are not.
- When including the possibility of abstinence as a viable alternative to sexual intercourse in adolescent relationships, it is often helpful to use the concept of 'complications'. More

specifically, when discussing the possibility of sexual intimacy, explore with the adolescent the degree to which life would become more or less 'complicated' as a result of his decision. It is crucial that the adolescent understands the implications of his choices and that the teenager is able to rehearse various scenarios as a strategy for decision making.

- Remember that for the most part, adolescents are acutely self-conscious, have a short future time perspective and varying abilities with abstract reasoning. It is imperative to work within these limitations with extreme sensitivity.
- Always explore with the adolescent the degree to which he has discussed the problem with parents. It is crucial to support and facilitate the adolescent/parental relationship, acting as a mediator if necessary.
- Adolescents often have problems accessing health services. Consider creative ways to improve access for them.
- Note that size and/or physical development is not an accurate predictor of chronological age. Be sure to manage the adolescent according to his age.

BIBLIOGRAPHY

Algranati PS. The pediatric patient: an approach to history and physical examination. Baltimore: Williams & Wilkins; 1992.

Coupey SM. Interviewing adolescents. Pediatr Clin North Am 1997; 44(6):1349–1364.

Department of Health. Seeking consent: working with children. London: Department of Health; 2001. Available: http://www.doh.gov.uk/consent.

Ehram W, Matson S. Approach to assessing adolescents on serious or sensitive issues. Pediatr Clin North Am 1998; 45(1):189–204.

Elster A, Levenberg P. Integrating comprehensive adolescent preventive services into routine medical care. Pediatr Clin North Am 1997; 44(6):1365–1377.

Gill D, O'Brien N. Paediatric clinical examination, 3rd edn. London: Churchill Livingstone; 2000.

Ginsburg K. Guiding adolescents away from violence. Contemp Pediatr 1997; 14(11):101–111.

Goldenring JM, Cohen E. Getting into adolescent heads. Contemp Pediatr 1989; 5:75–90.

Hillard P. Preserving confidentiality in adolescent gynecology. Contemp Pediatr 1997; 14(6):71–92.

Knight J. Adolescent substance use: screening, assessment, and intervention. Contemp Pediatr 1997; 14(4):45–72.

Neinstein LS. Adolescent health care, 3rd edn. London: Williams & Wilkins; 1996.

Nicholson D, Ayers H. Adolescent problems: a practical guide for parents and teachers. London: David Fulton; 1997.

Orr D. Helping adolescents toward adulthood. Contemp Pediatr 1998; 15(5): 55–76.

Prazar G, Friedman S. An office-based approach to adolescent psychosocial issues. Contemp Pediatr 1997; 14(5):59–76.

Taylor J, Muller D. Nursing adolescents: research and psychological perspectives. Oxford: Blackwell Sciences; 1995.

Viner R. Youth matters. London: Action for Sick Children; 1999.

CHAPTER **4**

General Principles in the Assessment and Management of the Ill Child

Katie Barnes

INTRODUCTION

- It is estimated that during the first 2 years of life, children will have 2–4 acute illnesses per year. Although the number of episodic illnesses will decrease as a child gets older, it is very likely that nurse practitioners (NPs) in most settings will be assessing and managing ill children.
- A large percentage of paediatric episodic illnesses are relatively benign, easily managed, of viral aetiology and almost always resolve completely. However, the implications of a missed diagnosis in cases which do not meet these criteria can be devastating and even life-threatening.
- Regardless of the illness, the basic information required for assessment and management of an ill child is, for the most part, the same for all children (adolescents excepted).
- A solid understanding of growth and development is the foundation upon which the history, physical examination, list of differential diagnoses and management plan are based. In addition, the assessment and management of ill children occurs within the family context (see Ch. 1).
- The primary objectives of the episodic paediatric consultation include identification of those conditions that are easily managed by the NP; accurate diagnosis and management; avoidance of missed pathology; appropriate and timely referral (if necessary); and delivery of health care within a context

that is age and/or developmentally appropriate.
- Remember that paediatric illnesses often have a developmental component (e.g. pathogenic organisms, peak ages of incidence, likelihood of sequelae, risk of complications, etc.) and that a child's age has important implications for her care.

PATHOPHYSIOLOGY

- Illness-specific, but it is important to place the pathophysiological processes within a developmental context as there are many physiological processes that are developmentally influenced (e.g. infants with a greatly decreased capacity to fight infection and, as such, at a greater risk for sepsis): see Chapter 2.
- It is very important to use age-appropriate values for vital signs and laboratory values.

HISTORY

- Parents/carers are often the historians (especially with younger children); however, do not exclude older children (and certainly not adolescents) from the information-gathering process. Remember to solicit information directly from them if developmentally appropriate.
- Precipitating factors, events or triggers.
- Location: often helpful to ask an older child to use 'one finger' to point to where it hurts most.

- Character/quality: assessment of pain can be difficult (see Sec. 13.3).
- Quantity/severity: number of episodes and degree to which the symptoms are affecting daily activities. Note that symptoms that awaken a child from a sound sleep are more worrying.
- Associated symptoms: request information regarding additional symptomatology (including presence or absence of fever); use a review of systems to organise the history to ensure no potential complaints are overlooked.
- Timing: onset, duration and frequency of symptoms. Include questioning about the order in which they appeared and the timing of any associated complaints: e.g. child had upper respiratory tract infection (URTI) symptoms for 3 days and was otherwise well but subsequently spiked a fever to 39°C and started vomiting.
- Setting: symptoms on Saturdays? Only in the mornings? Recent travel?
- Aggravating/relieving factors?
- Parent's (and child's) perception of illness?
- Treatments tried so far with results: home remedies, complementary therapies, prescription and over-the-counter (OTC) medications?
- Anyone else ill with same symptoms and/or exposures: siblings, nursery, school, play group?
- How is the family coping with the illness?
- Is the child eating, drinking, playing, urinating and to what degree are these affected by the illness?

- *Note: above points assume that the past medical history is known (allergies, immunisations, major illnesses, medications, etc.). If past medical history is unknown, this additional information must be obtained.*
- It is important to compliment parents on some aspect of their management and/or recognition of their child's illness. A sick child is anxiety-provoking for all parents, but especially those who are young, inexperienced, isolated or lacking support; thus, it is important to contribute to their development as competent parents. This can be as simple or basic as reassuring an anxious parent that she has done the correct thing in seeking care for the child.

PHYSICAL EXAMINATION

- A developmental approach to the physical examination is important (see Ch. 1) and, as such, keep parents in the picture (a potential exception is the physical examination of the adolescent).
- Careful observation is key: *a sick kid looks sick.*
- *Examination of all systems from head to abdomen is mandatory.*
- Repeat observations/examinations after fever relief.
- Special note should be taken of several areas:
  - *General appearance:* note the child's overall appearance (ill, well, alert, lethargic, altered consciousness, etc.), including their ease of movement, cry and colour. To assess nuchal rigidity in infants or small children, drop or move a brightly coloured object around and see if she watches or looks for it. Alternatively, ask the parents to move away and see if the child follows them (i.e. both manoeuvres are to get the child to move his neck). Ask older children to 'kiss' their knees while prone with knees flexed.
  - *Engagability:* the child's degree of interaction with the environment (i.e. smile, ability to turn head, consolability, activity, etc.).
  - *Respiratory effort:* the breath sounds of children with significant upper respiratory tract congestion are difficult to assess as upper airway 'noise' is transmitted to the chest. Listening with a stethoscope at the nose before listening to the lung fields allows aural accommodation to the upper airway sounds, hopefully making assessment of the lower airway easier (e.g. listening 'under' the noise). In addition, loud crying, while often obliterating the expiratory breath sounds, allows for assessment of air exchange/inspiratory effort when the child breathes in (the stronger the cry, the larger the inspiratory breath). However, it is important to be quick and focus on the inspiratory phase. *Beware the silent chest as this implies there is no air exchange and is a medical emergency.*
  - *Hydration:* check for skin turgor/tenting on abdomen. Palpate the oral mucosa in order to feel its texture: i.e. when rubbing the inside of the cheek, it should feel slippery.
  - *Temperature:* accurate measurement is very important, especially with younger children.
  - *Vital signs (including weight):* be sure to use age-appropriate normal values and it is very important to obtain the child's weight at the time of the episodic visit (if there is a return visit, the values will need to be compared). Note that a fever will increase the age-appropriate heart rate by approximately 10 beats/min for each 0.5°C elevation above normal core temperature.
  - *Skin:* carefully check for rashes all over the body, including the mucous membranes: i.e. check for rashes both inside and out.
  - *Perfusion:* note colour, texture and capillary refill (<2 s).

DIFFERENTIAL DIAGNOSES

- Numerous, so think very broadly.
- Consider age-specific pathogens and aetiologies.
- Consider the epidemiological features of different illnesses in your thinking (e.g. seasonality of some infections, likelihood of exposure, incubation periods, community outbreaks, etc.).

MANAGEMENT

Specific management of the ill child is aetiology-dependent, but the following are some basic principles to be considered.

- **Additional diagnostics:** availability of diagnostic testing is often dependent on setting. However, if available, both a full blood count (FBC) and urine dipstick (with leucocyte esterase and nitrites) are initial diagnostics that provide useful information for clinical decision making (see Sec. 14.1). This is especially true in young, febrile infants (see Sec. 15.1). Note that a butterfly needle is the easiest way to draw an FBC.
- **Pharmacotherapeutics:** usually not necessary. However, it is important to consider issues such as medication administration, refrigeration, scheduling, length of treatment and TASTE.
- **Behavioural interventions:** consider nutritional management and supportive care (including fever control). Give older children 'homework' or a 'special job to help themselves get better'. For example, explain to a 5 year old that their 'job' is to drink an extra glass of 'special water' each time they have diarrhoea. Use every consultation as an opportunity to promote appropriate interventions for self-care and healthy choices.
- **Patient education:** always review behavioural interventions related to the illness in addition to explaining to parents (and children) the aetiology of the illness; infection control instructions and 'expected' course of illness (including when to return to school or nursery); when to return/phone for 'unexpected' events during the course of the illness; and any follow-up instructions. Lastly, it is important to provide reassurance and praise where appropriate for the parent or carer's management.

MEDICAL CONSULT/ SPECIALIST REFERRAL

- Any child in whom presentation or history fall outside the NP's comfort level, expertise or scope of practice.
- Any child in whom there is a gravely ill appearance or whose clinical condition has deteriorated.
- Any child requiring specialist intervention or expertise.
- Young, febrile infants and neonates are at much greater risk of serious infection and as such, will likely require referral.

PAEDIATRIC PEARLS

- General appearance and engagability are important indicators; sick kids look sick—trust your instincts.
- You are not just treating the child, it is the whole family.
- The child's age and developmental level are the springboard from which the history, physical examination, differential list and management plan are launched; do not overlook these important considerations.
- Get some good paediatric reference books—keep them handy.
- Use age-appropriate vital signs and laboratory values.

- Develop good relationships with the paediatric professionals (registrars, consultants or NPs): they can be an important resource for paediatric-related questions and referrals.
- Don't overlook the urine as a potential source of infection.
- A head-to-abdomen physical examination is imperative in paediatric episodic illness.
- Don't forget to look 'inside' and 'outside' for rashes and always check perfusion and hydration status.
- Respiratory effort is a vital observation; listen 'underneath' the noise.

BIBLIOGRAPHY

Algranati PS. The pediatric patient: an approach to history and physical examination. Baltimore: Williams & Wilkins; 1992.

Algranati PS. Effect of developmental status on the approach to physical examination. Pediatr Clin North Am 1998; 45(1):1–23.

Boynton R. Manual of ambulatory pediatrics, 4th edn. Philadelphia: Lippincott; 1998.

Brundige KJ. Preparing pediatric nurse practitioners for roles in specialty practice. J Pediatr Health Care 1997; 11(4):198–200.

Burns C. Pediatric primary care: a handbook for nurse practitioners, 2nd edn. London: WB Saunders; 2000.

Callender D. Pediatric practice guidelines: implications for nurse practitioners. J Pediatr Health Care 1999; 13(3):105–111.

Engel J. Pocket guide to pediatric assessment, 3rd edn. St. Louis: Mosby; 1997.

Gaedeke MK. Advanced practice nursing in pediatric acute care. Crit Care Nurs Clin North Am 1995; 7(1):61–70.

Gill D, O'Brien N. Paediatric clinical examination, 3rd edn. London: Churchill Livingstone; 1998.

Jarvis C. Physical examination and health assessment, 2nd edn. Philadelphia: WB Saunders; 1996.

National Association of Pediatric Nurse Practitioners. The paediatric nurse practitioner (patient guide). Cherry Hill, New Jersey; 1997. Available: http://www.napnap.org/.

National Association of Pediatric Nurse Practitioners. Scope of practice for pediatric nurse practitioners. Cherry Hill, New Jersey: NAPNAP; 2000. Available: http://www.napnap.org/.

National Association of Pediatric Nurse Practitioners. Standards of practice for pediatric nurse practitioners in primary care. Cherry Hill, New Jersey; 2001. Available: http://www.napnap.org/.

Nazarian L. Practice parameters: what are they and why should we use them? Pediatr Rev 1997; 18(7):219–220.

Schwartz M. The 5 minute pediatric consult, 2nd edn. London: Lippincott, Williams & Wilkins; 2000.

Vessey JA. Developmental approaches to examining young children. Pediatr Nurs 1995; 21(1):53–56.

CLINICAL ISSUES IN PAEDIATRICS

CHAPTER 5

Pharmacology in Paediatrics

Katie Barnes and Sara Higginson

INTRODUCTION

- Adults and children respond to drugs differently. Disparities include the absorption, distribution, metabolism and elimination of the drug by the body as well as differences in formulation, dosage and administration.
- The field of paediatric pharmacology is relatively new and tremendous progress has been made in expanding paediatric pharmacology from an adult therapeutics 'add-on' into a recognised specialty. However, the development of a pharmacological evidence base in children has been hampered by the difficulties of conducting drug trials in paediatrics.
- Medications that are used commonly in paediatric practice do have well-articulated details such as age/weight dosing, implications for breast-feeding and important information related to drug absorption, distribution, elimination and adverse events. It is imperative that the clinician caring for children utilises this information to maximise the benefits of pharmacological agents.
- It is important to recognise that the nature, duration of effect and intensity of a drug's action are related not only to the intrinsic properties of the drug itself but also to the drug's interaction with the patient to whom it has been administered. Therefore, effective and safe drug therapy in neonates, infants, children and adolescents requires an understanding of the differences in drug action, metabolism and disposition that are determined developmentally.
- Nearly all pharmacokinetic parameters change with age and as a result, paediatric drug dosages must be adjusted accordingly. Likewise, issues such as medication administration and formulation have concordance implications in paediatrics.
- Although an in-depth analysis of paediatric pharmacology is beyond the scope of this book, important pharmacotherapeutic considerations are outlined.

DRUG ABSORPTION

- Among neonates and young infants, decreased intestinal motility and delayed gastric emptying time can result in a greater lag time between drug administration and a plasma concentration that is equivalent to that of an older child or adult. This is likewise true among older children with gastrointestinal problems (e.g. coeliac disease or cystic fibrosis). However, controversy exists as to the clinical significance of these factors outside of the neonatal and early infancy periods, as factors such as liquid administration, decreased gastric acid production and a relatively greater small gut surface area in young children contribute to potentially enhanced drug absorption.
- Reflux of gastric contents is very common during the first year of life: excessive reflux of medications can result in a variable and unpredictable loss of an orally administered dose.
- Rectal drug administration in paediatrics can be a useful alternative when conditions such as nausea, vomiting and status epilepticus preclude oral administration. Drugs administered rectally are absorbed directly into the haemorrhoidal vein (part of the systemic rather than portal system) and therefore, do not make a 'first pass' through the liver where a large fraction of the absorbed drug may be removed. However, rectal administration of drugs in suppository form is typically erratic, with the presence of stool and/or expulsion of the dose potentially affecting drug absorption through decreased bioavailability. Nevertheless, medications can be successfully administered rectally if in solution (e.g. diazepam and rectal corticosteroids). Note that rectal absorption of paracetamol can be variable, but that it is adequately absorbed, albeit more slowly than oral administration.
- The rate and extent of absorption from intramuscular and subcutaneous injection is influenced by characteristics of the patient—e.g. blood flow to the injection site, muscle mass, quantity of adipose tissue and muscle activity—as well as properties of the drug, such as solubility of the drug at the extracellular pH, ease of diffusion across capillary membranes and the surface area over which the injection volume spreads. In general, parenteral administration via injection is not an optimal route in hypoperfusion syndromes, dehydration, vasomotor instability or starvation, as absorption will be impeded. However for many drugs, including most aminoglycoside and penicillin antibiotics, intramuscular administration results in plasma

concentrations equivalent to those achieved with intravenous administration. Drugs for which intramuscular administration is not appropriate include those with an unacceptable degree of tissue reaction (e.g. erythromycin, some cephalosporins, digoxin) and those that are highly hydrophobic (diazepam and phenytoin). It is important to remember that intramuscular injection can be painful (especially relevant for children) and it can be unsuitable when a rapid response is needed as absorption can be slow and incomplete.

- It is important to recognise that absorption of topical medications is greater among infants and small children because of their (1) thinner stratum corneum, (2) greater total body surface area (TBSA) to weight ratio and (3) increased skin hydration. Amongst young children, the use of plastic-coated nappies can increase drug absorption in the nappy area (related to the occlusiveness of the plastic coating). All of these considerations have implications for the amount of drug absorbed transcutaneously and therefore, care needs to be taken with the use of high-potency medications (i.e. use of strong topical steroids in infants with severe eczema).
- The issue of drug absorption with regard to meals is also of importance in paediatrics. In order to facilitate ease of administration (and subsequent concordance) most orally administered drugs (isoniazid and narrow-spectrum penicillins excepted) should be given with meals.
- Sustained-release oral preparations are problematic in young children, as absorption may be unpredictable, incomplete and result in treatment failures. Dosing schedules may need to be adjusted depending on the rate of drug clearance and the effect of increased gastrointestinal transit time in infants and young children.

DRUG DISTRIBUTION

- Once absorbed, the distribution of a drug is related to host factors such as body compartment size and composition; protein-binding capacity (both plasma and protein); and blood–brain barrier permeability. Characteristics of the drug include its molecular weight and its degree of ionisation once absorbed. As a general rule, the volume of distribution of drugs tends to be greater among infants, with a subsequent decrease as the child matures into childhood (i.e. closer to adult values). However, there are many exceptions, including drugs such as theophylline and phenobarbital.
- Note that young children (especially infants) have a greater percentage of total body water and extracellular fluid for their size. Consequently, there may be increased distribution and dilution of water-soluble drugs (e.g. aminoglycosides) as the resultant concentration of the drug at the receptor site is reduced. This is the rationale behind increased milligrams of drug per kilograms of body weight (mg/kg) dosing of many medications (as compared to adult dosages).
- Reduced protein binding of drugs can be important in the neonatal period. The reduced albumin and displacement of drugs by bilirubin results in higher concentrations of the free drug, which is pharmacologically active. For example, ceftriaxone should be avoided in neonates with jaundice, hypoalbuminaemia, acidosis or impaired bilirubin binding.
- Among neonates, the blood–brain barrier is functionally incomplete so there may be an enhanced effect of some medications. In older children, relatively tighter junctions in the endothelial capillaries of the brain combined with the close proximity of the glial connective tissue to the capillary endothelium results in limited distribution of drugs to the brain tissue. However, with inflamed meninges (e.g. in meningitis), higher concentrations of a drug are attained in the cerebrospinal fluid (CSF) as a function of an increased vascular permeability and partial inhibition of the organic acid transport mechanism.

DRUG ELIMINATION: METABOLISM AND EXCRETION

- Differences in drug metabolism, which occurs primarily in the liver, are most acute in the immediate neonatal period, particularly in premature infants. They are related to the decreased ability of the liver and its microsomal enzyme system to metabolise a number of drug substrates. During the subsequent 3 months of life, the capacity of the liver to metabolise drugs increases rapidly. In the pre-school child, hepatic clearance actually exceeds adult levels, whereas in adolescence the metabolic capacity of the liver normalises to adult levels.
- In the kidney (the primary site of drug excretion) glomerular filtration and tubular function are less efficient in early infancy. However, creatinine clearance increases rapidly during the first year of life so that by 12 months of age, creatinine clearance—when adjusted for body surface area—equals adult clearance levels. In addition, there is some evidence that the average clearance in school-age children actually exceeds adult levels. Tubular function matures later than glomerular function but is essentially mature by 1 year of age. Clinical implications of decreased renal function are most pronounced in pre-term infants and among children with pre-existing renal pathology. Therefore, dose adjustment would be necessary for these groups when drugs dependent on renal excretion for cessation of their activity— e.g. penicillins, aminoglycosides, digoxin and thiazide diuretics—are administered. In brief, the half-life of a drug is prolonged among newborns, decreased during infancy and shortest in the school-age child.

DRUG CHOICE, DOSAGE, FREQUENCY, ADMINISTRATION ROUTE AND FORMULATION

- While many paediatric illnesses are self-limiting, if medication is required it is important that the drug choice is dictated by the pathophysiology of the illness and the most likely match between the causative agent/process and the pharmacological activity of the drug (e.g. penicillin V for treatment of streptococcal pharyngitis). Drug choice is also influenced by issues such as medication cost, safety of use in paediatrics and drug effectiveness.

- Drug dosages in paediatrics are most accurately calculated on a mg/kg basis (drugs calculated by total body surface area excepted). This is especially true for children <20 kg and for those medications with a narrow therapeutic range. However, the available concentration of a specific preparation will impact the clinician's ability to request a specific mg/kg dose. The commonly accepted method of paediatric dosing is to calculate the optimal mg/kg dose and subsequently adjust it to a *practical* dose and available preparation. Note that this is unlikely to be necessary when dosing older children and adolescents for whom standard formulations often apply.

- With regard to dose frequency, as a general rule the lowest number of daily doses of a drug is preferable. For example, once daily steroid dosing (orally) is associated with less toxicity and improved adherence than smaller, more frequently administered doses. Likewise, thrice (or twice) daily dosing of an antibiotic is preferable to one that is administered four times a day (assuming there is no decrease in drug effectiveness). This is especially relevant for school-age children who may be able to receive doses of medicine while at school.

- Oral administration is by far the most common route of paediatric drug administration. Topical preparations are largely reserved for dermatological conditions. Occasionally, there is an option of rectal or parenteral administration of a drug. Careful consideration of these routes is required as they are potentially more traumatic to the child (especially older children).

- Drug formulation can impact medication concordance. If the child is able to manage tablets or capsules,

they are often more easily stored, there is greater accuracy of dosing (compared to liquid preparations) and often a longer expiry date. If a child cannot manage solid preparations, then an oral preparation is often a better choice than 'crushing' tablets (although with unpalatable liquids, crushed medication may be more easily disguised). Sustained-release medication should never be crushed or chewed and likewise, medication should not be mixed into large quantities of food or drink (e.g. never put medication into a baby's bottle as there is no way to be assured that the complete dose has been administered). Useful foods for disguising medications include *small* quantities of yogurt, blackcurrant cordial, chocolate mousse and bananas (mixed immediately before administration).

- If a medication comes in two different strengths, a specific dosage may be maintained in a smaller volume of medication; this is especially helpful with uncooperative toddlers or pre-schoolers. In addition, many medications (especially liquid preparations) contain dyes, colouring agents and sucrose which children may be sensitive to (although the number who react is probably small).

- In paediatric asthma management it is vital that the drug delivery device and drug formulation are matched. In addition, it is important that the device and its mechanics of use are developmentally appropriate for the child (e.g. infants should not be using a spin inhaler).

- Many drugs used in paediatrics do not have a product licence for use in children. First choice should be a drug licensed for the age of the child being treated. However, as this is not always possible, it is inevitable that drugs will be used 'off label' (i.e. outside the product licence). In these cases, it is the prescriber's responsibility to select a drug where sound information is available (e.g. paediatric formularies). Use of unlicensed drugs can also present problems with supply and provision of the parent/patient information sheets (PILs).

CONCORDANCE AND PATIENT EDUCATION

- Difficulties with a particular medication regimen arise from uncooperative children, inaccurate measurement techniques, omission of doses and conflicts such as nursery or school attendance. The ideal medication is one that is: palatable, with the fewest number of doses, no special storage requirements, and available in an appropriate strength that is cheap, safe and effective.

- Parent and child education should include an understanding of (1) why a certain medication has been recommended, (2) what the medication should do (and what it shouldn't do), (3) for how long (and how many times a day) it should be administered, and (4) the importance of continuing the medication for the recommended length of time (even though symptoms may subside). In addition it is important to remind parents that all medications should be stored safely out of reach of children.

- Parents may need advice on administration techniques and equipment to ensure accurate measurement (a teaspoon is not a teaspoon is not a teaspoon). An oral syringe ensures accurate measurement and may be preferred in some patients.

- Administration of oral medication to infants requires (1) the head to be slightly elevated, (2) the correct dose measured in a dropper or oral syringe, and (3) placement of the drug in the back of the mouth on either side of the tongue. A gentle puff of breath onto the baby's face often elicits a swallowing reflex, which completes the process. Warn parents that if the infant starts to choke or cough, stop giving the medicine, sit him/her up and resume administration when the infant has settled.

- Positive reinforcement (stickers, praise, etc.) can be used in older children. It is often helpful to encourage a sense of autonomy with their medication: e.g. letting a child 'squirt' the medicine into their mouth or 'help' to measure. Children should be approached firmly with clear instructions on what is expected of them. If the medication has an unpleasant taste, use of a straw while simultaneously holding the nose is often helpful.

- Medications should not be put into juices or bottles, as there is no way to be assured that the complete dose has been administered.

PAEDIATRIC PEARLS

- Developmental changes in body composition, body proportions and relative mass of the liver and kidneys affect pharmacokinetics of a drug among different ages (e.g. neonates, infants, children and adolescents).
- The capacity for drug metabolism and elimination is the greatest between the first and second years of life when the size of the kidney and liver (relative to body weight) are at their maximum.
- Remember that body surface area (relative to body mass) is greatest in the infant and young child (as compared to the older child and adult) and thus, consideration must be given

to potential systemic absorption of topically applied drugs.

- The loading dose of a drug is primarily related to its volume of distribution, whereas the maintenance dose is a function of drug clearance.
- Clearance of most drugs is primarily dependent on hepatic metabolism, with the excretion of drug and metabolites completed by the kidneys (and to a lesser extent, the liver).
- In general, between 1 year of age and puberty, hepatic and renal function is not only equal to, but may exceed, normal adult levels of functioning.
- Children of the same age come in many different sizes. Always calculate drug dosages in mg/kg (especially among children less than 20 kg) and adjust the dose to the available preparations.
- In asthma management it is imperative to match the correct medication with the appropriate drug delivery device and the child's development.
- The ideal medication is one that tastes good, is only given once a day, does not require refrigeration, comes in the

right strength and is cheap, safe in kids and highly effective. Unfortunately, this combination does not exist; choose the closest option.

BIBLIOGRAPHY

Hein K. Drug therapeutics in the adolescent. In: Yaffe S, Aranda J, eds, Pediatric pharmacology. Philadelphia: WB Saunders; 1992: 220–230.

Kaufman RE. Drug therapeutics in the infant and child. In: Yaffe S, Aranda J, eds, Pediatric pharmacology. Philadelphia: WB Saunders; 1992: 212–219.

Loebstein R, Koren G. Clinical pharmacology and therapeutic drug monitoring in neonates and children. Pediatr Rev 1998; 19(12):423–428.

McGillis-Bindler R, Berner-Howry L. Pediatric drugs and nursing implications, 2nd edn. Stamford: Appleton Lange; 1996.

Niederhausen VP. Prescribing for children: issues in pediatric pharmacology. Nurse Pract 1997; 22(3):16–30.

Rylance GW. Prescribing for infants and children. BMJ 1988; 296:984–986.

Walson PD. 1997 Paediatric clinical pharmacology and therapeutics. In: Speight TM, Holford M, Nicholas HG, eds, Avery's drug treatment, 4th edn. London: Blackwell Science; 1997: 127–165.

CHAPTER **6**

Internet Resources for the Nurse Practitioner

John Walter

INTRODUCTION

- As information technology continues to offer greater promise in the delivery of health care, the computer may be the practitioner's best ally to enhance patient care. Through new emerging information systems, practitioners are accessing clinical information more efficiently, tapping into online repositories of medical information, communicating electronically with peers and finding new ways to simplify their work.
- This list of web sites is intended for use by advanced practice nurses and is for education and information purposes only. Accuracy of the information contained in individual web sites should always be verified through other sources before being applied to patient care. Browsing via the Internet to find up-to-date information is the wave of the future.
- To access the information on the Internet, it is assumed the reader can connect to online services. Each site was evaluated for current information, paediatric focus in the clinical practice areas, search features, international interest and parent/child resources.
- Individual sites are organised around broad subject headings: *Alternative and Complementary Medicine*; *Bioterrorism*; *Clinical Practice*; *Clinical Tools*; *Journals and Reference Tools*; *Literature Search Tools*; *Patient Information*; *Pharmacology*; *Practice Guidelines*; *Professional Organisations*; *Sports Medicine*; and *Travel Medicine*.

- *All the links are available on http://www.geocities.com/paediatric.*

ALTERNATIVE AND COMPLEMENTARY MEDICINE

http://www.mcp.edu/herbal/ default.htm The Longwood Herbal Task Force was organised in the autumn of 1998 to learn more about and teach other clinicians about herbs and dietary supplements. The group began with systematic reviews of the six most common supplements used by oncology patients. Work rapidly expanded to include approximately 85 herbs and dietary supplements. The site has in-depth monographs, clinician information summaries, patient fact sheets, toxicity and interactions, and resources.

http://www.altmedicine.com/ Alternative Health News Online offers a search engine, health news bulletins, diet & nutrition, mind/ body control, alternative medical systems, manual healing and many links to alternative and complementary medicine.

BIOTERRORISM

http://www.aap.org/advocacy/release/ cad.htm/ The American Academy of Pediatrics has a resource of material on bioterrorism, including anthrax and smallpox, and psychological support of children in disaster situations.

CLINICAL PRACTICE

- **Behavioural paediatrics:** http://www.aap.org/policy/ ac0002.html Practice guideline from the American Academy of Pediatrics on the 'diagnosis and evaluation of the child with attention deficit/ hyperactivity disorder'.

  http://www.psychiatry.ox.ac.uk/ cebmh/index.html Lots of information on behavioural health. The site is maintained by the Centre for Evidence Based Mental Health in Oxford, UK.

- **Breast-feeding:** http://lalecheleague.org/prof.html The LaLeche League International site has a database of over 15,000 breast-feeding-related professional articles. Registration is required.

- **Dermatology:** http://www.dermis.net/index_e.htm Dermatology Information System is a link to Paediatric Dermatology Atlas. There are over 2000 full-screen images available for viewing.

- **Diabetes:** http://www.childrenwithdiabetes.com/ index_cwd.htm Information for children, adults and professionals.

- **Down's syndrome:** http://www.ds-health.com/ Health issues on Down's syndrome for parents and professionals.

- **Gastrointestinal:**
  http://www.journals.uchicago.edu/
  CID/journal/issues/v32n3/001387/
  001387.html   *Practice guidelines for
  the management of infectious diarrhea*
  published by the Infectious Disease
  Society of America.

  http://www.cdc.gov/mmwr/
  preview/mmwrhtml/rr5002a1.htm
  *Diagnosis and management of
  foodborne illness: a primer for
  physicians*, published by the Centers
  for Disease Control and Prevention
  (CDC), is available for download.

- **General paediatrics:**
  http://www.omni.ac.uk/subject-
  listing/WS100.html   The UK's
  gateway to pediatric Internet
  resources.

  http://www.peds.umn.edu/divisions/
  pccm/teaching/acpcp.html   Acute
  paediatric primary care for the
  practitioner. A lecture series from
  the Pediatric Department at the
  University of Minnesota.

  http://www.pedinfo.org/   An index
  of the paediatric Internet. It has its
  own search function. Many categories
  and topics are listed.

  http://pedsccm.wustl.edu/All-Net/
  main.html   Paediatric critical care
  topics.

  http://www.vh.org/pediatric/index.
  html   Virtual Children's Hospital at
  the University of Iowa. Information on
  common paediatric problems,
  multimedia textbooks, teaching files,
  virtual patients, journals, grand
  rounds, practice guidelines and clinical
  references.

- **Immunisations:**
  http://www.health.state.mn.us/divs/
  dpc/adps/forgnvac1.pdf   Do you
  have difficulty understanding your
  patients' foreign vaccination records?
  If so, *Vaccines and biologics used in
  U.S. and foreign markets* can help you
  make sense of them. This is an 11-page
  guide to vaccine products that lists
  vaccines and biologics by their trade
  name as well as the manufacturer and
  country of manufacture. (Adobe®
  Acrobat® Reader™ is free software that

lets you view and print Adobe Portable
Document Format (PDF) files:
http://www.adobe.com/products/
acrobat/readstep2.html)

http://www.health.state.mn.us/divs/
dpc/adps/forgnvac2.pdf   Six-page
chart entitled *Translation of foreign
vaccine-related terms* (Adobe®
Acrobat® Reader™ is free software that
lets you view and print Adobe Portable
Document Format (PDF) files:
http://www.adobe.com/products/
acrobat/readstep2.html)

http://home.vicnet.net.au/~nmaa/
index.html   Comprehensive link to
the most up-to-date, expert
immunisation resources available via
the Internet. Use this site as the
jumping-off point for the best in
vaccine and antibody information.

- **Infectious disease—AIDS:**
  www.unaids.org/   Joint United
  Nations Programme on HIV/AIDS.

  www.iavi.org/   The International
  AIDS Vaccine Initiative.

  www.ama-assn.org/special/hiv/
  hivhome.htm   HIV/AIDS
  Information Center of the *Journal
  of the American Medical Association*.
  This site also has a collection of
  published guidelines for prevention
  and management of HIV/AIDS and
  related conditions.

  www.adolescentaids.org   Staff at the
  Adolescent AIDS Program at
  Montefiore Medical Center have
  developed the first comprehensive
  Gay and Lesbian Adolescent Health
  Resource Center.

- **Infectious disease—Tuberculosis:**
  http://www.journals.uchicago.edu/
  CID/journal/issues/v31n3/000549/
  000549.html   Practice Guidelines for
  the Treatment of Tuberculosis.

- **Neonatology:**
  http://www.neonatology.org/
  index.html   Can search for many
  neonatal topics.

- **Sickle cell disease:**
  http://www.scinfo.org   Sickle Cell
  Disease Information Center.

CLINICAL TOOLS

http://isabel.org.uk   Clinical decision
support software for paediatrics.
Requires registration, but access is
free and site is owned, updated and
developed by the Isabel Medical Charity.
Very valuable site for access to up-to-date,
detailed information on paediatric signs,
symptoms, differential diagnosis and
management.

http://www.intmed.mcw.edu/
clincalc.html   Clinical calculators from
the Medical College of Wisconsin.

http://www.toledo-bend.com/
colorblind/Ishihara.html   The Ishihara
test for colour blindness.

http://www.wilkes.med.ucla.edu/
intro.html   The Auscultation Assistant
provides heart sounds, heart murmurs
and breath sounds in order to help
students and others improve their
physical diagnosis skills.

JOURNALS AND REFERENCE TOOLS

http://www.thelancet.com/   *The
Lancet* site has free access to selected
full-text articles, unlimited search
facilities, Electronic Research Archive
(ERA) and full-text global news.

http://www.bmj.com/   *The British
Medical Journal* has free selected articles
and editorials for non-subscribers. Table
of contents for the journal can be viewed.

http://omni.ac.uk/subject-listing/
WS100.html   OMNI (Organising
Medical Networked Information) is a
gateway to evaluated Internet resources
in health and medicine. It is updated
regularly and has a great search function.
OMNI is created by a core team of
information specialists and subject experts
based at the University of Nottingham
Greenfield Medical Library. This web
address is for the paediatric section.

http://www.nice.org.uk/   The
National Institute for Clinical Excellence
was set up as a Special Health Authority
for England and Wales in 1999. It is part
of the National Health Service, and its
role is to provide patients, health
professionals and the public with

authoritative, robust and reliable guidance on current 'best practice'. This site includes Clinical Guidelines and information on the clinical management of specific conditions.

http://idinchildren.com/ *Infectious Diseases in Children*—free access to current and past issues.

http://www.priory.com/fam.htm Family Medical Practice On-Line have full-text articles. Only a few pertain to paediatrics.

http://content.nejm.org/ The *New England Journal of Medicine* has free registration access to full-text articles that have been published over 6 months ago. Abstracts are available for all current articles.

http://intl.pediatrics.org/ The American Academy of Pediatrics publishes the *Pediatrics* Electronic Page articles that are free and full-text. Free abstracts are available on all current articles in the printed journal.

http://www.nelh.nhs.uk/ National Electronic Library for Health in the UK.

http://pediatrics.medscape.com Medscape is a leading company for online medical information. Free registration is necessary for weekly medical news delivery via e-mail. Some full-text journal articles are online. MEDLINE abstracts, searches, guidelines, patient information and continuing education are available.

http://www.pedinfo.org/ PEDINFO: An Index of the Pediatric Internet. Dedicated to the dissemination of online information for paediatric health care providers and others interested in child health. MEDLINE searches, drug information, current health news and many more areas are available. Excellent site to search for specific health topics.

http://ww2.med.jhu.edu/peds/ neonatology/poi.html The Harriet Lane Links provide an edited collection of paediatric resources (5475 links) on the World Wide Web. Maintained and edited by physicians at the Johns Hopkins University, this site attempts to catalogue, review and score existing links to paediatric information on the Internet.

http://www.freemedicaljournals.com/ MedicalJournals.com Free full-text journals.

http://www.contemporarypediatrics. com *Contemporary Pediatrics* journal online.

http://www.emedicine.com/emerg/ index.shtml Full-text of *Emergency Medicine* textbook. Topics are listed alphabetically in the contents section.

http://www.merck.com/pubs/ mmanual/sections.htm *The Merck Manual of Diagnosis and Therapy* is online with a search function.

http://www.docguide.com/dgc.nsf/ge/ *Doctor's Guide*, global edition, scans 1500 peer-reviewed journals. Register to receive weekly medial news via e-mail. Numerous topics and specific disease information listed.

http://www.bartleby.com/107/ *Gray's Anatomy of the Human Body.*

http://www.nhlbi.nih.gov/index.htm National Heart Lung Blood Institute site, including articles, guidelines, and current clinical trials.

http://www.dynamicmedical.com/ DynaMed (Dynamic Medical Information System) is an interactive, real-time medical information system designed for use at the point of care. It consists mainly of a vast clinically organised reference covering basic information and is updated daily from developments in the literature. DynaMed is also designed to allow for user input and discussions. DynaMed is designed to provide quick and easy access to medical information and is a useful resource in clinical, educational and research settings. It contains basic information on over 2000 diseases, and provides an organised structure for finding disease-based information, including both standard medical knowledge and current developments.

http://www.ti.ubc.ca/pages/letter.html Full-text articles from the *Therapeutics Letter.*

http://www.ortho-u.net *Wheeless' Textbook of Orthopaedics* is an excellent online reference with many radiological views.

http://www.ornl.gov/hgmis/medicine/ medicine.html Latest news about medical genetics. The site has a large collection of articles and information on the Human Genome Project.

LITERATURE SEARCH TOOLS

http://gateway.nlm.nih.gov/gw/Cmd The NLM Gateway allows users to search in multiple retrieval systems at the US National Library of Medicine (NLM). The current Gateway searches MEDLINE/PubMed, OLDMEDLINE, LOCATOR*plus*, MEDLINE*plus* and DIRLINE.

www.tripdatabase.com The TRIP Database searches across 58 sites of high-quality medical information. The TRIP Database gives you direct, hyperlinked access to the largest collection of 'evidence-based' material on the web as well as articles from premier online journals such as the *British Medical Journal*, *Journal of the American Medical Association* and the *New England Journal of Medicine.*

http://nhscrd.york.ac.uk/darehp.htm Database of Abstracts of Reviews of Effectiveness (DARE). Supported by the University of York.

http://www.bmj.com/cgi/content/ full/315/7101/180 A full text article in the *British Medical Journal*: 'How to read a paper: the Medline database'. It's a how-to article on searching the MEDLINE database.

http://www.cochrane.org The Cochrane Collaboration is an international not-for-profit organisation. Its aim is to make up-to-date, accurate information about the effects of health care readily available worldwide. The Cochrane library can be accessed via a server in the UK, US or Germany.

PATIENT INFORMATION

http://www.nhsdirect.nhs.uk/about/ NHS Direct is a 24-hour nurse-led helpline providing confidential health care advice and information on what to do if you're feeling ill; health concerns; local health services; and self-help and support organisations. Its main purpose is to improve access to health information for patients and the public.

http://www.jr2.ox.ac.uk/bandolier/ *Bandolier* is evidence-based health care articles published on many topics, including a few on paediatrics.

http://www.patient.co.uk/ Patient UK is a directory of UK health, disease and related websites. It is edited by two general practitioners. Topics include child health, teenagers, student health, self-help groups and medicines.

http://www.chas.org.uk/ Children's Hospice Association Scotland is a charity committed to the provision of children's hospice services in Scotland, working exclusively with children with life-limiting conditions and their families.

http://www.ich.ucl.ac.uk/ The Great Ormond Street Hospital and the Institute of Child Health together form the largest paediatric training and research centre in the UK. The two institutions work in partnership to improve the health of children everywhere. The Hospital offers the widest range of paediatric specialties in the country. The Institute aims to define the scientific, epidemiological and clinical basis of childhood diseases and to promote child health across the country and internationally.

http://www.healthatoz.com/ Health A to Z 'search the web' feature that can search over 50,000 professionally reviewed health and medical Internet resources. Free registration for weekly personalised information on conditions or topics of interest. There is also online family health records organiser and free e-mail reminders about immunisations, checkups and appointments.

http://www.healthfinder.gov/ Guide to reliable health information sponsored by the US Department of Health and Human Services. There is a section for children—art contest, games, safe surfing and many health topics presented as cartoons and learning games.

http://kidshealth.org/index.html KidsHealth provides doctor-approved health information about children from birth through adolescence. KidsHealth

has separate areas for kids, teens and parents—each with its own design and age-appropriate content.

http://www.mayohealth.org/home? id=3.1.6 The children's page from the Mayo Clinic web site. Great resource for parents. Lists for specific conditions, medications, safety and first-aid.

http://www.nlm.nih.gov/medlineplus/childandteenhealth.html National Library of Medicine, MEDLINE Plus site on child and teen health topics.

PHARMACOLOGY

http://www.nppg.demon.co.uk/ Neonatal and Paediatric Pharmacists Group web site. Health professionals need to register to enter the electronic Medicines Compendium section.

http://cp.gsm.com/ Clinical Pharmacology 2000 provides up-to-date, peer-reviewed, clinically relevant information on all US drugs, as well as off-label uses and dosages, herbal supplements, nutritional products, new and investigational drugs, and can identify potential interactions. Nurse practitioners have free registration. Printouts are available for each product.

PRACTICE GUIDELINES

http://www.guideline.gov/index.asp The National Guideline Clearinghouse™ (NGC) is a public resource for evidence-based clinical practice guidelines. NGC is sponsored by the Agency for Healthcare Research and Quality (AHRQ) in partnership with the American Medical Association and the American Association of Health Plans. The site is searchable by keywords.

http://www.aap.org/policy/pprgtoc.cfm Current American Academy of Pediatrics policy statements through April 2001.

http://www.aap.org/policy/paramtoc.html Current American Academy of Pediatrics clinical practice guidelines.

http://www.med.umich.edu/pediatric/ebm Evidence-based paediatric web site at the University of Michigan.

http://cebm.jr2.ox.ac.uk/index.html The UK Centre for Evidence-based Medicine.

http://www.show.scot.nhs.uk/sign/guidelines/index.html The Scottish Intercollegiate Guidelines Network has full text and supporting material for many practice guidelines. Only a few pertain to paediatrics.

http://www.york.ac.uk/inst/crd/welcome.htm NHS Centre for Reviews & Dissemination. The purpose is to promote the use of research-based knowledge in health care.

PROFESSIONAL ORGANISATIONS

http://www.rcpch.ac.uk/ The Royal College of Paediatrics and Child Health site can be searched. Available are downloadable newsletters, growth references and paediatric news.

http://www.nursepractitioner.org.uk A website for and about NPs in the UK. Membership of the group is free. Excellent resource for access to a large listserv of NPs in the UK and around the world.

www.nmc-uk.org Nursing and Midwifery Council.

http://www.ukcc.org.uk/cms/content/home/ United Kingdom Central Council.

http://www.soft.net.uk/nursinguk/index.html UK Nursing Forum is a place where UK nurses can exchange comments, ideas, give support to each other and maintain direction. Specific areas include the UK Nurses Discussion Group, archives, a message board and links to other nursing sites.

http://www.nursingtimes.net/ *Nursing Times* on the Net—information for UK nurses.

http://www.doh.gov.uk/ UK Department of Health.

http://www.napnap.org/ The National Association of Pediatric Nurse Practitioners.

http://www.aanp.org American Academy of Nurse Practitioners.

http://www.nursingworld.org/
American Nurses Association.

http://www.nurse.org/acnp/
American College of Nurse Practitioners.

http://www.inurse.com/links/
default.htm   Links to US specialty
nursing organisations.

SPORTS MEDICINE

http://www.physsportsmed.com/
children.htm   The Physician and
Sportsmedicine Online has full-text
clinical and personal health articles. One
section is Guidelines for Parents of
Children in Sports with related articles.
The site has links to other sites in the
sports medicine community.

http://www.worldortho.com/   Full
text. Electronic version of *A simple
guide to orthopaedics* and *A simple
guide to trauma* are available. Other
orthopaedic resources are also online.

http://www.rad.washington.edu/
University of Washington online
teaching materials in radiology.

http://www.medscape.com/Medscape/
features/ResourceCenter/olympics/
public/RC-index-olympics.html

Medscape's Sports Medicine Resource
Center is a collection of the latest
news and information on the surgical
and non-surgical treatment of
musculoskeletal conditions affecting
athletes—from 'weekend warriors' to
elite competitors. This resource
includes news, conference summaries,
articles, MEDLINE abstracts, links to
government and professional
organisations, practice guidelines and
practical clinical tools.

TRAVEL MEDICINE

www.cdc/travel   This is the Centers
for Disease Control and Prevention
(CDC) traveller's health site. The CDC
sets the standard of practice for travel
health information and vaccination
recommendations. All other sites obtain
the majority of their information
and recommendations from the CDC.
Information and recommendations
can be obtained by region, by disease
and by travel risk or problem. Special
information and articles are also
featured.

www.medicineplanet.com/   Medicine
Planet is devoted to travellers' health for
international and adventure travellers.

There are sections with specific
information for travel of children,
women, seniors, etc. One can enter
an itinerary and some demographic
information and receive a list of
recommended immunisations and
preventative measures to avoid health
risks for which there is no immunisation.
There are also many timely articles on
travel health topics, as well as news
articles with commentary on the current
political situation, infectious diseases and
natural disasters. The entire site can be
searched.

www.travmed.com/   Travel Medicine
Inc. web site provides online full text of
the book *Travel health guide* by Stuart
Rose MD. Chapters cover all major
health risks, including environmental
problems, food and waterborne
problems and infectious diseases. The
last chapter, 'World Medical Guide',
provides a country-by-country disease
risk profile.

www.istm.org   The web site of the
International Society for Travel
Medicine is primarily for practitioners,
but has a list of the travel clinics of
their worldwide professional members.
The full text of the *Journal of Travel
Medicine* can be accessed online, but at
this time cannot be searched by topic.

CHAPTER 7

Paediatric Telephone Advice and Management for the Nurse Practitioner

Lynn Hunt

INTRODUCTION

- Telephone advice is increasingly being used as a tool to better manage service demand within primary care, NHS walk-in centres (WICs) and Accident and Emergency (A&E) departments. In addition, the potential efficiency of telephone advice has triggered the launch of NHS Direct. As such, the telephone is an important resource for nurse practitioners (NPs) to use in a variety of patient care settings.

- Parents/carers will phone the NP for a variety of reasons: for advice on how to manage a problem; to confirm that they are doing the right things; for reassurance generally and sometimes, to satisfy themselves that they are worrying unnecessarily.

- Common paediatric queries include abdominal pain, vomiting, diarrhoea, constipation, fever, rashes, dental queries, lacerations, insect/animal bites, respiratory system queries and questions regarding medications or ingestions.

- The goals of paediatric telephone advice and management are summarised in Box 7.1. In order to achieve these goals, it is important that the NP establishes a good rapport; avoids jumping to conclusions; excludes irrelevant detail; keeps the telephone call manageable (in terms of time and effort expenditure); and ensures documentation is thorough but concise.

- Two basic tenets of communication—body language and eye contact—are

---

> **Box 7.1   Goals of paediatric telephone advice and management**
>
> - To identify all significant pathology
> - To encourage good health practices in parents/carers (including management of the child's illness and healthy preventative behaviours)
> - To relieve the child's distress/discomfort and calm anxious parents
> - To limit or decrease unnecessary health care visits
> - To contribute to efficient administration (prescription renewals, laboratory results, scheduling, follow-up, etc.)
> - To contribute to good patient relations and quality of care

---

denied the NP managing a problem by telephone. In addition, there is no opportunity for physical examination or laboratory diagnostics to confirm clinical suspicions. Therefore, assessment, decision making and management are dependent on the NP's skills of listening and telephone data collection.

- Telephone rapport is very important for a successful telephone consultation. It can be conceptualised as the 4 R's, which are summarised in Table 7.1. A good rapport will help in establishing important details, increasing trust

---

Table 7.1 Telephone Rapport—The 4 R's	
Rapport characteristic	*Comments*
• **R**eceptiveness to the caller's concerns	• Most paediatric calls come from worried and/or inexperienced parents that need acceptance and reassurance in order to increase their confidence in managing their child's illness
• **R**eassurance regarding the illness/problem	• Parents call because they are worried • If the illness/problem has a name or diagnosis, explain this to the parent. Even if there is no definitive diagnosis possible (e.g. the illness is most likely due to a virus) avoid saying *'it's just a virus'* as this implies a lack of understanding of the parent's and child's distress
• **R**eassurance regarding parenting skills	• Compliment rather than criticise (even if their only attempt at treatment has been to call the NP for advice) • All reasonable attempts to care for the child should be praised • Less than ideal home management can be corrected by suggesting *'it is probably a better idea to... .'*
• **R**eassurance regarding the availability of additional support	• Remind the parents that if the situation does not improve or if they have further questions or concerns they can call back • It is also helpful to reassure parents that there is a back-up plan if the telephone advice is not sufficient (i.e. *'it is not a problem for your child to be examined, but first I need some information about his/her illness'* or *'I would like you to try ____ and then give me a ring back in... .'*

and it may help to reveal hidden agendas (calls concerning trivial problems that conceal an underlying issue).

- The discussion outlined below pertains to common paediatric complaints that are not of a life-threatening nature. If the NP receives a call that is a medical emergency, the emergency services should be dispatched immediately. In these situations, the NP should use a second telephone line to alert the ambulance, while keeping the parent (and hopefully someone else to help out) on the line in order to instruct them in the ABC's (**A**irway, **B**reathing and **C**irculation).

HISTORY (TELEPHONE DATA COLLECTION)

- If the caller is not known to the NP, it is important to identify yourself (i.e. your name), your role as a nurse practitioner (*not a physician*), and the organisation you are working for. Concluding the introduction with a direct query as to the problem (i.e. *How can I help?* or *What seems to be the problem?*) provides the parent/carer with the opportunity to state the presenting complaint.

- Child's name, age/date of birth and gender.

- Caller's name, phone number and relationship to the child.

- Information related to the illness/problem:
  - duration of the problem: 'When did it start?' or 'How long has it been going on for?'
  - location of the problem (including whether it is radiating or changing)
  - quality: intensity, duration, sharp, dull constant, intermittent
  - quantity: the degree to which the problem is interfering with sleep, play, appetite, behaviour and intake of food and fluids
  - temporality: gradual onset versus sudden onset or a recurrent complaint; 'What started the problem?'
  - triggers: 'What started the problem and does anyone at home, school, nursery have the same symptoms?'
  - exacerbating/alleviating behaviours: e.g. 'Has any medication helped or does a certain position provide relief?'

- Determine the parent's/carer's perception of the problem, as individual understanding of symptoms and conditions vary widely. The degree to which parents are confident and knowledgeable about their child's illness will influence anxiety levels. Ask: *'What do you think is causing the problem?'*.

- Ask important questions first and try to cluster symptoms together (e.g. presence of nausea, vomiting, diarrhoea).

- Obtain information regarding the general state of the child: *'What has she been doing for the last hour?'* (e.g. lying listlessly on the sofa, playing happily with toys, quietly watching television, etc.). Another useful question is to compare this episode of illness with previous episodes: *'Does she look sicker than the last time she had a fever?'*.

- Screen the parent's anxiety level, noting their tone and response during the history: *'Are you frightened by the way she looks?'*.

- If the parent is describing varied and unrelated symptoms, clarify what is most problematic to the parent/child at present: *'I need to know what is bothering her the most now?'* or *'What are you the most worried about?'*.

- Determine how the parent has treated the problem so far: *'What have you done at home to manage the … ?'*.

- Keep questions simple without medical jargon. Parents may have trouble assessing problems such as a stiff neck or breathing difficulties. Ask instead: *'Are her lips pink?'* or *'Does she move her head to follow you around the room?'* or *'Can she kiss her knees or nod her head?'*.

- If the patient is unknown to the NP, a brief medical and family history are necessary: chronic diseases, recent illnesses, operations, hospitalisation, medication use, allergies, and usual source of care; family history of asthma, diabetes, etc.

DIFFERENTIAL DIAGNOSES (TELEPHONE DECISION MAKING)

- By this point, the NP should have an understanding of the general state of the child, his symptoms, home management and parental anxiety level.

- In addition to deciding what the child's illness or problem is likely to be, the NP needs to determine if (or when) the child needs to be examined.

- Table 7.2 outlines these possibilities. As a general rule, approximately 3% of calls will require rapid evaluation (life-threatening, dangerous or semi-emergent complaints); 47% of calls will require the child to be evaluated (same day, next day or later in week) and the majority of calls can be managed at home (50%).

MANAGEMENT

- Establish a presumptive diagnosis. Given the absence of a face-to-face consultation and physical examination, it is often helpful to qualify the presumptive diagnosis by reminding the parent that it is *likely* that the child has a particular illness: *'I can't be sure without examining her, but it sounds like your daughter has … .'*. Give the parent a diagnosis if there is one: to tell a parent that *'it is just a virus'* implies a lack of sensitivity with regard to the family's distress.

- Compliment the parent's home management of the illness and supplement/correct it (if appropriate). Occasionally, the only accurate compliment of the parent's home management might be her decision to seek advice: *'You've done the right thing calling for advice, let's chat about some things you can do at home to treat the … .'*.

- Discuss the likely/expected course of the illness with specific management: *'Sometimes children with a cold also have some loose stool, if this happens … .'*.

- Review unexpected events in the illness (i.e. things to call back for). This includes (1) persistence of the symptoms; (2) a change in the child's condition or new symptoms; (3) worsening of symptoms or the child's

Table 7.2 Telephone Decision Making

Decision	Examples	NP action
EMERGENCY SITUATION *(approx. 3% of calls)*		
Life-threatening problem, emergency intervention required (care within 15 min)	• Anaphylaxis, choking, arrest, severe respiratory distress, etc.	• Organise emergency services • Keep parent on the line to talk them through Heimlich manoeuvre, CPR[a] or other applicable procedure
Potentially dangerous situation (care within 30–60 min)	• Significant wheezing, seizures, suspicious ingestions, suspected meningitis	• Emergency services may be required • Discuss recovery position, safety in the surroundings and advise on any additional procedures
Semi-emergent problem, urgent intervention required (care within 1–2 hours)	• Possible fractures, lacerations (that are deep, profusely bleeding or over joints), fever in a young infant	• Stress urgency of situation and importance of obtaining care
APPOINTMENT NEEDED *(approx. 47% of calls)*		
Appointment required (same day)	• Young child with a significant fever	• Remind parent of the importance of bringing child in to be seen
Appointment required (next day)	• Mild conjunctivitis	• Advise on actions to be taken at home until child is examined
Appointment required (1–2 weeks)	• Weight check	• Review management plan with family and rationale behind later appointment date
HOME MANAGEMENT *(approx. 50% of calls)*		
Home management should be sufficient	• Chickenpox, colds, flu, nappy rash	• Discuss home management with parent • See Management section

[a] CPR, cardiopulmonary resuscitation.

condition; (4) anxiety on the part of the parent; and/or (5) other symptoms specific to the illness that would be considered worrying (e.g. lesions on the eyes in chickenpox).
• Suggest a time frame for the advice to take effect, i.e. negotiate a reasonable time frame for a subsequent follow-up call: *'I would like you to telephone me back if there is no improvement in his activity level an hour after the paracetamol.'*. In emergency situations, it is likewise important to address the time frame parents should be working to: *'It is extremely important to get your child to A&E within 60 minutes.'*.
• Obtain immediate feedback on the telephone advice (i.e. ask the parent to repeat the instructions back to you); if the parent is anxious, it may be helpful to have her write the important parts down and read them back. Check that the parent understands the management instructions.
• Check that the parent is happy with the management plan as discussed and provide reassurance that she is able to call back if necessary.

FOLLOW-UP

• The need for continued telephone advice/management or a subsequent consultation is dependent on the parent, condition and judgement of the NP.

MEDICAL CONSULT/ SPECIALIST REFERRAL

• Any child with a medical emergency.
• Any child who appears gravely ill.
• Any child with an unreliable or extremely anxious carer/parent.
• Any child that is considered at risk in the opinion of the NP.

DOCUMENTATION

• Documentation is an important component of telephone advice and management as it contributes to consistency in patient care; allows for appropriate follow-up and review; and is important for liability/legal reasons. Therefore, it is vital that the documentation related to telephone

advice and management is easily stored, easily accessed and provides a clear 'picture' of the call.

• Many documentation formats are available (audio-taping, computer-assisted, pre-printed forms, multiple copy forms); the actual choice of documentation style/format is specific to the NPs using it.

• The content to be included:
  • date and time of call
  • patient's name and age (or date of birth)
  • caller's name and number
  • chief complaint/reason for the call
  • historical information obtained by NP
  • advice given or telephone protocol used
  • call-back instructions negotiated with the caller
  • referrals given to caller (if appropriate) with specific time frames (e.g. *'Your child's illness is very serious, it is important that you get her to A&E within 2 hours'*).
  • any warnings given (if appropriate).

PAEDIATRIC PEARLS

- Telephone triage is *not* telephone management.
- Most calls are not life-threatening emergencies; however, the NP must be prepared for emergency calls.
- Telephone management skills need to be learned, practiced and reviewed (regularly). It is often helpful to have regular audits/case conferences to discuss the consultation in a group with NPs learning from each other.
- Beware of asking too many questions, as the caller may feel criticised or interrogated. Sensitive questions need to be delayed to resist appearing intrusive. Also avoid leading questions; the caller may feel compelled to give an answer you expect, rather than one which is related to the problem. Ultimately this will not help in the decision-making process.
- Limit management to short-term objectives: *'Let's chat about things you can do tonight and we'll see how she is in the morning.'*.
- If you have any doubts or fears regarding parental understanding or reliability, or if parent/carer anxiety levels are high, the child should be seen.
- Do not overlook the importance of documentation and frequent updating of telephone skills.

BIBLIOGRAPHY

Brown A, Armstrong D. Telephone consultations in general practice: an additional or alternative service? Br J Gen Pract 1995; 45:673–675.

Brown JL. Pediatric telephone medicine: principles, triage and advice, 2nd edn. Philadelphia: JB Lippincott; 1994.

Coleman A. Where do I stand? Legal implications of telephone triage. J Clin Nurs 1997; 6(3):227–231.

Crouch R, Woodfield H, Dale J, et al. Telephone assessment and advice: a training programme. Nurs Stand 1997; 11(47):41–44.

Dimond B. Legal aspects of NHS Direct and walk-in centres. Br J Nurs 1999; 8(19):1313–1314.

Hallam L. Primary medical care outside normal working hours: review of published work. BMJ 1994; 308:249–253.

Henry P. Legal principles in providing telephone advice. Nurs Pract Forum 1994; 5(3):124–125.

Osterhaus J. Telephone protocols in paediatric ambulatory care. Pediatr Nurs 1995; 21(4):351–355.

Robinson DL, Anderson M, Acheson PM. Telephone advice: lessons learned and considerations for starting programs. J Emerg Nurs 1996; 22(5):409–415.

Robinson DL, Anderson M, Erpenbeck PM. Telephone advice: new solutions for old problems. Nurse Pract 1997; 22(3):179–192.

Schmitt BD. Pediatric telephone advice. Boston: Little, Brown; 1980.

Schmitt BD. Pediatric telephone advice, 2nd edn. New York: Lippincott-Raven; 1999.

Williams S, Crouch R, Dale J. Providing health care advice by telephone. Prof Nurse 1995; 10(12):750–752.

CHAPTER 8

Transcultural Nursing Care

Diane Norton and Sigrid Watt

INTRODUCTION

- In order to recognise and respect the uniqueness and dignity of every patient in our care, consideration needs to be given to their ethnicity, culture and religion; delivery of appropriate health care requires sensitivity to cultural diversity.
- Culture has four basic characteristics: (1) it is learned from birth through the process of language acquisition and socialisation; (2) it is shared by all members of the same cultural group; (3) it is adapted to specific conditions related to environmental and technical factors and the availability of resources; and (4) it is dynamic and ever-changing.
- Culture and illness are intrinsically linked; cultural heritage influences how we behave when well or sick and our expectations of health care. When children and their families require care, they will act and react within the context of their particular family, community and societal culture.
- Nurse practitioners (NPs) and other health care professionals are likely to encounter children, their parents and their wider family when they are at their most vulnerable. Therefore, an awareness of various cultural practices is essential. Health care providers need to ensure they are equipped with the insight and appropriate knowledge to reduce the stress associated with illness and, thus, able to carry out culturally appropriate care.
- Ignorance with regard to health care delivery will lead to assumptions, stereotyping and discrimination. Being misinformed, or relying upon information that is now considered out of date is also dangerous. Culture is never static, but constantly changing and evolving, and often involves the assimilation of aspects of two or more cultures.
- Consider the following points when gaining knowledge of a family's culture: (1) an understanding of the concept of culture; (2) an appreciation of the NP's own culture; (3) a desire to facilitate effective communication; and (4) an appreciation of the varying perceptions of health, illness and treatment across cultures.
- An extensive knowledge of the culture and customs of all patients accessing health care is neither possible nor desirable as it may reinforce stereotypes. The following good practice points are given to encourage the consideration and delivery of individualised care.

HISTORY

- A good practice point for obtaining the history is always to use open-ended questions that enhance a full response.
- Box 8.1 is a guide to the cultural assessment of the child and family within their community.
- Box 8.2 outlines important questions to elicit a family's perception of their child's illness: In some instances (e.g. when utilising an interpreter or translator and/or when advocating for the family) it may be necessary to use close-ended questions in order to ensure clarity of feedback and to

---

Box 8.1   Cultural assessment of the child and family

- Structure of the family, family roles and the dynamics within the family. Communication patterns and decision making
- Health beliefs and practices related to the cause of the disease. Treatment of altered health and the use of alternative therapies both within the home to treat the illness and/or within the community
- Patterns of daily living, including work and leisure activities
- Social networks, friends and neighbours. Does it influence health and altered health?
- National, ethnic identity of family and language used
- Nutritional practices and how they relate to cultural factors and health
- Religious preferences, health maintenance and the impact religion might have on daily living and influence health status or care
- Culturally appropriate behaviour styles, including what is manifested during anger. Also relationships with health professionals, between genders and relationships with groups in the community

---

Box 8.2   Assessment of illness perception

- What do you think caused the problem?
- Why do you think it started when it did?
- What do you think your child's illness does to him?
- How severe is your child's illness? Will it have a short or a long course?
- What kind of treatment do you think your child should receive?
- What results do you hope to receive from this treatment?
- What are the major problems that your child's illness has caused for you?
- What do you fear most about your child's illness?

maintain privacy (both of which are important).

- The NP should have an awareness of the complementary healing practices that are used within the community. Although it is dangerous to assume that *all* complementary/alternative/traditional approaches to healing are innocuous, the *majority* of practices are quite harmless (whether or not they are effective cures).

PHYSICAL EXAMINATION

- Sensitivity with regard to privacy during the physical examination is important for all patients. However, there can be cultural considerations that necessitate even greater attention to privacy and/or the possibility of same gender examination. If this is potentially an issue for an individual child or family, discuss with them how they would like the physical examination to proceed.
- Clear explanations of procedures and/or techniques used in the physical examination are good practice with all patients. However, families from other countries may or may not be familiar with medical and nursing practice as carried out in the United Kingdom. As such, care must be taken to ensure patients understand what will happen as part of the physical examination (and management plan). This is especially important for families who have a limited knowledge of English. In these instances, use of a translator is very important.

MANAGEMENT

- Nurse practitioners need to develop partnerships with families and acknowledge that family members provide care. There are three stages of interaction when working in partnership with a child and family: (1) family members should be encouraged to state the needs for caring as they see them; (2) the patient and carer, in conjunction with the NP, should identify the types and patterns of caring that are desired in relation to the child's needs; and (3) the patient, carer and NP should participate

Box 8.3	Cultural considerations regarding hospital admission

- There may be difficulty in comprehending the rules and regulations of life on a ward, either because these have not been explained, or the routines are implicit rather than explicit (so staff do not realise they need to be explained)
- Many cultures value the support of family and friends at a time of crisis and this is demonstrated by being at the patient's bedside. This can lead to tension around visiting times due to the number of visitors allowed at any one time
- Some women in the Asian, and particularly Bangladeshi, community may observe purdah and find it difficult to visit or stay with their child on the ward
- Sharing accommodation with other parents, observing prayer times, washing and eating an acceptable diet can all be difficult if resident in the hospital
- If treatment regimens are not adhered to, this can be interpreted as non-compliance or disinterest on the part of the parents, but may be due to lack of understanding of what is required or lack of support. For the parent of a minority ethnic group, this can be compounded by lack of information about their child's illness in their own language, either in written form or from health care professionals such as the nurse specialist
- There is a shortage of multilingual therapists in areas such as speech and language, occupational therapy, physiotherapy and social work. This can make it difficult for the family of a child requiring long-term care to get the support they need from the multidisciplinary team

in devising and agreeing upon a plan of care.

- After a symptom is identified, the first effort at treatment is often self-care. Home management is attractive for its accessibility, potential mobilisation of the child/family's social support network and provision of a caring environment in which to convalesce. It is important, therefore, to negotiate the family's preferences with regard to home care management (and follow-up).
- In negotiating a management plan, it is useful to consider the different communication styles displayed by the families: more specifically, the way they display fear, anxiety, concern and disagreement. In addition, it is important to appreciate the family's style with regard to responsibility and decision making.
- There will be specific values shared by the culture that need to be appreciated when formulating the management plan. For example, the emphasis on independence found in Western culture or the conformist qualities of Asian culture which include obedience and gender-appropriate behaviour.
- In addition, the NP must be sensitive to the difficulty some families will have in expressing their needs. This may be related to the intimidation parents feel in the strange health care environment or it may be due to the barriers created by health care jargon and/or the

reluctance of many parents to discuss their culture.

- The importance of translators cannot be overemphasised. If English is not spoken or understood, there is likely to be difficulty in understanding the care that is being given and the reason for it.
- Hospital admission presents special cultural considerations; these are outlined in Box 8.3.

FOLLOW-UP

- Follow-up needs to be negotiated with the same considerations used in formulating a management plan.

PAEDIATRIC PEARLS

- Try to know and understand what support is needed. It is helpful to have information available, for children and families, explaining the terminology used by NPs and others. It is helpful if this is available in other languages.
- Accommodate differences willingly and competently. Do not be afraid to ask the child or family if they require any particular help or care. You cannot know everything and most people are grateful to be asked.
- Show respect by being approachable and accessible. Coping with illness can be a frightening and confusing experience for the child and family. They may express anger, fear and

resentment or have many questions. Do not try to avoid them and their distress.

- Plan ahead to prepare for the care that may be required. Have access to contact numbers of local religious and spiritual leaders, or other members of the community whose support the family may desire.

- Do not take over roles or impose your own beliefs or agendas. Every family is unique and, although you may have cared for someone of that faith or cultural background before, it may not follow that they require identical care.

BIBLIOGRAPHY

Ahmann E. 'Chunky stew': appreciating cultural diversity, while providing health care for children. Pediatr Nurs 1994; 29(3):320–324.

Andrews MM, Boyle JS. Transcultural concepts in nursing care, 3rd edn. Philadelphia: Lippincott; 1999.

Bell D. Cross-cultural issues in prevention, health promotion and risk reduction in adolescence. Adolesc Med 1999; 10(1):57–69.

Brookins GK. Culture, ethnicity and bicultural competence: implication for children with chronic illness and disability. Pediatrics 1993; 91(5 Pt 2):1056–1062.

Chevannes M. Nursing caring for families—issues in a multiracial society. J Clin Nurs 1997; 6(6):1–7.

Edwards CP, Kumru A. Culturally sensitive assessment. Child Adolesc Psychiatr Clin N Am 1999; 8(2):409–424.

Enarson DA, Ait-Khaled N. Cultural barriers to asthma management. Pediatr Pulmonol 1999; 28(4):297–300.

Free C, McKee M. The new NHS: from specialist service to special groups: meeting the needs of black and minority groups. BMJ 1998; 316(7128):380.

Gates E. Culture clash. Nurs Times 1995; 91(7):42–43.

George M. Minority ethnic groups. Perceptions of health. Nurs Stand 1995; 9(28):18–19.

Guarnaccia P, Lopez, S. The mental health and adjustment of immigrant and refugee children. Child Adolesc Psychiatr Clin N Am 1998; 7(3): 537–553.

Holland K, Hogg C. Cultural awareness in nursing and health care, an introductory text. London: Arnold; 2001.

Kelley BR. Cultural considerations in Cambodian childrearing. J Pediatr Health Care 1996; 10(1):2–9.

Lynch MA, Cunninghame C. Understanding the needs of young asylum seekers. Arch Dis Child 2000; 83(5):384–387.

MacKune-Karrer B, Taylor EH. Toward multiculturality: implications for the pediatrician. Pediatr Clin North Am 1995; 42(1):21–30.

Miller S. Disability in Asian communities. Paediatr Nurs 1994; 6(1):17–18.

Papadopoulos I, Tilki M, Taylor G. Transcultural care: a guide for health care professionals. Lancaster: Quay Books; 1998.

Pearson M. Ethnic differences in infant health. Arch Dis Child 1991; 66:88–90.

Schwab-Stone M, Ruchkin V, Vermeiren R, et al. Cultural considerations in the treatment of children and adolescents: operationalizing the importance of culture in treatment. Child Adolesc Psychiatr Clin N Am 2001; 10(4):729–743.

Shah R. Practice with attitudes: questions for cultural awareness training. J Child Health Care 1994; 6:245–249.

Sheikh A, Gatrad AR. Caring for muslim patients. London: Radcliffe Medical Press; 2000.

Shuriquie N. Eating disorders: a transcultural perspective. East Mediterr Health J 1999; 5(2):354–360.

Slater M. Health for all our children. London: Action for Sick Children; 1993.

Sprott JE. One person's 'spoiling' is another's freedom to become: overcoming ethnocentric views about parental control. Soc Sci Med 1994; 38(8):1111–1124.

Stopes-Roe C, Cochrane R. Traditionalism in the family: a comparison between Asian and British cultures and between generations. J Compar Family Stud 1989; 21:141–158.

Swanwick M. Child-rearing across cultures. Paediatr Nurs 1996; 8(7):13–17.

Whiting L. Caring for children of differing cultures. J Child Health Care 1999; 3(4):33–37.

Wilkinson JA. Understanding patients' health beliefs. Prof Nurse 1999; 14(5):320–322.

Zahr LK, Hattar-Pollara M. Nursing care of Arab children: consideration of cultural factors. J Pediatr Nurs 1998; 13(6): 349–355.

COMMON PAEDIATRIC PROBLEMS

PART 2

CHAPTER **9**

Dermatological Problems

9.1 'MY CHILD HAS A RASH'

Jill Peters and Rosemary Turnbull

📖 INTRODUCTION

- Ill children often present with more than one symptom and one of the most common is a rash.
- Because children have a developing immune system, they can develop non-specific rashes to many things. Although most rashes are benign, self-limiting and resolve completely, it is important to identify additional clinical symptomatology and rule out serious pathology. As such, this may require a follow-up visit within 24 hours.
- Rashes can occur after an acute viral or bacterial infection, thus demonstrating that an infection has been present. For example, β-haemolytic streptococcal throat infection can trigger guttate psoriasis or a localised infection site can result in staphylococcal scalded skin syndrome (a serious infection with a mortality rate of 3% in children).
- Rashes can also occur as the main symptom of an infection—e.g. meningococcaemia, varicella (chickenpox), impetigo, etc. Some of these illness may be potentially life threatening and cannot be misdiagnosed.
- In addition, rashes can be an early indication of a developing dermatoses (e.g. a follicular keratotic rash that is subsequently diagnosed as psoriasis). These children frequently require re-evaluation, as the early presentation is unclear and it is not until the rash is more florid that a definitive diagnosis can be made.

- Once children enter nursery or school they will often pick up infections from their peers: e.g. chickenpox, impetigo, tinea capitis, etc.
- Older children may complain of rashes that are similar to adults in presentation: e.g. urticaria, pompholyx, prurigo and erythema multiforme.
- Management of skin diseases will require extra consultation time to: (1) explain the problem to the parent/carer and child; (2) outline the dermatoses; (3) discuss how the therapies will work; and (4) describe the progression to resolution/ improvement. Anxiety runs high because scratching can distress the child and disturb the whole family. Support from other professionals may be required as the skin care needs of the child may be labour intensive and, as such, the implications of this for the family will need to be considered within their individual dynamic.
- Inflammatory dermatoses can occur within hours but take days to weeks to resolve. This can be extra distressing to the parent/carer as well as the older child if the face and hands are affected. Parents/carers want 'a cure' and do not want to hear about a skin condition that can develop into a chronic disease.
- Skin diseases in ethnic patients can present a diagnostic challenge because of variations in clinical appearance that may be attributable to racial characteristics and/or inflammatory disease. In addition, certain disorders

can be unique to some populations. Examples include traction alopecia (the tight pleating of hair putting so much tension onto the hair that it breaks); or FACE, Facial Afro-Caribbean Childhood Eruption (monomorphic, flesh-coloured or hypopigmented papules which occur around the mouth, eyelids and ears, persist for several months and then resolve without scarring).

🔬 PATHOPHYSIOLOGY

- The newborn dermis is less mature. As such, there is less organisation of vascular and nerve structures and decreased collagen and elastic fibres. It is not until 2 years of age that the dermis has an adult-like form.
- A child's skin needs to be treated carefully, as many external factors make the skin vulnerable: e.g. soaps containing detergents, sunlight/heat and antigens in the environment like the house dust mite.
- The child's rash could be a manifestation of systemic illness.
- Skin changes occur in adolescence with the onset of puberty. The skin becomes greasier as the hormone androgen stimulates sebum production and the hair likewise becomes lankier and greasier.

⬅ HISTORY

- The subjective assessment of the patient should include the components of an episodic history, as outlined previously (see Ch. 4).

- Note that the family and child (if appropriate) should describe the skin condition in their own words and the history should include an assessment of the family's expectation of the consultation. The agenda that parents/carers have may be broader than solely the management of the rash. This is especially true when social issues are involved.
- Problem to be addressed in the consultation.
- How and when did the rash start?
- What did it look like at first, compared to now?
- What time lapse has occurred since the onset of the rash: hours, days or months?
- How long was the lesion present on the skin? e.g. hours as in urticaria or weeks as in eczema.
- Site of initial lesion (target lesion) and subsequent course of the rash (e.g. from where did the rash spread and in what kind of distribution). An example is pityriasis rosea, which has a herald patch (2–5 cm) occurring several days prior to the appearance of the main rash.
- Symptoms experienced: itch, dryness, redness, pain, and/or warmth. An analogue scoring mechanism can be useful with older children to assist in determining severity.
- Treatment tried at home (with results).
- Has this ever occurred previously and what was the outcome?
- Anything that happened prior to the development of the rash that could be considered a 'trigger' or precursor (e.g. tingling, pruritus, tenderness, trauma, localised increase in temperature, etc.).
- Accompanying systemic symptoms (fever, joint soreness, sore throat, nausea, vomiting, diarrhoea, etc.).
- Does the rash improve at the weekends or when on holiday?
- Recent travel, either abroad or outside of their normal environment (e.g. school trip to a forest).
- New activity or hobby.
- Activities that can no longer be done.
- Animals in the house.

- New medication or anything bought over the counter (including herbal or homeopathic remedies).
- Use of recreational drugs.
- Sun exposure: have they lived abroad, sun protection factor (SPF) used, influence of the sun on the skin condition in any way.
- Any family history of atopy, psoriasis or skin cancer.
- Any other members of the family with the same symptoms? Any classmates off ill?
- What initiated skin enquiry and any fears or anxieties regarding it?
- Changes in fluid or dietary intake?
- Recent and significant weight loss?
- Any lesions in the mouth?
- Is the sleep pattern disturbed, less attentive at school?
- Alcohol intake?
- Smoking?
- Any aggravating/relieving factors?
- What do they think is wrong with the child (or themselves) and expected outcomes (including any other agenda of the parent/carer).

PHYSICAL EXAMINATION

- A full skin examination should be carried out in a warm and private room with good natural lighting or artificial lighting that will not change the natural colour of the skin. A good magnified lamp is useful when assessing lesions as it allows for use of perpendicular lighting when looking for subtle skin changes. If the consultation takes place in the patient's home, use natural lighting where possible; otherwise, take a small portable light with a magnifying lens.
- If the rash is a symptom of a systemic illness, a complete physical examination will be required.
- Observe the child's overall appearance including physical bearing, posture and dress, as these may indicate unhappiness, loss of self-esteem or confidence, anger or embarrassment (adolescence). The skin is a window into the patient's inner feelings and is often reflected through their facial expression before any words are spoken. For example, an unhappy child who is distressed, irritated and appears

unwell is manifesting systemic effects of an inflammatory disease process (e.g. a child with acute atopic eczema is visually distressed whereas a child with seborrhoeic dermatitis is not).

- *It is essential to examine all the skin from head to toe (including skin folds).* Thus, undressing children down to their underclothes will likely require some explanation, especially if the lesion is on the face. It is often helpful to inform the child and family that affected skin needs to be compared with unaffected skin and that no lesion/rash should be looked at in isolation. In addition, parents often do not relate a rash on one part of the body to another part and/or there is a possibility that additional lesions may be identified (the chance of detecting a melanoma is 6.4 times greater with a complete skin examination than with a partial examination of just exposed skin). Note that there will need to be an awareness/sensitivity to cultural or religious differences as well as potential embarrassment.
- Use the fingertips to lightly run over the surface of the skin in order to appreciate subtle differences in texture and the changes that occur with pressure. Note that skin is more sensitive when inflamed and streptococcus infection is more painful than staphylococcus infection.
- Palpate around the edge of the lesion in order to identify infiltration, texture (i.e. hard, soft or encapsulated) and lesion depth.
- Flex the skin between finger and thumb to check for scale (tinea) or to induce scale in lesions where it is not readily apparent (e.g. pityriasis versicolor). Look for scaling in the skin creases of palms and soles as a possible indicator of fungal infection.
- Use a light source that is perpendicular to the lesions in order to highlight the lesion elevation and any epidermal changes.
- Look for signs of excoriation, as patients often do not admit to scratching.
- Note that the distribution of the lesions may assist in diagnosis (e.g. unilateral rash along a dermatome is likely to be herpes zoster).
- Examine the mucosa with good light.

- Check through the hair (parting it on a continuous basis all over the scalp) and look behind the ears (i.e. psoriasis and/or seborrhoeic dermatitis). Also press firmly on the scalp for texture. If it is boggy, think infection (depending on what you see on the scalp, either bacterial or fungal).
- Document findings on a body chart that can indicate the severity and distribution of the presenting rash. In the case of pigmented lesions or wounds, measurements should be taken. Record any analogue scores for comparison on future visits.

❓ DIFFERENTIAL DIAGNOSES

- The differential list is broad but it is helpful to organise commonly encountered rashes by their aetiological category (Table 9.1).

✚ MANAGEMENT

Specific management is aetiology-dependent. Basic principles are outlined below.

- **Additional diagnostics:** consider bacterial or viral swabs, fungal skin scrapings, nail clippings and hair debris. A rash that is possibly related to a systemic illness may require blood work, urinalysis or other diagnostics.
- **Pharmacotherapeutics:** depending on the diagnosis, medications can be topical or systemic. Note that it is important to be correct in your diagnosis if systemic therapies are to be used. Irrespective of route, a full discussion of the medication dose, technique of application (if topical), frequency and length of course is required. If antihistamines are used for itching, especially if scratching results in sleep loss and reduced concentration levels, the impact of potential drowsiness requires consideration, such as effect on school attendance. Likewise, the choice and preference of the parent/carer/child needs to be considered with regard to the emollient prescribed. In addition,

it is important that careful thought is given to the impact of the child's care on the family unit.

- **Behavioural interventions:**
  - Encourage frequent applications of topical emollients if the skin is hot, itchy or very scaly. Emollients in tubes or decanted (careful with infection control, small amounts, clean technique) would enable children to take them to school. Emollient application before and after swimming allows the child to safely participate in the activity and reduce exclusion by peers.
  - Psychological support for the family is important. A skin disease or cutaneous change due to systemic illness can be very distressing by its visual appearance and its perception by others. Lower self-esteem, embarrassment and feelings of social isolation can exacerbate or maintain a dermatoses and lead to poor concordance with topical therapies. Support may be required for the carer/parent who has to deliver the daily care; be sure to assess their needs as well as those of the child.
  - If the rash is not a self-limiting and benign condition, the expertise of other professionals may be required. For example, the school nurse may need to educate teachers/pupils and provide help with contact tracing and/or surveillance in an outbreak situation. Likewise, the paediatric community team may be required to support home care, assess the home environment and support the family.
- **Patient education:**
  - Discuss with the child and family the cause of the rash and the rationale for its management. Understanding the cause relieves guilt and feelings of shame with regard to the skin condition. Children with skin conditions can be targeted by bullies; health promotion to empower the child will disempower the bully.
  - Review with families the disease process, possible triggers (and strategies to deal with them) and the use of topical therapies to reduce

discomfort and minimise the appearance of the rash.
  - Remind families that they need to complete the full course of treatment rather than stopping as soon as things are starting to look better.
  - Complete the family-held Child Health Record in order to assist in the continuity of care. (All children under 5 years of age should have one.)
  - Provide written information to complement verbal instructions (essential).

➡ FOLLOW-UP

- Follow-up is aetiology-dependent with referral if the diagnosis is not clear. Some families will welcome a follow-up phone call if anxiety levels are running high. This is also true for children whose rash is associated with a systemic illness that may require monitoring.

⇄ MEDICAL CONSULT/ SPECIALIST REFERRAL

- Any child in whom the diagnosis is unclear.
- Any child with a gravely ill appearance.
- Any child who presents with a dermatological emergency, e.g. eczema herpeticum.
- Any child requiring specialist intervention or expertise.

👁 PAEDIATRIC PEARLS

- Dermatology is very visual: do not diagnose over the telephone as not everybody has the same skill for description.
- Always examine all of the skin; do not forget the hair, nails and mouth.
- Touch is a powerful tool.
- Purchase a good colour picture dermatology book and keep it handy as a reference.
- Develop a close link with your local paediatric dermatology nurse specialist; he/she is an invaluable resource.

Table 9.1	Commonly Encountered Rashes in Children
Consider	*Appearance and comments*

Bacterial aetiologies

Impetigo	• Superficial vesicles with yellow exudate and crusting or bullous blisters with easily ruptured roof • See Section 9.9
Staphylococcal scalded skin syndrome (Ritter's disease)	• A spectrum of exfoliative skin lesions which resemble scalding injuries • Can range from bullous impetigo to generalised spread • Caused by an epidermolytic toxin producing strain of *Staphylococcus aureus* • Infection usually preceded by upper respiratory tract infection or localised site of infection (e.g. umbilicus, ears, eyes, etc.) • Characterised by erythematous bullae on face and flexures • Skin is tender to touch and rubbing causes separation of the epidermis, leaving the red, shiny dermis resembling a scald • Requires urgent referral with emergency admission
Scarlet fever	• Group A β-haemolytic streptococcal infection that spreads systemically • Fine, maculopapular rash on erythematous background. Rash has sandpapery feel • Increased erythema at nape of neck and in skin folds of joints (Pastia lines) • May have bright red tongue (strawberry tongue) and palatal petechiae • Will require immediate antibiotic treatment in order to avoid renal and cardiac complications

Viral aetiologies

Herpes simplex (types I and II)	• Type I: characteristic clusters of vesicles on the skin surface and also buccal mucosa • Starts as small papule that develops quickly into a fluid-filled vesicle with subsequent crusting • Characteristic tingling prior to eruption enables early initiation of antiviral ointment. Systemic therapy also available (aciclovir) • If vesicles clustered near eyes, immediate referral to ophthalmology • Children with atopic eczema will likewise require referral (vesicles appear 'punched out') • Type II (genital herpes): potential child protection issues. Assess carefully and thoroughly
Molluscum contagiosum	• Small clusters of dome-shaped lesions with central punctum. Virus (poxvirus) contained in lesion fluid • See Section 9.15
Hand, foot and mouth	• Caused by the Coxsackie virus • Small greyish lesions on palms, soles and oral mucosa • Localised rim of erythema around each vesicle • Child may be febrile • Self-limiting and management is supportive
Erythema infectiosum (fifth disease)	• Caused by parvovirus B19 • Bright red erythema of the face (especially the cheeks) to give a 'slapped cheek' appearance • Erythema spreads across the shoulders, trunk and extremities • Body rash is reticulated with lacy pattern that becomes more intense with exertion. May have associated pruritus • Usually resolves in 7 days but may last up to 20 days • Self-limiting and management is supportive
Pityriasis rosea	• Aetiology unknown, assumed to be viral in origin or a postviral immune response • Single, round/oval, salmon-coloured patch (herald patch) that is scaly with central clearing and erythematous border, 3–6 cm in diameter. Located on trunk and precedes development of macular, papular, scaly rash of discrete lesions of varying sizes. Lesions typically on trunk and usually in a Christmas tree configuration • Rash lasts 2–10 weeks • Self-limiting and management is supportive
Roseola infantum	• Common in pre-school children • Characterised by fever for 3–7 days followed by rapid defervescence and the appearance of a blanching maculopapular rash (usually on fourth day of illness) that lasts 1–2 days • See Section 15.5

Fungal infections

Candida infection	• Caused by *Candida albicans*, a normal part of the flora of the gastrointestinal tract • Shiny erythematous areas usually in moist warm areas such as flexures and napkin region with satellite papular lesions or pustules • See Section 9.8
Pityriasis versicolor	• Caused by yeast (*Malassezia furfur*) which multiplies on the skin surface when there is high sebum production, increased humidity, immunosuppression, increased cortisone levels and/or when the normal environment of the skin surface changes • Characterised by discrete hyper- or hypopigmented macules usually on the upper trunk and upper arms. Most noticeable after sun exposure • See Section 9.8

(continued)

Table 9.1 *continued*

Consider	Appearance and comments
Tinea infections	• Caused by dermatophytes which produce an annular infection • Classification depends on location • Single or multiple erythematous plaques with an active edge and central clearance as it enlarges in size • If organism invades hair shaft, corresponding inflammatory response in its severest form results in a boggy, painful inflamed area of the scalp known as a kerion, subsequent scarring can cause permanent hair loss • See Section 9.8

Other

Lyme disease	• Multisystem illness caused by the tick-borne spirochaete *Borrelia burgdorferi* • Most patients with typical annular rash (erythema chronicum migrans) for 1–2 weeks after tick bite (50–80%) • Begins as small red macule or papule that expands to an annular lesion 20–30 cm in diameter with partial central clearing • May also have non-specific flu-like symptoms • Common after trips to forested areas and endemic in the northeast, north central and Pacific coastal parts of the United States • Lymphadenopathy is not uncommon • If typical rash present, requires systemic antibiotics
Kawasaki disease	• An idiopathic, multisystem disease of young children characterised by vasculitis of the small and medium-sized blood vessels • Aetiology is uncertain but speculation as to possible immunological response to an infectious agent • Characterised by pyrexia for 10–14 days followed by an erythematous, non-vesicular, polymorphous rash with a predilection for the perineum. Rash usually appears 6 days after initial symptoms. Changes to the extremities include erythema of the soles and palms with periungual desquamation. Often accompanied by conjunctivitis and involvement of the oral mucosa (strawberry tongue) • Children can be very ill and often are admitted to hospital for management
Atopic eczema	• Presentation can vary • See Section 9.3
Seborrhoeic dermatitis	• Yellow to erythematous scaly greasy lesions on scalp, fontanelle and skin folds • Complicated by the yeast *Pityrosporum ovale* • See Section 9.10
Guttate psoriasis	• Discrete, well-demarcated lesions appearing after Group A β-haemolytic streptococcal infection • See Section 9.13
Urticaria	• Immune-mediated reaction very common after insect bites • Characterised by well-circumscribed localised (or less commonly generalised) erythematous, raised skin lesions (i.e. wheals or welts) of varying sizes • Intensely pruritic • Can be chronic or acute; acute form can be life-threatening • Managed by avoidance of triggers and antihistamines
Scabies	• Infestation of the stratum corneum by the human mite *Sarcoptes scabiei* • Characterised by intense pruritus • Areas commonly infected include web spaces of the hands, neck and heel and soles of feet (especially in infants), wrist, axillae, gluteal cleft and genitals • Burrows present in 90% of symptomatic cases and are 'S' shaped with a broad base and punctate brown–black dot at the leading edge
Miliaria rubra	• Also known as heat rash or prickly heat • Characterised by erythematous papular rash distributed across areas where sweat glands are concentrated • Treatment is symptomatic and includes trying to maintain cool dry environment • Reassure parents regarding the self-resolving nature of the rash

BIBLIOGRAPHY

Camilleria M, Pace JL. Disorders of the perineum and perianal regions. In: Parish LC, Brenner S, Ramos-e-Silva M, eds, Women's dermatology from infancy to maturity. Carnforth: Parthenon; 2001; Ch. 30.

Child FJ, Fuller LC, Higgins EM, Du Vivier AWP. A study of the spectrum of skin disease occurring in a black population in south-east London. Br J Dermatol 1999; 141:512–517.

Craft JC. Bacterial, rickettsial and viral diseases. In: Parish LC, Brenner S, Ramos-e-Silva M, eds, Women's dermatology from infancy to maturity. Carnforth: Parthenon; 2001: Ch. 23.

Epstein E. Crucial importance of the complete skin examination. J Am Acad Dermatol 1985; 13(1): 150–153.

Fitzpatrick TB, Johnson RA, Wolff K, et al. Colour atlas and synopsis of clinical dermatology, 3rd edn. New York: McGraw-Hill; 1997.

Frieden IJ. Childhood exanthems. Curr Opin Pediatr 1995; 7(4):411–414.

Higgins E, du Vivier A. Skin diseases in childhood. Oxford: Blackwell Science; 1996.

Hughes E, Van Onselen J. Dermatology nursing: a practical guide. Edinburgh: Churchill Livingstone; 2001.

Lawton S. Assessing the skin. Prof Nurse 1998; 13(4):S5–7.

Mackie R. Clinical dermatology, 3rd edn. Oxford: Oxford Publications; 1991.

Mairis E. Four senses for a full skin assessment: observation and assessment of the skin. Prof Nurse 1992; 7(6):376–380.

Mancini AJ. Exanthems in childhood: an update. Pediatr Ann 1998; 27(3):163–170.

Noble W. Impetigo and related diseases. Dermatol Pract 1996; Jan/Feb:11–12.

Peters J. Assessment of patients with a skin condition. Pract Nurse 1998; 15(9):525–530.

Peters J. Assessment of the skin. In: Cross S, Rimmer M, eds, Nurse practitioner manual of clinical skills. Edinburgh: Baillière Tindall; 2001.

Retzback M. Bullying and eczema. Dermatol Pract 2001; 9(3):18–20.

Rigel DS, Freidman RJ, Kopf AW, et al. Importance of complete cutaneous examination for the detection of malignant melanoma. J Am Acad Dermatol 1986; 144(5):857–860.

Roberts R. Paediatric dermatology. Dermatol Pract 2001; 9(3):9–11.

Steen A. Staphylococcal scalded skin syndrome. Pract Nurs 2000; 11(11):9–12.

Turnbull R. Skin assessment in children: a methodical approach. Nurs Times 2000; 96(41):33–34.

Van Onselen J. Age-specific issues. In: Hughes E, Van Onselen J, eds, Dermatology nursing: a practical guide. Edinburgh: Churchill Livingstone; 2001:146–167.

Weston WL, Lane AT. Colour textbook of pediatric dermatology. St. Louis: Mosby; 1991:223–230.

9.2 ACNE

Julie Carr

📖 INTRODUCTION

- Acne is a term derived from the Greek word '*acme*' meaning prime of life. It is almost universal in teenagers, with an estimated 85% of people experiencing some degree of acne during their teenage years.
- It comes at a time when body image is of great importance and any deviation from being 'less than perfect' can provoke anxiety. Acne patients are often described as being self-conscious and having a low self-esteem. Consequently, they may also become dissatisfied with other aspects of their body image such as their weight or shape (dysmorphophobia).
- Acne can persist into adulthood and, left untreated, may cause physical and psychological scarring. Fortunately, modern treatment is effective, and teenagers with acne are no longer dismissed or told they will 'grow out of it'. Treated appropriately and quickly, acne can be controlled or even cured with good cosmetic results.
- Health care professionals have an important role in recognising the psychological impact of acne on a young person. Optimising management through good communication and support before, during and following therapies is essential.

📑 PATHOPHYSIOLOGY

- Acne is a disease of the sebaceous follicle which occurs predominantly on the face, chest and upper torso. The normal pilosebaceous unit consists of sebaceous glands, a rudimentary hair and a wide follicular duct lined with stratified squamous epithelial cells (Fig. 9.1).

- During normal epidermal desquamation (shedding), epithelial cells are transported via the follicular duct by sebum secreted from the sebaceous glands. The glands require androgens to stimulate sebum secretion and there is a significant increase of androgenic hormone during puberty.

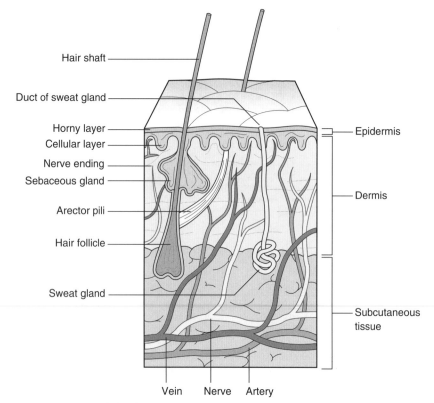

Figure 9.1 Anatomy of the skin.

Hair shaft
Duct of sweat gland
Horny layer
Cellular layer
Nerve ending
Sebaceous gland
Arector pili
Hair follicle
Sweat gland
Epidermis
Dermis
Subcutaneous tissue
Vein Nerve Artery

- With acne, there is hyperproliferation of the cells lining the follicular duct. The cells adhere to the duct walls and, combine with sebum and bacteria, which results in a partial obstruction of the follicular duct. This process is visible on the skin surface as a comedone, which has either a black (open) or white (closed) head; and is commonly referred to as a 'blackhead' or a 'whitehead'. The black colour of the plugs is due to pigment (not dirt), as comedones are the precursors of both non-inflamed and inflamed acne lesions.
- In addition, the obstructed ducts become colonised by propiono-bacterium (*Propionibacterium acnes*). This dilates the ducts further, due to the release of inflammatory mediators such as cytokines. The ducts will continue to dilate until the rupturing process discharges the contents into the surrounding tissues. These foreign bodies are an irritant and contribute to the inflammatory response seen in most forms of acne.

◁ HISTORY

- Age of onset (commonly appears during Tanner stage II).
- Areas affected.
- Current skin care regimens and previously tried regimens with outcomes (including results of prescriptions and over-the-counter products used).
- Presence of androgen-related symptoms (amenorrhoea, hirsutism, obesity) and age at menarche (females).
- Perceived triggers: cosmetics and/or occupational exposures (note that chocolate, nuts, sweets, shellfish and fatty foods have not been shown to have an effect on acne severity).
- Medications: oral contraceptives, phenytoin or steroids.
- Family history of acne.
- Degree of emotional upset or effect that the acne has on the individual (including interpersonal relationships, employment/school, self-image/ self-esteem and general body image).

◔ PHYSICAL EXAMINATION

- **General observation:** dress, interpersonal communication, eye contact, etc., may give indication of self-esteem issues.
- **Skin:** inspection of affected areas (face, neck, chest, back, etc.) to determine the degree of skin greasiness; types of lesions present (open/closed comedones, papules, pustules and cysts); number of each type, distribution and intensity of inflammation. Examine for presence of scarring, keloid formation or hyperpigmentation (post-inflammatory changes). Note that there can be involvement of thighs, buttocks and upper arms.
- Assess adolescent females with severe acne for potential androgenic disorder (e.g. polycystic ovary syndrome): evaluate for obesity, hirsutism and alopecia.

⍰ DIFFERENTIAL DIAGNOSES

- The diagnosis of acne vulgaris in adolescents is usually clear-cut; however, consider the possibility of obstructed sebaceous follicles caused by *cosmetics* (this is called *cosmetic acne*, when moisturising creams or oil-containing hair products cause acne); *occupational exposures* (mineral oil, petroleum, coal tar and pitch are triggers); and *medications* (androgens, steroids, lithium, phenytoin, isoniazid, rifampin and some combined oral contraceptives that contain an androgenic progesterone component, e.g. norethisterone).

- In addition there are numerous acne variants:
  - *Acne excoriée* is an acne variant usually associated with young female patients who relentlessly pick at their skin; it requires psychological input as it can be obsessional and/or destructive in nature.
  - *Infantile acne* is quite common in early infancy and is probably related to transplacental stimulation of sebaceous glands; it resolves spontaneously.
  - *Nodulocystic acne* (acne conglobata) is a severe type of acne more commonly affecting males. This form is characterised by nodules, sinuses and abscesses; it is more prone to scarring and requires oral retinoids.
  - *Acne fulminans* (rare) is largely seen in males who have extensive truncated lesions (that may be an immune reaction to *P. acnes*). Patients can be unwell with malaise, fever and general systemic upset; this form of acne requires oral retinoids.

✚ MANAGEMENT

Management decisions are guided by the type of acne lesions present (Table 9.2) in addition to the extent/number of each type, intensity of inflammation and degree of scarring and/or pigment changes. However, although this approach is helpful in clinical decision making, it does not necessarily reflect the amount of emotional upset the adolescent may be suffering. Treatment regimens need to balance the extent of the acne with the effect it is having on the adolescent's quality of life, self-image and self-esteem.

Table 9.2	Type of Acne Lesions
Type	Characteristics
Papule	• Inflammatory lesion (<5 mm) that occurs (usually superficially) within the follicle; can present as a 'bump' under the skin surface
Comedone	• Blocked follicular duct; can be open (blackhead) or closed (whitehead)
Pustule	• Inflammation and exudate around the comedo; lesion has a visible central core of purulent material
Nodule	• Inflammatory lesion (≥5 mm) occurring with deeper inflammation within the follicle; more likely to scar
Cyst	• A sac containing pus or other products from deep inflammation of the follicle; more likely to scar

Table 9.3 Pharmacotherapeutic Management of Acne

Product	Use	Mechanism of action	Advantages	Disadvantages	Comments
Topical treatments					
Benzyl peroxide: • Available in numerous strengths and preparations (aqueous gel, creams and washes)	• Mild to moderate acne	• Bactericidal effect of *Propionibacterium acnes* • Mild comedolytic action	• Used for many years in the management of acne • No evidence of bacterial resistance developing • Available over the counter	• Can cause bleaching and staining of clothes • Can be irritating to skin (redness and peeling)	• Important to build up tolerance gradually so as to avoid redness and irritation • Initially apply once daily; increase to twice daily if no irritation occurs and further improvement is required • Apply after washing with mild soap • Aqueous gels may be better tolerated than alcohol-containing products and may also have better penetration
Topical antibiotics: • Clindamycin, 1% lotion/solution • Erythromycin, 2% gel/solution • Erythromycin/zinc • Erythromycin/benzyl peroxide	• Mild to moderate acne	• Antibacterial and anti-inflammatory • Addition of zinc is thought to lower bacterial resistance and assist absorption of erythromycin	• Allow for direct application of antibiotics to localised areas with negligible systemic effect	• Resistance to *P. acnes* may develop • Can cause dryness and irritation if alcohol-based • Cannot replace systemic antibiotics for more severe acne • Available on prescription only	• Apply once or twice daily after washing with mild soap • Can alternate with benzyl peroxide or tretinoin (or use instead of benzyl peroxide) • Erythromycin/zinc appears to be more effective than pure topical antibiotics • Erythromycin/benzyl peroxide can also be very effective • Topical antibiotics are not initial choice in treatment preparations because of risk of resistance
Topical retinoids: • Numerous formulations available • Cream: 0.025%, 0.05% and 0.1% • Gel: 0.01%, 0.025% • New generation: adapalene (Differin)	• Mild to moderate acne	• Prevent formation of comedones by de-plugging follicle • Reduces the amount of inflammatory lesions (vitamin A analogues)	• Very useful in comedonal acne • Use of benzyl peroxide in the morning and retinoids at night effective combination • Gel helpful with oily skins • Cream better with sensitive skin	• Potential skin irritation • Photosensitivity can occur • Contraindicated in pregnancy • Daylight can break down retinoids to less active form • After 1–2 weeks some irritation may occur • After 3–4 weeks pustular eruption can occur	• Close supervision and instruction are required • Important to build up tolerance, especially those with fair skin • Apply gradually in small amounts (pea-sized amount only) • Various strengths and products available; newer preparations released frequently • Creams are less irritating, followed by gels and liquid • Start with 0.025% cream or 0.01% gel every other night (after mild soap wash); increase gradually to nightly use. If not effective (and no irritation) increase strength; if too irritant try next strength down • Patients will need encouragement if inflammation temporarily increases (unplugging of follicles) • Use with caution on darker pigmented skins as can cause hyper- or hypopigmentation • New-generation topical retinoids may be less irritant than other topical retinoids (see *BNF*ª)

Systemic treatments

Oral antibiotics • Oxytetracycline (most common) • Minocycline • Doxycycline • Erythromycin • Trimethoprim	• Moderate to severe	• Decreases population of *P. acnes* • Anti-inflammatory effect in sebaceous follicle	• Less expensive	• Side-effects include: gastrointestinal upset and candidal infections • Resistance can develop • Interactions with other medications (including oral contraceptives) can occur	• Not indicated for non-inflammatory comedonal acne • Oxytetracycline: absorption affected by food, milk, etc.; give 30 min before or 4 hours after last meal; contraindicated in children <8 years of age or pregnancy • Minocycline: use if resistant to tetracycline • Use over 4–6 month period and if effective continue for longer • Reduce dose of antibiotics after 6–8 weeks to lowest dose that maintains clear skin
Oral retinoids • Isotretinoin (Roaccutane)	• Severe, nodulo-cystic acne • Acne resistant to other therapies	• Reduce inflammation by 90% in 1 month • Reduce bacterial colonisation by 90% in 1 month • Reduce sebum production by 90% in 1 month	• Useful when self-esteem and self-image issues are affecting quality of life • Useful with cystic acne or if scarring is problematic • Single 16-week course gives 75% cure rate	• Only available under consultant dermatologist supervision and after all other treatments have failed • Numerous side-effects which require in-depth discussion with adolescent and parents • Highly teratogenic	• If relapse occurs, another course can be attempted or a retry of other treatments • Side-effects to be discussed include teratogenicity, mucous membrane dryness, increased liver enzymes and cholesterol levels, blurred vision, headaches, photosensitivity, pruritus and worsening of eczema, possibility of mood swings and depression (rare) • Requires regular growth monitoring if younger adolescent • Requires regular full blood test (FBC), fasting lipids and liver function test (LFT) prior to commencing treatment and then monthly • Females require counselling with regard to effective contraception
Hormonal therapy • Cyproterone acetate/ethinylestradiol (Dianette)	• Acne related to endocrine disorder (polycystic ovaries)	• Blocks androgen receptors • Provides contraception	• Especially effective with adolescents with polycystic ovaries and mild hirsutism	• Can only be used with females	• Careful consideration required when treating young women with acne • Provides simultaneous contraception

ª BNF = *British National Formulary*, published by British Medical Association and Royal Pharmaceutical Society of Great Britain.

- **Additional diagnostics:** none generally required. Consider evaluating adolescent girls with severe acne (with or without evidence of hirsutism) for an androgenic disorder (polycystic ovaries, adrenal hyperplasia). Evaluation includes luteinising hormone (LH), follicle-stimulating hormone (FSH), free and total testosterone and dehydroepiandrosterone (DHEA).

- **Pharmacotherapeutics:** See Table 9.3; note that numerous preparations are available, with new generations released frequently.

- **Behavioural interventions:**
  - Skin should be washed a maximum of twice a day with a mild soap or non-astringent cleanser. The areas should not be scrubbed with abrasive cleansers or pads. Likewise avoid alcohol, astringents and oil-based cosmetics and/or moisturisers.
  - Strict adherence to treatment regimen is vital.
  - Do not pick, squeeze or scratch at lesions and try to keep hair off the face/forehead.

- **Patient education:**
  - Reassure adolescents that acne is treatable, even curable, but that it takes work and strict adherence to treatment regimens. Let them know that sometimes things get slightly worse before getting better, but they can usually expect improvement after 3–6 weeks.
  - Review treatment instructions and behavioural interventions; provide written information for reinforcement and a contact phone number for future questions/concerns.
  - Discuss acne 'myths' (such as chocolate, fats, sugar or poor hygiene causing acne). Additional support can be gained from the acne support group (tel: 0208-561-6868 or www.stopspots.org).

- Remind adolescents to return immediately for additional help if they feel their acne is interfering with their ability to 'enjoy life' or they are unhappy with how their treatment is progressing.

FOLLOW-UP

- The adolescent will probably require follow-up contact, support and encouragement throughout his treatment. In addition, subsequent visits allow for potential side-effects to be assessed; fine-tuning of skin care regimes; and monitoring of the psychological impact that acne can have on adolescents.

MEDICAL CONSULT/ SPECIALIST REFERRAL

- Any adolescent with moderate to severe acne, which is non-responsive to topical treatments and/or courses of antibiotics taken for at least 6 months.
- Any adolescent with nodulocystic acne (acne conglobata).
- Any adolescent who presents with scarring.
- Any adolescent who presents with psychological problems related to their acne.
- Any adolescent female whose acne may be related to an ovarian or endocrine abnormality such as polycystic ovary syndrome.

PAEDIATRIC PEARLS

- Acne is a very treatable skin disorder that should always be taken seriously and never trivialised. Early referral to a GP or dermatologist is essential to prevent scarring and psychological problems; the short- and long-term consequences to an adolescent's psychological and emotional well-being should not be underestimated.
- Patient compliance with all acne treatments is vital and should be monitored and discussed on a regular basis.

- Frequent, vigorous washing or excessive scrubbing of the face with abrasives is unnecessary and may lead to dermatitis.
- Although astringents and alcohols make the skin's surface less oily, they have minimal effect on acne and may irritate the skin and/or stimulate oil production.
- The combination of benzyl peroxide in the morning and topical retinoid at night may be beneficial when either agent alone has been unsuccessful.
- Both soap and previous applications of topical medicines must be thoroughly washed off the skin before any further topical applications.
- Stress has a reciprocal effect on acne: it seems to make it worse, which further heightens the adolescent's anxiety, decreases self-esteem and creates more stress.

BIBLIOGRAPHY

Boston M. Treating patients with acne vulgaris. Pract Nurs 1997; 8(15):27–29.

Buxton PK. ABC of dermatology, 3rd edn. London: BMJ Publishing; 1998:47–51.

Chu T, Munn S, Basarab T. Acne. In: Maxim M, ed., Current issues in dermatology, 2nd edn. London: Imperial College of Science, Technology and Medicine; 1998:19.

Cooley S, Atkinson P, Parks D, et al. Management of acne vulgaris. J Pediatr Health Care 1998; 12(1):38–40.

Eady EA. Bacterial resistance in acne. Dermatology 1998; 196:59–66.

Gupta MA, Gupta AK, Schork NJ, et al. Psychiatric aspects of the treatment of mild to moderate facial acne: some preliminary observations. Int J Dermatol 1990; 29:719–721.

House of Lords Select Committee on Science and Technology. Resistance to antibiotics and other antimicrobial agents: evidence and report. London: HMSO; 1998.

Poyner T. How do we manage acne. Kent: Magister Consulting; 1999.

Vivier A. Dermatology in practice. London: Grower Medical Publishing; 1990: 181–188.

9.3 ATOPIC ECZEMA

Jean Robinson

📖 INTRODUCTION

- Atopic eczema is a chronic pruritic inflammation of the epidermis and dermis with a strong genetic aetiological component that is associated with other atopic conditions (asthma, rhinitis and seasonal allergies).
- Also known as atopic dermatitis (synonymous term often used interchangeably with atopic eczema) it affects all ethnic groups and current estimates suggest that somewhere between 5 and 20% of children in developed countries will develop eczema. The prevalence appears to be increasing, probably due to a combination of genetic and environmental factors.
- The main types of eczema seen in childhood are atopic and seborrhoeic eczema. Other inflammatory skin conditions (irritant eczema, contact dermatitis and pompholyx) are seen less commonly (see Sec. 9.10).
- Atopic eczema usually starts in the first year of life (often on the face) before spreading to the limbs; up to 90% of these children will grow out of it by the time they reach their teens. The prognosis is less optimistic for those who develop it after the age of 1 year.
- The condition is chronic and may be exacerbated by infection (bacterial and/or viral) as well as by irritants. Atopic eczema can have tremendous physical, psychological and social effects on children and their families; these should not be underestimated.

📝 DIAGNOSIS

- There is no specific laboratory test available, so diagnosis is made on clinical grounds. For a diagnosis to be made, the child must have *pruritus, plus three or more of the following*. Note that itching is such a prominent feature of eczema that if it is not present, another diagnosis should be considered (see list of differential diagnoses).
  - History of itchiness in the skin creases such as folds of the elbows, behind the knees, fronts of the ankles and/or around the neck, the cheeks and behind the ears (in children under 4 years of age).
  - History of asthma or hay fever or history of atopic disease in a first-degree relative of a child less than 4 years old.
  - General dry skin in past year.
  - Visible flexural eczema or eczema involving the cheeks or forehead and outer limbs in children under 4 years. Note that Asian, Black African or Afro-Caribbean children sometimes show a reverse pattern of extensor eczema and are also more likely to produce lichenification, papular or follicular eczema and marked areas of hypo- or hyperpigmented, post-inflammatory pigment changes.
  - Onset of symptoms in the first 2 years of life (not always diagnostic in children under 4 years of age).

🔬 PATHOPHYSIOLOGY

- The aetiology of eczema is multifactorial, with genetic, environmental, physiological and immunological factors all playing a role. The skin is chronically dry with decreased pliability, most likely related to changes in lipid content (which allow increased epidermal water loss). The resultant skin barrier becomes less effective, with a greater risk of irritant penetration.
- Inflammation of the epidermis (with associated oedema) leads to the formation of intraepidermal blisters, which can rupture and give rise to exudation and crusting (acute phase). In addition, concomitant pruritus (the aetiology of which is poorly understood) results in an itch–rub–scratch cycle which causes increased epidermal regeneration and thickening (subacute and chronic phases).
- Meanwhile, the upper dermis becomes flooded with white blood cells (that leak out of the vessels and pass up into the epidermis), thus exacerbating the inflammation. It is thought these T cells drive the epidermal inflammatory process, although many patients also have elevated levels of immunoglobulin E (IgE).

⬅ HISTORY

- Age of onset, distribution and characteristics of the eczema.
- Family history of atopic-associated conditions (asthma, allergies, hay fever and/or others with eczema) or history of these in patient.
- General growth and development.
- Sleep patterns (especially whether itching awakens at night).
- Diet history, including whether any particular food(s) seems to trigger a flare-up.
- Bathing history/habits, including frequency and use of soaps, moisturisers, bubble bath, etc.
- Details of previous treatments and their effectiveness.

🩺 PHYSICAL EXAMINATION

Systematic head-to-toe examination of the skin with inspection of all areas of the body. Note:
- Distribution and pattern of dryness and lesions (often age-related, see Diagnosis).
- Detailed examination of lesions, noting the presence of erythema, scaling, crusting, exudate and excoriation. In addition, examine lesions for blisters, pustules, papules and lichenification. Compare lesions for differences and note size.
- Other associated findings include pityriasis alba (scattered, dry white patches), infraorbital darkening, facial

Table 9.4   Differential Diagnoses of Atopic Eczema

Consider	Distinguishing features
Allergic/contact eczema (dermatitis)	• Erythema, oozing and vesicles as in atopic eczema but distribution is usually limited • History provides clue to trigger • Elimination of irritant usually initiates resolution
Histiocytic disorders (rare)	• Reddish papules may appear purpuric (in groins, neck and axillae) • Signs of systemic illness • Lymphadenopathy
Nummular (discoid) eczema	• Characterised by well-defined, coin-shaped lesions that may be dry and scaly or oozing and crusted • Usually on limbs, rarely on face
Psoriasis	• Silvery scales prominent feature in well demarcated, thickened areas (see psoriasis)
Scabies	• Extremely pruritic papules (may be increased at bedtime) • Commonly found in interdigital spaces, palms of hands, soles of feet and penis • Scrapings may reveal mites, eggs and/or faeces • Symptoms often present in other family members and of fairly recent onset
Seborrhoeic dermatitis	• Itching is not prominent or may be absent; greasy yellow scales

pallor and keratosis pilaris (dry rough hair follicles on extensor surfaces of upper arms and thighs), hyperlinear palms and ichthyosis vulgaris (marked scaling in the absence of inflammation).

🛈 DIFFERENTIAL DIAGNOSES

• See Table 9.4.

➕ MANAGEMENT

It is vital that health care providers work in partnership with parents/carers, as management is not curative but rather aims to achieve symptom control. Atopic eczema is characterised by periods of flare-up and remission, both of which require interventions tailored to the severity of the symptoms. A triple therapy approach is suitable for most children: (1) bath oils and soap substitutes for cleansing; (2) regular and liberal use of moisturisers and (3) intermittent use of the least-potent steroid preparation.

• **Additional diagnostics:** no tests are diagnostic for atopic eczema. Skin biopsy can be used to rule out other papulosquamous disease (e.g. psoriasis). Consider cultures (viral, Tzanck smear and/or bacterial) if lesions appeared infected. Patch testing can help to differentiate atopic eczema from allergic or contact eczema. Blood results often reveal elevated levels of IgE, especially in cases of severe eczema. Full blood count (FBC) may show eosinophilia.

• **Pharmacotherapeutics:**
  • Bath oils include products such as Oilatum, Hydromol Emollient and Balneum Plus.
  • Soap substitutes for bathing include aqueous cream and/or emulsifying ointment.
  • Moisturisers/emollients include: Diprobase, Oily cream and white soft paraffin/liquid paraffin (50% WSP : 50% LP).
  • Topical steroids are used to control flare-ups (Table 9.5), with higher potency preparations used in the acute phase and tapering to lower potency when control is achieved. Once the skin has cleared, judicious emollient use may be all that is needed.
  • Antihistamines are used for their sedative effect. They don't control the itch as it is not histamine-mediated. They can be successfully used 1 hour before bedtime. While not addictive, use should be monitored and administered only when necessary (Table 9.6).
  • Systemic steroids are rarely indicated and generally reserved for when control of the eruption is very difficult (and then for short-duration use only).

• **Behavioural interventions:** compliance/adherence to treatments is a mainstay of daily control; it is vital that parents understand their role and the importance of the following:
  • *Cleansing routines:* daily bath in warm (not hot) water with added oil and use of a soap substitute to cleanse the skin of dry scales and crusts. Avoid all soaps and bath additives as they can irritate the skin. These will make the bath slippery so children need to be supervised. After soaking in the water the child should be patted, not rubbed dry.
  • *Moisturisers:* should be applied as often as needed in order to stop the skin drying out. This may need to be up to 5 or 6 times daily. They should be applied in a thin layer with sweeping motions (in the direction of hair growth) and allowed to soak in. In general, the more occlusive the topical product, the more effective it is at sealing in moisture; thus, the best moisturiser is the greasiest the child and family will tolerate and use. However, older children may find lighter moisturisers more aesthetically acceptable to use. Children may need up to 500 g, every 1–2 weeks. Occlusive moisturisers (applied after the skin is hydrated in the bath) seal water in and are very important. Lotions are the least helpful of moisturisers as they often contain more water, alcohol, preservatives and fragrance.
  • *Occlusive bandages:* applied over topical steroids, they increase steroid absorption to improve effectiveness; provide a barrier to scratching; and maintain a constant environment for the skin (which reduces pruritus). They are helpful in treating areas of

Table 9.5 Topical Steroids

General considerations of use

- Use as second-line intervention (after hydration and moisturising) and to control flare-ups.
- Use only on red, itchy inflamed areas and lowest potency possible.
- Do not use more than twice daily; some newer steroids are designed for once daily use.
- Apply sparingly: e.g. 'only enough to make the skin look shiny'.
- Use ointment formulations in preference to creams as they are greasier; the exception is wet or weepy eczema (use creams).
- Apply steroid 20–30 min after applying moisturiser to prevent dilution of steroid effect.
- Topical steroids are classified by potency; in older children mild or moderate potency steroids may be used on the body; use only mild steroids on the face and nappy area.
- Long-term use can lead to skin atrophy, telangiectasia and, occasionally, interference with growth; this is not a concern with mild or moderate potency steroids.

Group potency	Chemical name
Mild	• 0.5% hydrocortisone • 1% hydrocortisone
Moderate	• 0.05% clobetasone butyrate (Eumovate) • 0.025% betamethasone valerate (Betnovate-RD)
Potent	• 0.1% betamethasone valerate (Betnovate) • 0.1% mometasone furoate (Elocon)
Very potent	• 0.05% clobetasol propionate (Dermovate)

Table 9.6 Antihistamines

Name	Dosage
Hydroxyzine	• 6 months to 6 years: 5–15 mg once at night (maximum dose = 50 mg) • 7–12 years: 15–25 mg once at night (maximum dose = 50–100 mg) • 12–18 years: 25 mg once at night (maximum dose = 100 mg) • *Note: increase dose as necessary (in 3–4 divided doses). Do not exceed maximum daily dosages*
Promethazine	• 1–12 months of age: 5–10 mg at bedtime • 1–5 years: 10–20 mg at bedtime • 6–10 years: 20–25 mg at bedtime • 10 years: 25–50 mg at bedtime • Usually needs to be given 2 hours before desired onset of effect • *Cautious use in infants <1 year of age due to a possible association with sudden infant death syndrome*
Trimeprazine	• >6 months of age: 1 mg/kg/day in 3–4 divided doses • In chronic eczema an increased dosage may be needed (1.5–3 mg/kg/day) but **omit** daytime doses

lichenification on limbs (they cannot be used on the trunk) and, as such, are not a first-line treatment. Children requiring this level of intervention need medical referral. Impregnated paste bandages (e.g. Ichthopaste or Viscopaste PB7) are applied in a pleating fashion over an application of topical steroid. The pleating allows for shrinkage and drying of the bandage, which otherwise could cause constriction of the limb and blood supply. A second outer bandage of Coban is applied to keep the paste bandage in place. The bandages can be left in place for up to 3 days. Close supervision (and support) are needed with treatment and there is some risk of steroid absorption.

- *Wet wraps:* can be used to treat all of the skin, including the face. It is a very time-consuming procedure and is generally used in hospital to treat children with erythrodermic eczema (a large area of the child's body is abnormally red, flaking and thickened). It involves the application of a double layer of tubular gauze bandage (cut to fit the child's legs, arms, trunk and in some cases, face) applied over a topical steroid cream (either applied to the skin or the inner layer of bandage). The inner layer is wet in warm water and then applied; the outer layer is dry. The whole process is repeated every 12 hours and the bandages have to be kept wet in between.

- **Patient education:**
  - Discuss the rationale and importance of all skin care routines with parents and children. Practical demonstration is vital, as is the use of interpreters if the first language is not English. All information should be reinforced with printed materials as appropriate.
  - Stress the importance of frequent moisturising and include the significance of skin hydration (by sealing water in with emollients) as dry skin will itch more. Reinforce with parents that moisturising is the fundamental therapy for eczema and should occur 3–4 times per day (minimum).
  - Review the lack of a 'cure' for eczema, stressing that it is a chronic disease controlled through good skin care (although a large percentage of children will 'outgrow' their eczema after the age of 6 years).
  - Outline the instructions for steroid use (e.g. apply 20–30 min after emollients, use sparingly only on affected areas, with a frequency as directed). Include information on any other medications (e.g. antihistamines) that may be part of the child's regimen.
  - Discuss the controversy that exists with regard to dietary management of eczema and explain there is little evidence that dietary changes in children over 1 year of age are of any benefit. Even in those children less than 1 year old, dietary restriction is rarely recommended and would require supervision by a dietician: therefore, it is not considered a first-line treatment.
  - Complementary treatments (reflexology, hypnotherapy, homeopathy, herbalists and Chinese herbal treatments) have been used

COMMON PAEDIATRIC PROBLEMS

2

for the management of atopic eczema and many parents wish to discuss them. For the most part, the evidence base is largely anecdotal and while some children may benefit from these therapies, their families should be advised to think carefully before embarking on them. Some oral Chinese herbal treatments can damage the liver and kidneys, so regular blood tests are needed.

- Additional measures that are important to review include use of non-biological washing powder; avoidance of fabric conditioners; keeping nails short; avoidance of synthetic fibres, wool and pets with fur, hair or feathers; keeping house dust down; and maintaining a cool temperature in the home.

➡ FOLLOW-UP

- None required if symptoms settle with supportive care.
- For children with significant involvement (that requires time-consuming and complicated treatments), both the child and family will require consistent support, reinforcement of knowledge and encouragement.

⇄ MEDICAL CONSULT/ SPECIALIST REFERRAL

- If doubt exists regarding the diagnosis.
- Any child who is erythrodermic (a large area of the child's body is abnormally red, flaking and thickened) needs immediate referral.
- Suspected bacterial infection (weeping, crusted eczema often yellow/honey-coloured).
- Suspected eczema herpeticum (rare but serious complication due to herpes simplex virus). Consider if sudden, dramatic eczema flare, an unwell/ pyrexial child, and a 'punched out' appearance to the lesions (especially around the eyes).
- Any child where first-line treatment fails despite adequate explanation, demonstration and adherence.

◉ PAEDIATRIC PEARLS

- Symptoms can only be controlled if families understand how (and when) to use treatments and if they keep using them; always provide written information (if appropriate) to accompany verbal instruction and practical demonstrations.
- The importance of emollients/ moisturisers cannot be overemphasised.
- A triple therapy approach is suitable for most children (bath oils and soap substitutes for cleansing; regular and liberal use of moisturisers; and intermittent use of the least-potent steroid preparation).
- Support, encourage and educate; support, encourage and educate; support, encourage and educate … .
- Eczema has social and emotional implications and can seriously affect interpersonal relationships.

Consequently, children can experience alienation from peers as a result of the disfigurement and may fall behind in school because of absences; the disease can be especially devastating for adolescents. Provide families with information on support groups and consider referral for psychological services if significant pathology is presenting.

- **National Eczema Society**, Hill House, Highgate Hill, London N19 5NA. Tel: (020) 7281 3553.
- **Eczema Information Line**: tel: (0870) 241 3604 or www.eczema.org

目 BIBLIOGRAPHY

Atherton DJ. Eczema in childhood: the facts. Oxford: Oxford University Press; 1995.

Dennis H, Watts J. Skin care in atopic eczema. Prof Nurse 1998; 13(4):S10–S13.

Donald S. Atopic eczema: management and control. Paediatr Nurs 1997; 9(8):29–34.

Elliott BE, Luker K. The experiences of mothers caring for a child with severe atopic eczema. J Clin Nurs 1997; 6:241–247.

Heer-Nicol N. Managing atopic dermatitis in children and adults. Nurse Pract 2000; 25(4):58–76.

Lawton S. Assessing the skin. Prof Nurse 1998; 13(4):S5–S7.

Lynn S. Managing atopic eczema: the needs of children. Prof Nurse 1997; 12(9):622–625.

McHenry PM, Williams H, Bingham EA. Management of atopic eczema. BMJ 1995; 310:843–847.

Mitchell T, Paige D, Spowart K. Eczema and your child: a parent's guide. London: Class; 1998.

9.4 BIRTHMARKS

Jane C. Linward

📖 INTRODUCTION

- The term 'birthmark' refers to a wide variety of conditions, some more common than others.
- For the most part, birthmarks that are seen commonly in paediatric practice can be divided into *vascular* or *pigmented* lesions.
- The incidence of the individual lesions varies, with some considered almost a normal variant (e.g. mongolian spots which can affect more than 80% of newborns).
- Likewise, the management and prognosis of the lesion may vary from a transient phenomenon of minimal significance (e.g. stork marks) to a permanent cutaneous abnormality that may be associated with significant systemic complications (port-wine stains).
- Commonly encountered birthmarks included in this section are summarised in Table 9.7.

Table 9.7 Common Birthmarks in Children

Lesion	Appearance	Comments
Hyperpigmented Lesions		
Mongolian spots	• Blue-grey or blue-black patches most commonly on the sacrococcygeal area of infants but can occur on the buttocks, dorsal trunk and/or extremities • Size ranges from a few millimetres to >10 cm • Can be single or multiple	• The most common congenital pigmented lesion • Affect >80% of black and Asian infants • Prevalence among white infants is much less (ranging from 0.5 to 13%) • Benign • Colour stabilises in infancy and disappears before puberty (in most patients)
Café au lait macules (CALMs)	• Round or oval, flat, distinct and uniformly light-brown pigmented lesion(s) • Size ranges from a few millimetres to >20 cm • Can occur anywhere on the body (more often on the buttocks of newborns) • Can be single or multiple	• Affect approximately 10–28% of individuals • Solitary lesions are common and non-specific • Multiple CALMs (more than 6 that are >0.5 cm) and/or inguinal and axillary freckling will require further investigation to rule out neurofibromatosis type 1 • Neonates with multiple CALMs should be carefully evaluated
Congenital melanocytic naevi (CMNs)	• Brown/black pigmented areas of skin • CMNs can be macular, papular or plaque-like • Textures vary and may be with or without hair	• Lesions grow proportionately with child and are categorised by size • Lesions <2.5 cm occur 1:100 births • Large CMNs (>20 cm in diameter) occur 1:10,000 births • Clinically significant because of their association with childhood malignant melanoma • Removal is problematic as their full-thickness depth would cause scarring • Partial thickness removal will result in re-pigmentation and recurrence of hair growth
Vascular Lesions		
Stork marks	• Bright red or dark pink blanching patch with irregular borders • Usually involves the forehead above the nose but may also involve the upper eyelids, bridge of the nose, upper lip and nape of neck • Appear redder when crying or straining and lighter when at rest	• Most common capillary malformation • Present at birth and may initially be attributed to birth trauma or port-wine stain • Nape lesions often persist (while others usually resolve within 2 years)
Haemangioma	• Classified according to clinical appearance (i.e. superficial, deep, or mixed) • Superficial lesions appear dark red, slightly raised from the surrounding skin and with a convoluted surface • Deeper lesions appear bluish in colour and can stand proud of the skin (sometimes several centimetres) • Some lesions with a combination of superficial and deeper elements	• Benign vascular tumour that affects 1:20 births • An area of skin (anywhere on the body) which becomes red or raised during the first few weeks of life should always flag up the possibility of a proliferating haemangioma • More common in females, premature and multiple births • Complications of haemangiomas are a result of their size, location or proliferation • No known genetic factors • Usually excellent cosmetic results after natural involution but some residual cutaneous findings possible (redundant skin, hypopigmentation, slight scarring, etc.) • Numerous haemangiomas noted in neonates can be associated with internal malformations and will require investigation • Approximately 30% have spontaneously involuted by 3 years of age, 50% by 5 years, 70% by 7 years and 90% by 9–12 years of age
Port-wine stain	• A flat, well-defined, pink to red area that is present at birth • Blanches with pressure • Darkens in colour with mood and environment (e.g. hot or cold) • May lighten during first few months and grows proportionately with the child • Darkens with age and skin can become thicker with papules which can bleed if scratched	• Affect approximately 3:1000 births • Initially thought to be related to birth trauma and/or the use of tape for intravenous lines (but lesions persist) • If lesion involves eyelids there is an increased risk of glaucoma • Port-wine stains on the scalp may have brain involvement, resulting in convulsions and/or motor delays

PATHOPHYSIOLOGY

- Vascular birthmarks can be grouped into *vascular malformations* (capillaries, veins, lymphatics or arteries that have undergone errors of morphogenesis) or *vascular tumours* (benign tumours that demonstrate endothelial hyperplasia, the most common being *haemangiomas*).
- *Vascular malformations* are present at birth and are (usually) classified according to vascular flow characteristics and predominant vessel type (i.e. capillary, venous, lymphatic, arterial or mixed), although there is controversy with regard to the classification of vascular lesions. Common capillary malformations encountered in paediatric practice include *stork marks* (which are caused by distended dermal capillaries) and *port-wine stains* (which are the result of thin-walled capillary to venular-sized channels located in the papillary and upper reticular dermis).
- *Haemangiomas* may be present at birth, although more commonly they develop over the first 2–3 weeks of life. These benign tumours involve endothelial tissue that grows rapidly with a high expression of proliferating cell nuclear antigen. The lesions undergo a rapid proliferative phase (usually 3–9 months, rarely beyond 18 months) in which they increase rapidly in size and colour. This is followed by a spontaneous, slow involution (that typically lasts from 2–9 years). Approximately 30% of haemangiomas have spontaneously involuted by 3 years of age, 50% by 5 years, 70% by 7 years and 90% by 9–12 years of age.
- Hyperpigmented birthmarks may be macular, papular, plaque-like, evenly coloured, speckled or spotty. Often a morphological approach is used for classification, description and diagnosis.
- *Mongolian spots*, a frequently encountered hyperpigmented birthmark, are thought to result from interrupted embryonic migration of melanocytes from the neural crest to the epidermis. It is not well understood why the lesions typically appear in the same places (most commonly the lower back and sacrum). The characteristic bluish hue of the lesions is a result of the Tyndall effect; more specifically, the optical scattering of light as it passes through a turbid medium (i.e. the dermis).
- *Café au lait macules* (CALMs) are regularly seen in paediatric practice. They result from epidermal collection of heavily pigmented melanocytes that are of neural crest origin. CALMs can occur anywhere on the body (and are often located on the buttocks of newborns). Multiple CALMs (6 or more that are >0.5 cm in diameter) and/or inguinal/axillary freckling are associated with neurofibromatosis type 1. Infants and children meeting these criteria will require further investigation.
- *Congenital melanocytic naevi* (CMNs) are uncommon birthmarks that have important implications for later life. They result from collections of melanocytes that are present at birth or develop within the first year. CMNs are clinically significant because of their association with childhood malignant melanoma (especially intermediate or large CMNs). Typically, the lesions grow proportionately with the child and are usually classified according to their size. The majority of CMNs are unsightly and may or may not have hair growth.

HISTORY

- Antenatal and birth history.
- When the lesion(s) was first noticed and whether it has changed or grown in size.
- Any other systemic symptoms?
- History of skin lesions in the family.
- Treatment and advice received elsewhere.

PHYSICAL EXAMINATION

- Head-to-toe examination of all skin. It is imperative to note size, colour, distribution and extent of any lesion(s).
- Texture of lesion and whether it is easily compressed, blanched and/or is emptied of blood.
- Complete physical examination of the remaining systems (e.g. cardiovascular, pulmonary, gastrointestinal, neurological and musculoskeletal) in order to rule out any additional findings.

DIFFERENTIAL DIAGNOSES

- Be sure to rule out other aetiologies for the lesion(s): more specifically, acute infections, trauma, child protection issues, soft tissue tumours, etc.

MANAGEMENT

- **Additional diagnostics:** see Table 9.8.
- **Pharmacotherapeutics:** see Table 9.8.
- **Behavioural interventions:** see Table 9.8.
- **Patient education:** Lesion-specific information is outlined in Table 9.8. However, in general, it is important to address the following broad categories:
  - Review cause of the birthmark.
  - Discuss the likely course (i.e. what will happen to the lesion as the child grows and when it will go away). Include the importance of watching for changes.
  - Inform parents of the potential association of the birthmark with other problems (if applicable).
  - Outline what to do and what will happen if the lesion is touched, scratched or cut.
  - Discuss with parents the possibility of other children having this birthmark.
  - Outline the skin care necessary for the lesion.

FOLLOW-UP

- Lesion specific: see Table 9.9.

MEDICAL CONSULT/ SPECIALIST REFERRAL

- Lesion-specific: see Table 9.9.

Table 9.8 Management of Common Birthmarks

Lesion	Additional diagnostics	Pharmacotherapeutics	Behavioural interventions	Patient education
Mongolian spots	• None unless persistent and/or atypical lesion	• None	• None	• Mongolian spots are benign and very, very common (especially in infants with darker pigmented skin) • Colour will stabilise in infancy and lesion usually disappears by puberty • Lesion can be mistaken for bruising
Café au lait macules (CALMs)	• Histological examination can distinguish them from melanocytic naevi	• None	• Family to watch for increase in number or appearance of lesion(s)	• Very important to watch for changes in appearance
Congenital melanocytic naevi (CMNs)	• Histological examination may differentiate from other lesions	• None	• Family to watch for a change in the appearance of lesion(s)	• Full-thickness removal will cause scarring • Partial-thickness removal will result in re-pigmentation and hair regrowth
Haemangiomas	• Imaging and subspecialty diagnostics—(e.g. ocular ultrasound, ENT assessment, ECG and abdominal ultrasound)—may be necessary if >3 lesions or involvement of eyes, ears or upper respiratory tract	• Systemic steroids considered with large lesions and infants with multiorgan involvement (e.g. eyes, neck or others) • Interferon-alpha given by daily injection considered for life-threatening lesions (used with caution due to long-term side-effects) • Antibiotic ointment for ulcerated lesions and/or to prevent infection of traumatised lesion(s)	• Observation and natural involution for small, inconspicuous lesions • Laser treatment considered for early stage lesions (e.g. when only slightly raised and red). Note laser therapy not effective for blue, deeper lesions • If lesion ulcerated, swabbing, antiseptic bath cleansing and non-adherent dressings required daily • Laser therapy and twice daily dressings used for persistent ulcerations (provides pain relief and promotes healing)	• Treatment often involves a combination of therapies • Skin care of haemangioma is very important • Oral steroids given over a period of weeks (will slow growth and even reduce size of lesions) • Possibility of immune suppression if oral steroids used (review risk of illness and to seek care immediately) • Protect from trauma (skin of haemangioma is very fragile and if traumatised, slow to heal) • Infection of traumatised skin will prolong ulceration • If trauma causes bleeding, apply pressure for 5 min and seek care • Keep nails short and skin moisturised (skin tends to be dry) • Management of ulcerated lesions • Support group information
Stork marks	• None usually required	• None	• Observation	• Reassurance with regard to the likelihood of resolution without intervention
Port-wine stains	• Eye examination with intraocular pressures if lesion involves eyelids (yearly checks) • Neuroimaging possible if involvement of scalp	• None	• Pulsed laser therapy (started between 6 and 12 months of age) will significantly lighten (also may lessen skin thickening and papule development in later life) • Numerous treatments required (every 4–6 months) in order to obtain best results before school-age	• Support group information • Clear and accurate information regarding treatment and prognosis • Complete removal is not possible and treatments usually performed under light general anaesthetic (and a day in hospital) • Skin care post-laser therapy very important (i.e. high factor sun block) to prevent skin hyperpigmentation

Table 9.9 Follow-up and Indications for Referral of Common Birthmarks in Children

Lesion	Follow-up	Referral/consult
Mongolian spots	• None usually required	• Any child with an atypical and/or persistent lesion(s)
Café au lait macules (CALMs)	• If isolated and singular lesion, none required • Lesions with cosmetic significance may benefit from laser therapy	• Any neonate with multiple CALMs • Any child with >6 CALMs of 0.5 cm or larger • Any infant or young child with inguinal and axillary freckling
Congenital melanocytic naevi (CMNs)	• Yearly monitoring for development of childhood malignant melanoma	• Any neonate with a significant lesion (refer in first weeks of life) • Any child in whom a lesion has changed in appearance
Stork marks	• None required unless redness persists for more than 2 years	• Any child with redness persisting after 2 years (rule out port-wine element)
Haemangioma	• If oral steroids are used as part of the treatment regimen, there needs to be regular monitoring of blood pressure and weight • Due to immune suppression among children treated with oral steroids, live vaccines (oral polio) should not be used (substitute inactivated vaccine) and exposure to varicella will require varicella zoster immunoglobulin (VZIG) to be given	• Any neonate with numerous lesions (rule out internal lesions). This includes ophthalmology assessment with orbital ultrasound (rule out orbital involvement); ENT assessment if auditory or respiratory involvement; and ECG and abdominal ultrasound if >3 lesions. Beware thrombocytopenia and cardiac failure with large internal lesion(s) • Any child with lesions on the eyelids, nostrils, throat or around the ears as these need careful monitoring • Any child with significant lesions (treatment needs to be started early, before rapid growth occurs) • Any child with a lesion around the eye as there is a risk of amblyopia
Port-wine stain	• Annual eye checks for children with eyelid stains • Yearly reevaluation of lesions treated with lasers (check for repigmentation)	• Any child with a port-wine stain should be evaluated for possible intervention • Any child with a port-wine stain on the eyelid will require ophthalmology referral (rule out glaucoma) and yearly rechecks • Any child with a port-wine stain of the scalp will require neurology referral (rule out brain involvement, seizures or other problem)

PAEDIATRIC PEARLS

• Advice on skin care always available from specialist units.

• An area of skin (anywhere) on the body of a neonate that becomes red or raised during the first few weeks of life should flag up the possibility of a proliferating haemangioma. Likewise, if there were any treatments that involved the use of tape, the skin may have developed red areas. If normal skin cleansing and moisturisers do not clear (or if ulcerations occur) haemangioma should be considered.

• Nappy rash can sometimes be confused with telangiectatic haemangiomas (bilateral, flat, red/pink areas without a clearly defined edge). Cleansing and barrier cream should clear if nappy rash.

• Occasionally, deep haemangiomas that are not identified as such and are subsequently confused with malignancies (and referred to an oncologist). This is probably related to the significant swelling and mass-like consistency of deep haemangiomas.

• Port-wine stains that occur in conspicuous places can cause great distress to parents and relatives. Significant support and correct advice on treatments is imperative from diagnosis (i.e. birth). Likewise, put parents in contact with support groups (see below).

• **Birthmark Support Group** (PO Box 3932, Weymouth, DT4 9YG, e-mail: birthmarksupportgroup@btinternet. com) will always give names and numbers of a specialist nurse either to a parent or health care professional. In addition, the Birthmark Support Group has parents who will always be happy to talk to other parents.

• Cosmetic camouflage is available from some specialist units or the Red Cross. It may be requested after completion of treatments or for special occasions.

BIBLIOGRAPHY

Dohil M, Baugh W, Eichenfield L. Vascular and pigmented birthmarks. Pediatr Clin North Am 2000; 47(4):783–808.

Dover JS. Pulsed dye treatment of port wine stains. J Am Acad Dermatol 1995; 32:237–240.

Lacour M. Role of pulsed dye laser in the management of ulcerated haemangiomas. Arch Dis Child 1996; 74(2):161–163.

Lanigna SW. Treatment of vascular naevi in children. Hosp Med 2001; 62(3):144–147.

Rasmussen J. Vascular birthmarks in children. Dermatol Nurs 1998; 10(3):169–230.

Wahrman J, Honig P. Hemangiomas. Pediatr Rev 1994; 15(7):266–271.

9.5 BURNS

Paulajean Kelly

📖 INTRODUCTION

- Accidents are a significant cause of childhood mortality; they account for the highest proportion of deaths in children greater than 1 year of age. Thermal injuries and burns are second only to road traffic accidents as the most common cause of accidental death (50% mortality attributed to smoke inhalation and 50% from thermal skin damage).
- The Department of Trade and Industry estimate that 4675 children (i.e. those under the age of 18) with thermal injuries attend hospital Accident and Emergency (A&E) departments and specialist burns units each year. Pre-school children account for 75% of these admissions (almost 10 per day).
- Health promotion directed at primary prevention of burn injuries is a major public health concern. In addition, it is vital to address the issues of immediate burn management and reduction of burn complications with both carers and health care professionals.
- This section will focus primarily on minor burns and scalds that would be appropriately managed in the primary health care setting or within the scope of care provided by district general hospitals. However, given the significant number of children sustaining thermal injuries, nurse practitioners (NPs) may be involved in the management of severe burns in the intensive care setting and/or they may provide long-term follow-up care from specialist burns centres. The severity of the injury notwithstanding, NPs require knowledge of appropriate initial management of paediatric burns.

🔬 PATHOPHYSIOLOGY

The pathophysiology of burns can be considered in three parts:

- *Local damage* to the cutaneous membrane and related structures as a result of contact with the thermal agent (heat, radiation, electrical shock or chemical agent). Impairment of skin function is dependent on the depth and extent of injury. In light sunburn, for example, wide dilation of the capillaries in the dermis causes erythema and fluid loss into the tissues, which manifests as swelling. The subsequent rise in interstitial pressure stimulates nerve endings and causes pain. More severe burns increase the fluid loss, which appears as blistering, and results in damage to the overlying epidermal cells. Once the dermal layer is compromised (either fully or partially) associated nerve endings are destroyed and there is a concomitant reduction in sensation. Subsequent regeneration of epithelial elements in glands and hair follicles will be slow and, without surgical intervention, may result in thin skin. Damage to the pulmonary system results from inhalation of hot gases and irritants (e.g. smoke or chemical byproducts of combustion). Upper airway obstruction occurs as a direct result of oedema of the respiratory structures, whereas oedematous bronchioles and alveoli result in poor perfusion.
- *Systemic effects* of burns often pose a greater threat to the child's life than local effects. Attempts to maintain cardiovascular homeostasis drive the systemic pathophysiology. Loss of plasma-rich fluid from the burn site (especially in large percentage burns) can lead to hypovolaemic shock in the paediatric patient. Electrical burns, in particular, are characterised by minimal local effects and potentially devastating systemic effects. More specifically, the systemic effects of an electrical current passing through body tissues (especially those with the lowest resistance: nerves, vessels and muscle) can be considerable. The extent of damage depends on several factors, including the voltage and amperage of the source, site of injury and duration of contact. The majority of the children with systemic effects, secondary to thermal injury, will require management in a high-dependency facility.
- Children with burns are especially vulnerable to *infection* due to the loss of their protective skin barrier and invasive management techniques. Even children with relatively mild burns can suffer fever and malaise. Wound infections can delay healing and adversely affect the cosmetic results of healing. *Staphylococcus aureus* is the most common pathogen colonising burn wounds. Children with staphylococcal wound infections are vulnerable to toxic shock syndrome (TSS), a rare and potentially life-threatening complication of an *S. aureus* infection. TSS is primarily seen in children with small burns; it is thought to be a result of bacterial toxin production and its effect on the immune system.
- Thermal injuries are classified by the depth of the burn(s): see Table 9.10.

⬅ HISTORY

- Type of thermal exposure/agent of injury (e.g. scalding water, hot oil, battery acid, etc.) and length of time agent was in contact with the skin: if the burn is from a chemical source, a description of the packaging and purpose (if known) will aid identification if a sample has not been brought to the A&E or clinic.
- The circumstances of the injury, including interpretation of the incident within the context of the child's developmental stage: e.g. scalds to the head and trunk from pulling cups/mugs containing hot drinks are more common in the 9-month to 2-year age group and relate to the developing gross motor skills of late infancy and toddlerhood. Note that it is important that the history and the clinical findings are compatible and plausible.

Table 9.10	Burn Classification		
Type of burn[a]	Appearance	Key management principles	Estimated healing time
Superficial	• Involve the epidermis only • Characterised by erythema, pain and dryness	• If no blister formation can be left exposed • Application of cool compresses and analgesia • Important to avoid further thermal exposure until well healed	• Painful for 3 days with healing in 5–10 days • Healing usually without significant scarring

Partial thickness	• Involve the epidermis and the dermis
	• May vary in appearance:
	  ○ erythematous blisters with decreased sensitivity
	  ○ diffuse erythema that blanches with pressure
	  ○ white and dry
		• Monitor daily for first few days to ensure proper healing and to assess for infection
		• Irrigation, cleansing and debridement of wound prior to initial dressing (rinse thoroughly)
		• Dressing management is wound-dependent
		• Electrical and chemical burns will require hospitalisation for observation as will children with involvement of upper airway, fractures, uncertain parental follow-up and/or severe pain
			• Usually healed in 10–14 days; however, this is dependent on tissues involved
			• Extent and duration of pain and scarring is variable
			• Can develop into full-thickness burn with infection

Full thickness	• Involve the dermis and underlying tissues • Avascular and, as such, appear waxy, with a brown leatherish surface • Numb to touch	• Will likely require treatment in hospital setting that includes surgical management • Grafting required • Fluid resuscitation and supportive management required for all apart from very small percentage burns	• Prolonged healing time (can be several months) • Likely to spend considerable period of time receiving inpatient care and will require multidisciplinary follow-up • Usually some degree of permanent impairment

[a]Note that differentiation between deep partial-thickness and full-thickness injury is sometimes difficult on initial assessment.

- Time that injury occurred (the time lapse post-injury can be determined).
- Treatment given to burn (initial and subsequent).
- Possibility of any additional exposures (e.g. inhalation, ingestion, etc.).
- Previous history of burn injuries.
- Immunisation status (especially tetanus).

PHYSICAL EXAMINATION

- Initial assessment of the burned child always will prioritise airway, circulation and breathing (ABCs) and neurological status.

- Assessment of pain with appropriate analgesia (see Sec. 13.3) is vital once the ABCs are stabilised. Cling film applied to the burned area reduces pain (caused by exposure of burnt skin to the air) and the potential for airborne contamination during the initial history taking and while awaiting relief from oral analgesics.

- The location, depth and extent of the thermal injury are the foundation upon which the management plan is based. In general, deeper and more extensive burns require greater intervention. However, some superficial burns may be problematic because of their location (e.g. near the eyes). The classification and appearance of different depths of thermal trauma is summarised in Table 9.10.

- **Skin:** starting with head, the entire body should be examined in order to evaluate the surface area affected, the depth of the injury and any pattern of distribution. The percentage of total body surface area (TBSA) burned should be estimated using an accepted tool: e.g. Lund and Browder chart, 'rule of nines', etc. Note that a child's age will affect the TBSA calculations (e.g. the head of young children/infants comprises a greater percentage of TBSA than an older child, whereas the reverse is true for the thigh). In making the calculation of TBSA affected, simple erythema should be ignored. Any child with 10% of their TBSA affected will be classified as a major burn and requires immediate intravenous fluid management and referral to a paediatric burns centre. Observe for any areas that are or have the potential to become circumferential (e.g. wrists, ankles and neck).

- **Head and ear, nose and throat (ENT):** check for any evidence of smoke inhalation, such as soot around the nasal passages or mouth in addition to identifying head, neck or facial burns that will require plastic surgery referral/evaluation.

- **Cardiopulmonary:** evaluate and monitor trends in order to identify early signs of shock.

- **Neurological:** monitor for changes signifying shock or impending shock.

DIFFERENTIAL DIAGNOSES

- The differential diagnoses to be considered relate to the reported absence of contact with heat. Both staphylococcal scalded skin syndrome (SSSS) and toxic epidermal necrolysis (TEN) present with erythema, blisters, bullae and exfoliation that may suggest contact with a thermal substance. However, there is no history of thermal injury in SSSS and with TEN there is often a history of commonly reactive drugs (e.g. phenobarbital, phenytoin, allopurinol, sulphonamides and penicillin).

- Note that the possibility of non-accidental injury needs to be considered in the differential diagnosis of paediatric thermal trauma. Parents, carers and children may all be reluctant to disclose the source of injuries caused either deliberately or through neglect of the child. Careful history taking may reveal inconsistencies in explanations, whereas the shape and distribution of the burn or scald may provide alerts that the injury was not an accident. Causes include burns where there has been prolonged contact with a hot object (e.g. cigarette burns, domestic irons and immersion scalds of the feet or buttocks). Any suspicion of a child protection issue requires careful investigation and activation of local child protection pathways.

✚ MANAGEMENT

Basic principles of burn management are outlined in Tables 9.10 and 9.11.

- **Additional diagnostics:** dependent on burn severity; however, consider full blood count (FBC), haematocrit, sickle cell screen, urea and electrolytes, cross matching and possibly wound cultures.

- **Pharmacotherapeutics:** Pain management may require significant analgesia, especially during initial assessment and dressing changes. Consider short-acting sedation (e.g. intranasal midazolam) to reduce distress when dressing injury. Superficial burns remain painful for approximately 3 days, so regular analgesia will be required (see Sec. 13.3). For injuries managed at home, mild analgesia is usually effective (e.g. ibuprofen or paracetamol). Routine or prophylactic use of antibiotics is not recommended. Update tetanus immunisation if appropriate.

- **Behavioural interventions:** the mainstay of burn management (post-injury) is wound management (assuming pain is under control).

Table 9.11	General Principles of Burn Management
Topic	*Comments*
Intravenous (IV) cannula	• Will be required if fluid replacement or IV medication required • IV fluid replacement and maintenance as per local protocols
Cleansing of burn site	• Objective is to remove any embedded debris (e.g. chemicals, clothing fibres, devitalised tissue) • Sodium chloride (0.9%) is usually first-line irrigation solution as it is non-toxic to tissues and isotonic (thereby decreasing the risk of tissue damage during irrigation)
Care of blisters	• Wounds without blisters and/or small superficial burns (e.g. minor sunburn or scalds) can be left exposed • Small blisters should be left intact • Large blisters management is controversial as serous fluid is potential bacterial growth medium; but intact blisters can provide protection from external pathogens • Blisters over flexures should be punctured and drained (with sterile technique) to improve patient comfort

Table 9.12	Commonly Used Dressings
Dressing type	*Comments*
Silver sulfadiazine dressings	• Apply 1% silver sulfadiazine to wound margins, cover with fine-mesh paraffin tulle and gauze • Secure with crepe bandage or tubi gauze (dependent on location). Avoid using adhesive tape to secure as this increases discomfort and distress at dressing changes • Cautious use if large areas of skin are treated (risk of sulphonamide-related adverse effects)
Hand dressings	• Manage with liberal application of liquid paraffin or silver sulfadiazine (above) and place in sterile bag or glove • Paraffin gauze beneath a thick gauze dressing at wrist will absorb the exudate • Better tolerated by older children
Non-porous silicone dressings (e.g. Mepitel)	• Can be used as alternative to traditional silver sulfadiazine as it is thought to decrease healing time • Is thought to provide a moist environment for wound healing; adhere only to healthy skin; and be less painful to remove than paraffin gauze • It can be left in place for several days (dependent on the amount of exudate) which reduces damage to areas of new epithelialisation • Use with caution on darker pigmented skins (e.g. Afro-Caribbean children) as there have been reports of pigmentation abnormalities
Clear film dressings (e.g. Dermoclear)	• Additional alternative to traditional silver sulfadiazine that allows for visualisation of wound without removal of dressings
Dressings after surgical intervention	• Dressing management dependent on surgical intervention performed • Objectives of dressing selection are to maximise wound healing and prevent postoperative infection

Choice of dressing will need to take account of the burn extent, location and anticipated exudate. The products used in dressing the burns and the schedule of dressing changes need to provide an appropriate environment for wound healing and to protect the burn from contamination. A summary of commonly used dressings for the management of minor to moderate burns is provided in Table 9.12.

- **Patient education:**
  - Review with parents (and the child) the expected management course and sequelae of the burn, including post-injury follow-up care.

- Discuss wound management and dressing care, including the importance of preventing infection and the role of nutrition to promote healing (adequate protein and calories).
- Teach carers about the signs and symptoms of complications (e.g. infection, toxic shock, fever, foul-smelling dressings, increased pain, etc.). Stress with them a rapid return for care if the child's condition deteriorates or if the child appears unwell.
- Inform parents that additional sun protection will be required for newly healed burns (for at least 12 months) as the burns are more sensitive to the sun and will sunburn more severely.
- Warn parents that as the burn heals it may become itchy (treat with liberal use of moisturisers).
- Discuss the issue of scarring, including the difficulty of predicting potential outcomes with any certainty. Tell parents that many factors influence the healing (and scarring) process. More specifically, the extent of scarring is dependent on the depth of the burn, length of time needed for healing, need for grafting, child's age, skin colour and the role of infection on the healing process. Let them know that scars change over time (remaining immature for 12–18 months post-injury) and that the scar will go through colour and texture changes as the child grows.
- Talk to families about the prevention of further injury. This should not be limited only to a discussion of the initial injury but should encompass a range of child safety issues, including smoke alarms, sun safety, water safety and storage of hazardous substances. Families in this situation are highly receptive to information. Although the under-5s are the most at-risk group for thermal injuries in the home setting, older children are vulnerable outside the home (e.g. Guy Fawkes Day celebrations, playing with matches, etc.).

➡ FOLLOW-UP

- All burns should be re-evaluated in 24 hours, as depth of injury is not always apparent immediately after the injury.
- Frequency of dressing changes will vary with material used. Note that paraffin tulle should not be allowed to dry as it will adhere to new tissue, causing pain and distress on removal.
- Lanolin-based creams (Diprobase or aqueous cream) should be gently massaged into the newly healed burn site 3–4 times daily to help minimise scarring.
- Specific follow-up is dependent on the extent and depth of the injury. It is likely that follow-up will continue until the burn is healed completely. This may be done in the community (e.g. GP surgery, community children's nursing service) or hospital-based clinic.
- For children requiring significant pain relief and/or sedation for dressing changes, the hospital setting may be the most appropriate. Dressing changes are often identified as the most painful and psychologically distressing aspect of burn management. Consider the need for post-trauma psychological support, referring as necessary.

⇄ MEDICAL CONSULT/ SPECIALIST REFERRAL

- Any child with full-thickness and/or significant burns should be referred for hospitalisation to a paediatric burns centre or a service that can provide plastic surgery support.
- Any child with an inhalation, chemical and/or electrical burn requires referral to services that can provide high-dependency and/or intensive care.
- Any child with a burn that could potentially result in loss of function or significant scarring (e.g. serious burns to the hands, fingers or face) should be referred to a paediatric burns centre with plastic surgery and rehabilitation support.
- Any child that is identified during follow-up as having an increased risk of disfigurement will require scar management services.

- Any child in whom there is suspicion of a child protection issue (both deliberate child harm or injury through neglect). As such, referral should be initiated with local child protection team.
- Any child with circumferential burns or burns to the head, neck, face, hands or feet.

🔍 PAEDIATRIC PEARLS

- Organise dressing changes to maximise the analgesic effects of pain medication.
- The child's palm, as 1% of TBSA, can be used as a quick guide to estimate the extent of a thermal injury.
- Telephone advice can be obtained from any of the 23 UK burns centres that regularly manage children.

📖 BIBLIOGRAPHY

Bosworth C. Burns trauma. London: Ballière Tindall; 1997.

Bruce E, Franck L. Self-administered nitrous oxide (Entonox®) for the management of procedural pain. Paediatr Nurs 2000; 12(7):15–19.

Bugmann PH. A silicone coated nylon dressing reduces healing time in burned paediatric patients in comparison with standard sulfadiazine treatment: a prospective randomised trial. Burns 1998; 24(7):609–612.

Coleshaw S, Reilly S, Irving N. Management of burns. Paediatr Nurs 1997; 9(7):29–36.

Edwards-Jones V, Dawson MM, Childs C. A survey into toxic shock syndrome (TSS) in UK burns units. Burns 2000; 26(4):323–333.

Kelly H. Initial nursing assessment and management of burn-injured children. Br J Nurs 1994; 3(2):54–59.

Kent L, King H, Cochrane R. Maternal & child psychological sequelae in paediatric burn injuries. Burns 2000; 26(4):317–322.

Lund CL, Browder NC. The estimation of burns. Surg Gynecol Obstet 1944; 79:352.

O'Neill JA. Advances in the management of pediatric trauma. Am J Surg 2000; 180(5):365–369.

Orr J. Thermal injuries in children: nursing and related care. J Child Health 1997; 1(2): 68–73.

Rodgers GL. Reducing the toll of childhood burns. Contemp Pediatr 2000; 17(4):152–173.

Teare J. A home care team in paediatric wound care. J Wound Care 1997; 6(6):295–296.

Williams G, Withey S, Walker CC. Longstanding pigmentary changes in paediatric scalds dressed with a non-adherent siliconised dressing. Burns 2001; 27(2):200–202.

Additional Resources

Child Accident Prevention Trust, 4th Floor, Clerks Court, 18–20 Farringdon Lane, London, EC1R 3UA.

www.rospa.co.uk: Royal Society for the Prevention of Accidents web site. Details of child safety issues, including developmental fact sheets that can be adapted as a teaching and health promotion tool for families and children at risk of accidents from thermal or other hazards.
www.peds.umn.edu/divisions/pccm/teaching/acp/burns.html: University of Minnesota Department of Pediatrics teaching page on the management of moderate and severe burns.

ACKNOWLEDGEMENT

The author would like to acknowledge the expertise of Aine Ennis, Paediatric Emergency Nurse Practitioner, Homerton University Hospital NHS Trust, in the preparation of this section.

9.6 CELLULITIS

Sara Burr

📖 INTRODUCTION

- Cellulitis is an infection of the skin and subcutaneous tissue.
- Any area of the body can be affected and, therefore, cellulitis is usually classified by body area involved (e.g. periorbital, orbital, extremity, breast, etc.).
- Cellulitis often develops secondary to local trauma: the legs are the most common sites of infection.
- Complete recovery without complications is dependent on prompt recognition, with administration of appropriate antibiotics in a timely fashion.

🔬 PATHOPHYSIOLOGY

- The most common pathogens responsible for cellulitis are *Staphylococcus aureus* and *Streptococcus* spp. (especially group A β-haemolytic and *S. pneumoniae*). The incidence of *Haemophilus influenzae* type B (Hib) infection, formerly a common cause of invasive disease, has declined dramatically since widespread vaccination with the Hib vaccine. Other less common causes of cellulitis include *Pseudomonas aeruginosa* and other Gram-negative bacilli; anaerobic bacteria (especially among immunocompromised children); and *Erysipelothrix rhusiopathiae* (if injury was secondary to a puncture wound from freshwater fish or shellfish, infected turkeys and/or pigs).
- Cellulitis as a consequence of damage to the integument (e.g. laceration, abrasion, bites, excoriated dermatitis, etc.) is by far the most common cause of cellulitis in children. However, cellulitis less commonly may develop as a result of (1) local invasion or infection (e.g. sinusitis leading to orbital cellulitis) or (2) through haematogenous dissemination of an invasive organism (classically *H. influenzae* type B).
- The localised, rapid spread of the bacteria into subcutaneous tissue and the lymphatic system results in an expanding, red, hot, swollen and painful area of inflammation. There is often a history of local trauma and systemic complaints such as fever and malaise. There may be a red lymphangitic streak (sign of lymph involvement) and regional adenopathy is common.
- Complications of cellulitis include spread of the infection, abscess formation, extension into deeper tissues (to produce an arthritis or osteomyelitis) and, in the case of orbital cellulitis, visual loss.

← HISTORY

- History of local trauma to the integument, pre-existing skin conditions and/or condition of the skin prior to symptoms developing.
- History of contact with animals and situations of potential trauma (woodland or beach trips without shoes, football/hockey without shin guards) over the last week.
- Onset, location and appearance of inflamed or tender area (including original area of redness, presence of any 'red streaking' and rate at which size of area is or is not increasing).
- Systemic symptoms (fever, malaise, swollen glands, etc.).
- History of systemic infection prior to onset of redness.
- Treatment(s) used and results.
- Coexisting disease (especially immunocompromise).
- Immunisation status (especially Hib vaccine if <6 years old).

🔍 PHYSICAL EXAMINATION

- As systemic symptoms can be present, a full physical examination should be performed, noting abnormalities.
- **Head and ENT:** routine examination, noting any areas of inflammation (warmth, redness, pain and/or swelling). Careful assessment of eyes and cranial nerves if orbital cellulitis suspected.
- **Lymph:** assess for regional lymphadenopathy in nodes that drain the affected area.

- **Cardiovascular and respiratory:** routine examination—note abnormalities.

- **Skin:** head-to-toe assessment of all skin is important. Note extent of inflammation, appearance and presence of lymphangitic streaking. It is useful to encircle the borders of the inflammation (in pen) in order to monitor the size of the area.

- **Musculoskeletal:** note any swelling, pain or tenderness of joints.

DIFFERENTIAL DIAGNOSES

- Consider non-infectious cause of localised inflammation (allergic angio-oedema; contact dermatitis and traumatic contusion). However, with these diagnoses there should be historical clues that rule out cellulitis (e.g. history of allergic reactions and exposure, etc.). In addition, there is likely to be an absence of systemic signs.

- Severe conjunctivitis may mimic periorbital cellulitis; however, the conjunctival injection, chemosis and discharge provide clues to the diagnosis of conjunctivitis. Likewise, the pathophysiology of some childhood malignancies (e.g. retinoblastoma, rhabdomyosarcoma, neuroblastoma and leukaemia) may give an appearance of a periorbital or orbital cellulitis.

MANAGEMENT

- **Additional diagnostics:** dependent on the clinical presentation and suspicion of complications. Consider full blood count (FBC), erythrocyte sedimentation rate (ESR), C-reactive protein (CRP), blood cultures and lumbar puncture (very ill infants and young children to rule out sepsis). X-ray studies can be used to rule out complications such as osteomyelitis and arthritis. Head computed tomography (CT) is considered in orbital cellulitis to delineate the extent of disease or when a distinction between periorbital and orbital cellulitis is clinically difficult. If

a malignancy is suspected, additional diagnostics are aimed at confirming suspicions.

- **Pharmacotherapeutics:** choice of antibiotics is dictated by local antibiotic policy. However, most cases of uncomplicated cellulitis can be treated with oral antibiotics that are effective against *Staphylococcus* spp. and *Streptococcus* spp. (e.g. flucloxacillin, amoxicillin-clavulanic acid, cefalexin, erythromycin). Ill-appearing children or those with extensive involvement will require intraveneous (IV) antibiotics (usually in hospital). Initial IV therapy should be directed against *S. aureus* and *Streptococcus* spp. (e.g. IV benzylpenicillin, IV flucloxacillin, cefazolin). If haematogenous dissemination is suspected, an agent active against *H. influenzae* should be added (e.g. ceftriaxone, cefotaxime, cefuroxime, chloramphenicol). Infants <7 weeks of age should have Gram-positive and Gram-negative coverage as should immunocompromised children (obtain infectious disease consultation). As the child is likely to be uncomfortable, analgesia should be administered and adjusted as the clinical condition indicates. The same is true of antipyretics (including the monitoring of temperature); administer as needed and monitor response.

- **Behavioural interventions:** adequate skin care of the infected area to avoid further compromise of the integument (emollients, soap substitute washes); good nutrition and hydration to promote healing and the body's own immune system; rest and elevation of the affected area to promote circulation and observation of the affected area for rapid resolution. Monitor response to antipyretics and analgesic medications.

- **Patient education:**
  - review with parents the importance of good wound care (i.e. soap and water cleansing, appropriate dressing) in order to prevent the development of cellulitis
  - stress the importance of completing the full course of antibiotics and daily observation for improvement of the affected area

- let parents know that cellulitis is not contagious, although proper handwashing should be a part of good health practices.

FOLLOW-UP

- Rapid and steady resolution should occur with appropriate antibiotic selection. If daily improvement is not seen, further investigation is required (i.e. to rule out deeper infection, abscess or other complication).

MEDICAL CONSULT/ SPECIALIST REFERRAL

- Any child with a gravely ill appearance or in whom a more serious infection is suspected.
- Any child who has developed a complication of cellulitis.
- Any child who does not respond to appropriate initial treatment.
- Any infants or young children or any child with a less than competent immune system.

PAEDIATRIC PEARLS

- To monitor the progress of an area of inflammation, outline the edges with a marker pen and follow the borders of the erythema (very useful for parents to assist in monitoring).
- Do not try to make a distinction between a streptococcal or staphylococcal aetiology for the infection by clinical observations. Antibiotics should cover both organisms.
- If there is abscess formation, incision and drainage is usually required.
- If serious systemic symptoms are present, suspect bacteraemia.

BIBLIOGRAPHY

Darmstadt G. A guide to superficial strep and staph skin infections. Contemp Pediatr 1997; 14(5):95–116.

Darmstadt G. Oral antibiotic therapy of children with uncomplicated bacterial skin infections. Pediatr Infect Dis J 1997; 16:227–230.

Darmstadt G. A guide to abscesses in the skin. Contemp Pediatr 1999; 16(4):135–145.

Fulton B, Perry CM. Cefpodoxime proxetil: a review of its use in the management of bacterial infections in paediatric patients. Paediatr Drugs 2001; 3(2):137–158.

Hurwitz S. Clinical pediatric dermatology: a textbook of skin disorders of childhood and adolescence. St. Louis: WB Saunders; 1981.

Jain A, Daum R. Staphylococcal infections in children: part 1. Pediatr Rev 1999; 20(6):183–191.

Rook D, Wilkinson S, Ebling D. Textbook of dermatology, Vol 2, 6th edn. London: Blackwell Science; 1998.

Ruiz-Maldonado R, Parish LC, Beare JM. Textbook of paediatric dermatology. London: Grune and Stratton; 1989.

9.7 FOOD ALLERGY

Maureen Lilley

INTRODUCTION

- Food allergy is an abnormal immunological response to a specific food protein (allergen) that results in illness. This is in contrast to *food intolerance*, which is related to a non-immunological reaction (e.g. lactose intolerance).
- The exact incidence of food allergy in children is unknown but it appears to be on the increase. The prevalence of true food hypersensitivity ranges between 1 and 3% of children.
- Common allergenic foods are age-related and include milk, eggs, wheat, soya, peanuts, tree nuts, fruits and white fish. Factors which influence a child's predisposition to allergic disease include:
  - a family history of atopy
  - increased atmospheric pollutants such as tobacco smoke and pollen
  - foods eaten during pregnancy and breast-feeding in atopic mothers
  - weaning patterns and exposure to certain offending food allergens in predisposed infants (e.g. peanut butter introduced in the first year of life).
- The vast majority of children outgrow the common childhood food allergies such as milk and eggs by 6–7 years of age. Peanut allergy, however, is usually lifelong and is the most likely food to cause severe anaphylaxis and death in children.
- Clinical presentation varies from localised symptoms (e.g. urticaria, facial, lip and eye swelling, tingling of lips, tongue or throat, vomiting and abdominal pain) to life-threatening wheeze, stridor, hypotension and collapse (anaphylaxis). Many of these children will present to their general practitioner (GP) with localised reactions; more severe reactions will likely present directly to the A&E.

Table 9.13	Clinical Symptoms of the Allergic Response
Reaction	Symptom
Skin reactions	Urticaria, pruritus, oedema, erythema
Respiratory reactions	Sneezing, laryngo-oedema, wheeze, stridor
Gastric reactions	Abdominal pain, vomiting, diarrhoea
Generalised reactions	Unconscious, hypotension, shock (anaphylaxis)

PATHOPHYSIOLOGY

- To develop an allergy to a particular food protein the child must first be exposed to the allergen. This initial exposure leads to sensitisation, so that when the child comes into contact with the allergen again a damaging immune response occurs and the result is illness.
- The most common allergic response is type I hypersensitivity: IgE-mediated. This occurs within minutes of contact either through touch, ingestion or inhalation of the offending food protein (allergen). The allergen reacts with IgE antibodies on the surface of mast cells and basophils, which degranulate, releasing potent chemical mediators (e.g. histamine, prostaglandins and leukotrienes).
- The chemical mediators trigger vascular leakage, mucosal oedema, vasodilatation and smooth muscle constriction; the processes responsible for the clinical symptoms of the allergic response can affect all body systems (Table 9.13). The resulting reaction varies from mild, to moderate or severe.
- Note that delayed type I hypersensitivity can present in a small proportion of children hours after initial exposure (particularly in children with asthma who present with increasing wheeze).
- In addition, a type IV delayed hypersensitivity reaction is possible in some children. This non-IgE-mediated reaction often occurs 12–72 hours post-exposure to an offending allergen. It is a cell-mediated response, caused by activation of macrophages that stimulate an inflammatory response (e.g. Mantoux skin test for tuberculosis).

HISTORY

A thorough history is the key to diagnosis in food allergy. Although time consuming, the benefits of allergen identification far outweigh time spent in obtaining an in-depth history. It is often fairly easy to identify the food allergen if the reaction occurs within minutes of contact with the offending food, more difficult when the reaction is delayed. Consequently, it is important to establish a temporal relationship between when the offending food was ingested and the onset of symptoms:

- Date of first exposure.

- Nature of exposure, including symptoms, in the patient's/parent's own words, specifically in relation to:
  - tongue, mouth tingling or itch
  - urticaria/pruritus
  - swelling
  - vomiting/nausea, cramping and/or diarrhoea
  - breathing problems, choking, cough, stridor or wheeze and/or chest tightness
  - shock, feeling faint, lightheadness, loss of consciousness.

- Time between ingestion of food and development of symptoms.

- Action taken by child/parent (including medication use) and response.

- Outcome and time lapse to improvement (if any).

- Previous and subsequent exposures/ related allergens (peanut allergic children can be allergic to other nuts, peas, beans, lentils, sesame and coconut).

- History of eczema and asthma with treatment regimens.

- Family history and history of atopy/ allergy in other family members (e.g. asthma, hay fever, eczema, food allergy).

PHYSICAL EXAMINATION

- It is often difficult to examine first hand the results of the allergic response, as many children present in between exposures or symptoms may have subsided by the time of the consultation. Note that the physical examination of most food allergic children is unremarkable, especially if the patient presents after symptoms have subsided.

Table 9.14   Differential Diagnoses of Paediatric Food Allergy

Condition	Diagnosis
Gastrointestinal conditions	• Cows' milk, soya or gluten intolerance/coeliac disease, overfeeding/reflux (which can cause vomiting and abdominal pain), infection, food poisoning, colitis, food toxins, irritable bowel syndrome, Behçet's syndrome
Enzyme deficiency/metabolic conditions	• Phenylketonuria (PKU)
Food additive reactions	• Dyes, chemicals; e.g. tartrazine
Food fads/pseudoallergenic conditions	• Aversion to certain foods, anorexia, foods containing vasoactive mediators

- **General observation of the child:** colour, respiratory effort and rate, stridor (related to swelling of the larynx), angio-oedema, heart rate and blood pressure.

- **Skin:** careful inspection for discoloration, erythema, wheals (note size and contour), rash (note type and distribution), and skin temperature.

- **Head and ENT:** rhinoconjunctivitis, oropharyngeal oedema.

- **Respiratory:** wheezing and/or cough (which can be delayed signs of allergic response, especially in children who have asthma).

- **Abdomen:** discomfort, hyperactive bowel sounds and/or distension.

DIFFERENTIAL DIAGNOSES

- Adverse reactions to foods can be produced by many medical conditions, including infectious diseases; other important conditions are outlined in Table 9.14.

MANAGEMENT

Immediate management will depend on clinical presentation and severity of symptoms. Any child requiring intramuscular adrenaline/epinephrine should be transported immediately by ambulance to hospital.

- **Additional diagnostics:**
  - *Skin prick tests with dietary allergens:* helpful when there is a high index of suspicion for food allergy (IgE-mediated). If a positive result is obtained to the suspected food allergen, these tests are 90–100% sensitive. They are not useful in non-mediated reactions and must be carried out by appropriately trained personnel as there is a slight risk of anaphylaxis.
  - *Radioallergosorbent testing (RAST):* used to measure elevated IgE levels to specific allergens. The results must be interpreted with caution as a positive result cannot predict how severe a reaction could be if the child is subjected to future exposures.
  - Hospital admission for food challenge: day case admission may be undertaken by specialist centres.

- **Pharmacotherapeutics:** use of medication for symptom management is dependent on the severity of the symptoms (Table 9.15).

- **Behavioural interventions:**
  - Severe hypersensivity reactions: the main course of action is avoidance of the offending food allergen (if known) until seen by an immunologist or specialist in food allergy.
  - Mild hypersensivity: attempt an elimination trial of 1–3 months. If symptoms resolve, offending food(s) should be reintroduced to see if symptoms reappear. If symptoms persist, consider specialist referral. Note care should be taken in elimination trials that the child's diet is not compromised; therefore, any trial should only be under the supervision of a paediatric dietician.

Table 9.15   Pharmacotherapeutic Management of Food Allergy

Symptom	Treatment
Mild reaction	
Urticaria, pruritus, angio-oedema, erythema, sneezing, runny nose and eyes	• Oral antihistamine, e.g. Piriton syrup (chlorphenamine/chorpheniramine): 1 month to 2 years 1 mg 2–5 years 2 mg 6–12 years 2–4 mg >12 years 4 mg Dose can be repeated after 10–15 min if no improvement (two doses only: if no improvement seek medical assistance)
Moderate reaction	
Wheeze (no airway compromise)	• Piriton syrup (as above) • Nebulised salbutamol: <1 year 1.25 mg 1–5 years 2.5 mg >5 years 5 mg Nebulise once and if no improvement after 10–15 min seek medical assistance
Severe reaction	
Wheeze, stridor, compromised airway	Intramuscular (IM) adrenaline/epinephrine (1:1000) As below
Loss of consciousness, collapse	Seek assistance immediately and administer: IM adrenaline/epinephrine (1:1000) Under 6 months 0.05 ml 6 months to 6 years 0.12 ml 6–12 years 0.25 ml adolescent 0.5 ml If no improvement after 5 min repeat adrenaline/epinephrine dose Adrenaline/epinephrine pen: EpiPen Junior autoinjector 0.15 mg (15–30 kg) EpiPen Adult autoinjector 0.3 mg (>30 kg)

- **Patient education:**
  - Oral chlorpheniramine/chlorphenamine (Piriton) should be prescribed and the parent/child given clear verbal and written instructions on when it should be used (e.g. at the first sign of lip tingling, swelling or contact with the known offending food).
  - Piriton should be carried by the parent/child at all times and should be available at the child's school/nursery where personnel should be appropriately trained in its use.
  - Children carrying EpiPens should have them available at school as well as at home.
  - Children should be educated from an early age to ask if food offered is allowed, especially if they are not under the care of their parents/guardians. Instilling this from an early age gives the child some control and aids the prevention of accidental exposures.
  - During the elimination trial or when the potential allergen is being investigated, a food diary which lists foods ingested, time of ingestion, time of onset of symptoms, symptoms and relieving measures can be useful.
  - If referral is made for paediatric allergy testing, the child and family should be counselled on the services available from the allergy/immunology team. These include diagnosis of mild, moderate and severe allergies, nutritional counselling and longer-term follow-up.

⇨ FOLLOW-UP

- A prolonged elimination diet is usually not necessary as tolerance to allergens usually develops over time; even children with severe allergic reactions can eventually outgrow them. However, IgE-mediated disease tends to persist longer. As such, follow-up on a yearly basis is usually all that is required. The follow-up visit should review management instructions and adjust if necessary (moderate/severe reaction occurs or new allergen is suspected).

✐ MEDICAL CONSULT/SPECIALIST REFERRAL

- Children who have had an allergic response related to an identified or unknown food substance should be referred to a Paediatric Allergy Centre (particularly those with a severe reaction). In addition, all children who have experienced a moderate or severe reaction will require an adrenaline/epinephrine pen (EpiPen) and long-term follow-up. The paediatric allergist or immunologist will be able to offer a comprehensive service, including skin prick testing, RASTs and a food challenge under strict hospital supervision (if this is deemed appropriate).
- Consultation with a paediatric dietician may help in identifying foods with offending allergens and will likewise provide appropriate advice regarding a diet that avoids the identified allergens and yet maintains adequate growth and development.

☗ PAEDIATRIC PEARLS

- Only severe reactions require intramuscular adrenaline/epinephrine.
- Diagnosis of food allergy is made on a thorough clinical history, which may be supported by other investigations, i.e. skin prick testing, RAST and IgE.
- Food allergy cannot be diagnosed on RAST alone; they are a small piece of a 'big' picture.
- Any child who is allergic to a single nut should avoid all nuts. Children cannot distinguish between different sorts of nuts but they can understand a simple message: avoid 'all nuts'.
- If a child has eczema, make sure that the presenting/described rash is not a flare of the child's eczema.

- The shorter the time interval between food ingestion and reaction, the more likely it can be confirmed to be the trigger of the adverse reaction.

BIBLIOGRAPHY

Anonymous. ABC of allergies. London: BMJ Books; 1998.

Bock SA, Sampson H. Food allergy in children. Pediatr Clin North Am 1994; 41(5):1047–1067.

Bury T, Rademecker M. Histamine: from neurone-mast cell to allergy. Liege: The UCB Institute of Allergy; 1990.

David TJ. Food and food additive intolerance in childhood. London: Blackwell Science; 1993.

Department of Health. Peanut allergy: report on toxicity of chemicals in food, consumer products and the environment. London: Crown; 1998.

Fox D, Gaughan M. Food allergy in children. Paediatr Nurs 1999; 11(3):28–31.

The Project Team of Resuscitation Council. Consensus guidelines: emergency medical treatment of anaphylactic reaction, 41. London: The Project Team of Resuscitation Council; 1999.

Young RT. A population study of food intolerance. Lancet 1994; 343:1127–1130.

9.8 FUNGAL SKIN INFECTIONS

Annabel Smoker

INTRODUCTION

- Superficial fungal infections or mycoses are common in childhood, affecting both sexes and all socio-economic groups. Although such infections rarely compromise a child's life, they can be unpleasant, embarrassing and very difficult to eradicate.
- The nature and severity of the inflammatory response to the infection is dictated by the strain of the invading fungi. Fomites and animals (especially domestic pets and cattle) may be a source of infection, with the host response to zoophilic infections (those that normally colonise animals) generally more severe. Geophilic dermatophytes contaminate soil and can infect both humans and animals; while anthropophilic fungi are those transmitted by humans or fomites to other people.
- Certain fungi prefer specific sites of the body. In addition, the prevalence of different types of infection vary with age (Table 9.16).
- A number of factors increase a child's susceptibility to fungal infections (Table 9.16). Fungal infections thrive on skin that is either excessively moist and macerated or dry and chapped. Likewise, changes in skin temperature and normal acid balance (pH) can encourage opportunistic infections to flourish. Babies and immunosuppressed children—especially those with human immunodeficiency virus (HIV) or organ transplants—are at particular risk. Other predisposing factors include diabetes mellitus, the use of broad-spectrum antibiotics (increased *Candida* risk), long-term glucocorticosteroids and the use of potent topical steroids or cytotoxic therapy.
- Accurate diagnosis requires distinguishing fungal infections from other conditions such as contact dermatitis, atopic eczema or psoriasis. Misdiagnosis, lack of information and poor concordance with treatments inevitably results in avoidable transmission and reinfection.

PATHOPHYSIOLOGY

- Human fungal skin infections are caused by either dermatophytes (e.g. species of *Epidermophyton*, *Microsporum* and *Trichophyton* which are responsible for tinea infections); or yeasts (such as *Candida* or *Pityrosporum* that result in candidiasis and pityriasis versicolor, respectively). Distinguishing dermatophytes from yeasts is imperative, as clinical presentation and treatment varies considerably according to the species of fungi and location of the infection. The nature and severity of the inflammatory response is dictated by the strain of invading fungi.
- Dermatophytes are thread-like hyphae that colonise skin, hair and/or nails, resulting in a tinea infection. They are temperature-sensitive and, therefore, do not penetrate beyond the stratum corneum into living tissue. Dermatophytes have a unique enzymatic capacity that enables them to digest keratin (the chemical protein abundant in dead skin cells). As keratin is destroyed, scale forms and debris (that contains viable infectious elements) is shed. Infected nails crumble and hair becomes fragile and breaks off. Two of the three dermatophyte species (e.g. *Microsporum* and *Trichophyton*) colonise the skin and hair of the scalp (Table 9.16).
- *Candida* is a yeast that commonly lives as a commensal organism in the gastrointestinal tract, vaginal tract and mucocutaneous areas. However, in the right environment, opportunistic infections can occur in the mouth, perineum, genitalia, skin folds (groin, axilla, neck and submammary) and between fingers, toes and nails. *Candida* can also cause disseminated fungaemia in an immunocompromised host. *Pityrosporum orbiculare* is the yeast responsible for pityriasis versicolor (a superficial, non-infectious condition) and pityrosporum folliculitis. It is also considered to be the cause of seborrhoeic dermatitis and pityriasis capitis (dandruff).

Table 9.16 Common Fungal Infections in Children and Adolescents

Location and type of infection	Common causative agent(s)	Age group commonly affected	Predisposing factors	Typical appearance	Comments
Scalp					

• Tinea capitis	• Dermatophytes:
	  ◦ *Microsporum* (especially *M. canis*)
	  ◦ *Trichophyton* sp. (*T. tonsurans*)
		• Pre-adolescents	• Direct contact with infected animal, person and/or fomites	• Early indicators are patchy hair loss with or without inflammation
				• Appearance varies depending on whether infection is confined to the interior of hair shaft (endothrix) or involves the outer hair shaft surface, skin and scalp (ectothrix)
				• In endothrix (*T. tonsurans*), hair breaks off at scalp leaving areas of alopecia with 'black dots'; there can be diffuse or minimal scaling and the extent of alopecia likewise can vary
				• In ectothrix (*M. canis* and *M. andouini*), there is patchy, scaling, erythema, multiple pustules and crusting; pustules can be confused with bacterial folliculitis
				• Can also present as an inflamed, boggy pustular and ulcerating area (usually associated with animal ringworm of the scalp) and referred to as a kerion
					• One of the most common superficial fungal infections affecting children
					• Child likely to complain of an itchy scalp and hair looks lustreless
					• Non-inflammatory endothrix infections more common in children between 3–8 years of age
					• Infections acquired from cattle and pets can provoke an intense inflammatory response and cause a painful, hairless and boggy lesion that enlarges rapidly (kerion)
					• Risk of secondary bacterial infection, tinea corporis and alopecia secondary to permanent scarring
					• Will not respond to nystatin; treat with griseofulvin and antifungal shampoo (e.g. ketaconazole)

Mouth					
• Candida (thrush)	Candida albicans	• Newborns and infants up to 6 months of age	• Mother with history of vaginal candidias	• White, curd-like plaques on inflamed oral mucosa • Plaques located on tongue, buccal mucosa, gingivae and pharynx • Early lesions start as pinpoint size and subsequently grow • Differentiated from milk plaques by inability to be wiped off with gauze pad	• Often associated with cutaneous candidiasis in the nappy area • Newborns can be infected during passage through the birth canal • Nursing mothers may have concomitant infection of nipples • Will not respond to griseofulvin or terbinafine; treat with nystatin oral suspension
Body					

• Tinea corporis (ringworm)	• Dermatophytes:
	  ◦ *Trichophyton* (especially *T. rubrum*, *T. tonsurans*, *T. mentagrophytes* and *T. verrucosum*)
	  ◦ *Microsporum* (*M. canis*)
	  ◦ *Epidermophyton* (*E. floccosum*)
		• All ages	• Direct contact with infected animal, person or fomite
			• Can also spread from infected body site (e.g. feet)
				• Annular, expanding plaque with a well-defined active edge
				• Lesion can be flesh-coloured, erythematous or violet to brown
				• The slightly raised, scaly, vesicular edge becomes more prominent as the infection resolves and the centre heals/clears
					• Child may complain of itch but the infection is often asymptomatic
					• Spreads rapidly in nurseries and schools due to high contagion and relative asymptomy
					• Will not respond to nystatin; treat localised lesions with topical agents (clotrimazole or other imidazole)
					• For persistent cases or more extensive disease treat with griseofulvin (children <12 years of age) or for those >12 years of age (terbinafine or itraconazole)[a]

(continued)

Table 9.16 continued

Location and type of infection	Common causative agent(s)	Age group commonly affected	Predisposing factors	Typical appearance	Comments
• Pityriasis versicolor	• Pityrosporum yeasts (ubiquitous in environment)	• Postpuberty	• Warm humid climate • Seborrhoea • Hyperhidrosis • Immunosuppression	• Well-demarcated hypo- or hyper-pigmented patches; degree of hypo- or hyperpigmentation dependent on skin type • Patches typically appear on trunk, shoulders, and arms; often covered with a fine scale (unlike vitiligo) and usually are oval shaped (varying sizes)	• Uncommon in childhood • Recurrence is a problem • Usually asymptomatic although there may be some complaints of itch • Will not respond to nystatin, griseofulvin, terbinafine or itraconazole,[a] treat with antifungal shampoo (e.g. selenium sulphide) diluted 1:10 with tap water, the resultant lotion applied daily for 10–14 days)
• Pityrosporum folliculitis	• Pityrosporum yeasts	• Adolescents	• Warm humid climate • Occlusion • Seborrhoea • Hodgkin's disease • Diabetes mellitus	• Itchy papules and pustules result from yeasts that are trapped in hair follicules • Usually localised to the chest, back, upper arms but may extend to the neck and face	• Easily mistaken for acne, especially as it is commonly seen in adolescence • Treat as for pityriasis versicolor (as above)
Skin folds					
• Intertrigo (*Candidiasis*)	• Candida	• All ages but more common in neonates and infants	• Occlusion, moisture, heat and maceration • Poor hygiene or overzealous cleansing • Obesity • Diabetes • Systemic antibiotics • Oral contraceptives • Long-term use of glucocorticosteroids (inhaled or systemic)	• Erythematous, scaling rash that is diffuse and without central clearing (unlike tinea) • Bilateral areas affected (unlike tinea which is usually unilateral, except for tinea cruris) • Often with creamy-white pustules along border and multiple 'satellite' lesions • Eruption is brick-red and appears excessively moist and raw • Often accompanied by distracting intense pruritus or burning sensation	• Commonly affects interdigital spaces, neck, axillae, submammary, umbilicus, genital and anal areas • Intriginous candida refers to an infection on two opposing surfaces • Eroded skin encourages secondary bacterial infection • Will not respond to griseofulvin or terbinafine; treat with nystatin cream • See also Section 9.11
Hands					
• Tinea manuum	• Dermatophytes: • *Trichophyton* (*T. rubrum* and *T. mentagrophytes*) • *Epidermophyton* (*E. floccosum*)	• Postpuberty	• Tinea pedis	• Palmar rash (usually unilateral); dry and scaly at the edges	• Scratching of feet (tinea pedis) may transfer infection to hand ('one hand/two feet syndrome') • Will not respond to nystatin; treat with topical imadozoles initially, reserving griseofulvin, terbinafine or itraconazole[a] if no improvement

Condition	Organism	Age group	Clinical features	Predisposing factors	Notes
Nails • Tinea unguium (onychomycosis)	• Dermatophytes (as above)	• Postpuberty	• Distal edge and side of nail plate become detached with discoloured (white, yellow or silver), thickened (hyperkeratotic) and friable nail	• Pre-existing tinea pedis, tinea capitis • Trauma • Diabetes • Down's syndrome	• Nails may harbour fungus present in tinea infections of scalp and feet • Difficult to eradicate • Will respond to griseofulvin, terbinafine, itraconazole[a] or amorolfine (topical)
• Paronychia	• Candida (C. albicans and C. parapsilosis)	• All ages	• Inflammation of the nail bed with loss of cuticle, painful swelling of proximal nail fold and potential secondary bacterial infection (a whitlow) • If distal nail involved, presents as onycholysis, hyperkeratosis and temporary dystrophy (difficult to differentiate from dermatophyte infection)	• Nail 'pickers' • Finger or thumb-sucking • Frequent immersion in water • Diabetes	• Proximal infection of nail generally caused by Candida; distal nail infection usually tinea • Rare to have mixed nail infection • Skin between fingers and toes should be examined for infection • Will not respond to griseofulvin. Treat topically with nystatin or imidazole. Systemic itraconazole,[a] can be used for recalcitrant cases
Groin • Tinea cruris (jock itch)	• Dermatophytes: *Trichophyton* (T. rubrum, T. mentagrophytes) *Epidermophyton* (E. floccosum)	• Adolescents (exceedingly rare in infants)	• Sharply demarcated (usually unilateral but occasionally bilateral) eruption in groin, perineum or perianal regions • Active margin is irregular, red, raised and scaly • Complaints of pain with activity and pruritus	• Tinea pedis • Friction and occlusion (tight-fitting underpants and wet swimming trunks) • Shared sports gear • Obesity	• Also known as 'jock itch' • Predominantly male disorder and very uncommon before adolescence • Often simultaneous infection of feet • Diagnostic clue: rash does *not* spread onto scrotum • Will not respond to nystatin; treat with topical imadazoles; griseofulvin for persistent infections
Feet • Tinea pedis (athlete's foot)	• Dermatophytes: (as tinea cruris)	• Mainly postpubertal	• Itchy, dry scaly rash (especially on edges) that often starts between fourth and fifth toes • Surrounding skin can become inflamed, macerated and fissured (which increases risk of secondary bacterial infection) • May be accompanied by foul odour and burning sensation • Can also affect the plantar and lateral surfaces ('moccasin foot')	• Occlusive, abrasive footwear, poor hygiene • Communal swimming and sports facilities • Diabetes • Down's syndrome	• Do not discount as a cause of foot dermatoses in prepubescent children • Scratching can transfer infection to dominant hand ('two foot/one hand syndrome') • Trainers and socks made of synthetic fibres should be avoided • Disinfectant footbaths in communal bathing and changing areas do not eradicate the fungus • Will not respond to nystatin; treat with topical imadazoles; griseofulvin for persistent infections

[a]Note: terbinafine and itraconazole are newer, systemic, antifungals (with the same spectrum of activity as griseofulvin) that are licensed for use in children over 12 years of age. As such, they are feasible for older children requiring systemic therapy. Terbinafine has limited data to suggest use in children under 12 and has an adverse event profile that is no greater in children than adults; no evidence of new, unusual or more severe reactions to those seen in the adult population. However, due to the limited extent of the data it remains unlicensed for use in children under 12 years of age.

- Dermatophytes and yeasts disseminate through fragmentation and spore formation.

← HISTORY

- Onset (which typically is gradual, candidal nappy rash excluded), spread and distribution of rash.
- Appearance of lesion or rash (including whether there has been any change in appearance).
- Associated pruritus and/or any other symptoms (fever or others).
- Past history of skin disorders and/or medical conditions (including immunodeficiency).
- Similar symptoms in family members or other contacts.
- Exposure to animals (patients are often unaware that pets or farm animals have fungal infection).
- History of foreign travel.
- Treatment used so far (including over-the-counter and prescription drugs) with response of rash to treatment.

PHYSICAL EXAMINATION

Clinical presentation varies considerably according to the species of the fungi and location of the infection (Table 9.16). Careful examination of the skin (and scalp) is required. Note:

- Distribution and pattern of lesions with associated pustules, scaling, crusting, erythema exudate and/or excoriation. Compare lesions for differences and note size.
- Regional lymphadenopathy is a common finding; however, other symptomatology is not and if discovered requires more thorough investigation.
- Previous treatments may have changed the appearance of the rash, making identification during physical examination more difficult.

DIFFERENTIAL DIAGNOSES

- The differential diagnosis is complicated by conditions that mimic fungal infections. The most common are outlined in Table 9.17. It is essential that a correct diagnosis be

Table 9.17 Differential Diagnoses of Common Fungal Infections

Fungal infection	Consider	
Tinea corporis	• Granuloma annulare • Discoid eczema	• Pityriasis rosea • Psoriasis
Tinea cruris	• Candidiasis • Contact dermatitis • Erythrasma	• Prickly heat • Psoriasis • Seborrhoeic dermatitis
Tinea capitis	• Alopecia areata • Psoriasis • Pyoderma (with or without lice) • Staphylococcal abscess	• Seborrhoeic dermatitis • Trichotillomania • Lichen planus • Systemic lupus erythematosus (SLE)
Tinea pedis	• Atopic eczema • Candidiasis • Contact dermatitis • Discoid eczema	• Hyperhidrosis • Juvenile plantar dermatosis • Scabies • Psoriasis
Tinea manuum	• Atopic eczema • Contact dermatitis • Granuloma annnulare	• Psoriasis • Lichen planus
Tinea unguium	• Bacterial infections • Paronychia • Nail injury	• Psoriasis • Lichen planus • Eczema
Candidiasis	• Bacterial infection • Burns • Contact dermatitis • Herpes simplex	• Lichen planus • Psoriasis • Seborrhoeic dermatitis
Pityriasis versicolor	• Pityriasis rosea • Seborrhoeic dermatitis	• Tinea corporis • Vitiligo
Pityrosporum folliculitis	• Acne	• Bacterial folliculitis

obtained prior to commencing treatment. Tinea infections can be mistaken for contact dermatitis or atopic eczema and inappropriately treated with topical steroids. This masks the characteristic features of the ever-present ringworm infection and produces a condition known as tinea incognito.

✚ MANAGEMENT

- **Additional diagnostics:**
  - *Wood's ultraviolet light examination:* small-spored ectothrix infections (e.g. *M. canis*) will fluoresce a blue/green colour and pityriasis infections, a pale green colour. However, other species (e.g. *T. tonsurans*) are non-fluorescent. Likewise, Wood's lamp fluorescence is not helpful with nail infections.
  - *Microscopy:* distinguishes dermatophytes from yeasts, but will not assist in identifying the specific species involved (only fungal culture will accomplish this). Infected hair roots should be plucked from the edge of the scale and sent for examination. Skin scrapings can be obtained by (1) using a round-bladed scalpel; (2) using a sterile toothbrush; or (3) applying Sellotape to the lesion, removing and sticking tape onto a slide. Samples should be taken from the active edge of the lesion, avoiding any area treated in the past 7 days with topical antifungals. Nail samples require full-thickness clippings of damaged nail and as much subungal debris as can be obtained.
  - *Mycology culture:* the only definitive method for identifying causative organism. Specimen collection as above. Note that routine swabs for bacterial culture are useless in fungal infections.

- **Pharmacotherapeutics:**
  - *Topical antifungals:* polyenes, nystatin and broad-spectrum imidazoles are usually well tolerated and effective. However, they should

only be used after confirming diagnosis with laboratory samples (see Additional diagnostics). Note that nystatin is only effective against yeasts with no activity against dermatophytes. In addition, terbinafine (Lamisil) is not currently approved for use in children, whereas itraconazole is only approved for use in children over 12 years of age. Combinations of imidazoles and hydrocortisone may be used for a few days only to alleviate symptoms in severe tinea infections. Continue to treat all affected areas for 1 week after clinical signs of the infection have gone, in order to prevent reoccurrences. Antifungal powders should be used conservatively in conjunction with creams or sprays. Treat pityriasis versicolor by rubbing selenium sulphide shampoo (diluted 1:10 in tap water) onto lesions until lathered; leave on for 10–20 min, then rinse thoroughly. Treat in this manner daily for 10–14 days (monthly retreatment may help to prevent reoccurrences); use a bland moisturiser if skin becomes dry or cracked. Systemic treatment in pityriasis versicolor is rarely required.

- *Systemic antifungals:* Griseofulvin is the only licensed oral systemic antifungal available for use in children. Recommended dose for children under 25 kg is 10 mg/kg in divided doses 3–4 times daily; dose for children over 25 kg is 250–500 mg/dose 3–4 times daily. Griseofulvin should be administered with food. Therapy needs to be continued for 6 weeks or until the infection is cleared, which may be up to 2 years for severe toenail infections. Note that griseofulvin has no activity against yeasts (i.e. *Candida* or *Pityrosporum*). Scalp infections **always require** griseofulvin as do areas where the keratin is thickest (palms, soles and nails), although, in children, topical preparations (imidazole) may clear these areas (scalp excepted). Oral thrush is treated with nystatin suspension.

- *Antibacterial preparations*: used only for secondary bacterial infections; treat accordingly.

- **Behavioural interventions:**
  - Advise patient and household contacts to use an antifungal shampoo (selenium sulphide or ketoconazole) to reduce cross-infection.
  - Bedding, clothing, towels, toys and personal items such as hairbrushes and combs (i.e. all objects that come in contact with infected skin and hair) should be washed in hot, soapy water at the start of treatment and should not be shared. This is important as fomites are a common source of reinfection and spread.
  - Cleanse affected skin at least twice daily with an unperfumed soap (or soap substitute) and dry thoroughly with a clean towel or tissues.
  - Keep nails short and treat pruritus with bland moisturisers or calamine lotion.
  - Wash hands thoroughly after touching affected areas and after applying antifungal creams.
  - With tinea pedis, dry feet last and change footwear daily. Shoes should be worn in communal areas to prevent cross-infection. Cotton socks and leather footwear should be encouraged as they allow sweat to evaporate and decrease the humidity.
  - With candidal nappy rash, disposable nappies are preferable to cotton ones. If used, the latter should be boil washed (in addition see Sec. 9.11).
  - All contacts should be notified and screened regularly; in addition, treat infected pets to avoid reinfection.

- **Patient education:**
  - Fungal infections may leave families feeling distressed, embarrassed and stigmatised. Correct any misconceptions that ringworm is caused by a 'worm' and/or any misplaced blame that parents may express.
  - Review medication administration, behavioural interventions, issues of communicability and infection control measures. Include a discussion of the possibility of social activity limitation (day-care/

school attendance and/or after-school/recreational activities). This is especially important for highly infectious diseases (e.g. tinea capitis due to *M. audouinii*).
- Warn parents that dermatophyte infections may take several weeks to resolve although the inflammation should improve within several days. Nail infections may take 6–12 months to resolve. Pityriasis versicolor may take weeks to improve; repigmentation requires exposure to sunlight and often takes months. Candidal lesions improve within 1–2 days and usually are cleared in 1 week.
- Teach parents the signs of secondary bacterial infection and remind them to call if some improvement does not occur within 2 weeks.

⇨ FOLLOW-UP

- Not necessary if symptoms clear; given the length of treatment in some infections, periodic telephone contact may be helpful. Further care should be sought if symptoms reappear or persist.

⇄ MEDICAL CONSULT/ SPECIALIST REFERRAL

- Any child in whom symptoms persist (especially tinea capitis or tinea unguium) despite correct treatment.
- Any child with symptoms of secondary bacterial infection.
- Any child who develops a fungal infection and is also immunosuppressed.
- *Any child in whom there is widespread and/or severe infection (think possible immunocompromise).*
- *Any child in whom there is concern of neglect and/or abuse.*

⊘ PAEDIATRIC PEARLS

- Never discount fungal infections, particularly if the child presents with an unresponsive asymmetrical 'eczema'.
- Mycology is a cheap, painless and very simple method of organism identification.

- If symptoms persist, review correct use of the antifungals; emphasise the importance of completing treatments, even after the symptoms have disappeared.
- *Use of steroids or other creams/ treatments can change the appearance of the infection, making diagnosis difficult (especially without culture). However, mild topical steroids (used only for a couple of days) can be helpful for infections with marked inflammation.*
- *Tinea capitis always requires systemic treatment.*
- *Repeated infection may be indicative of an undiagnosed source (pet or family contact); if severe, systemic and/or recurrent, consider potential immunocompromise.*

BIBLIOGRAPHY

Buxton PK. ABC of dermatology, 3rd edn. London: BMJ Publishing Group; 1998.
Grant JS, Davis M. Neuroscience patients: under attack by fungi. J Neurosci Nurs 1991; 23(4):241–246.
Guenst BJ. Common pediatric foot dermatoses. J Pediatr Health Care 1999; 13(2):68–71.
Hall JC. Sauer's manual of skin disease, 8th edn. Philadelphia: Lippincott, Williams & Wilkins; 2000.
Hunter J, Savin J, Dahl M. Clinical dermatology, 2nd edn. Oxford: Blackwell Science; 1995.
Leppard B, Ashton R. Treatment in dermatology. Oxford: Radcliffe Medical Press; 1993.
Lesher J, Levine N, Treadwell P. Fungal skin infections: common but stubborn. Patient Care 1994; 28(2):16–44.
Rudy SJ. Superficial fungal infections in children and adolescents. Nurse Pract Forum 1999; 10(2):56–66.
Suhonen R, Dawber R, Ellis D. Fungal infections of the skin, hair and nails. London: Martin Dunitz; 1999.
Verbov JL. Handbook of paediatric dermatology. London: Martin Dunitz; 2000.
Winsor A. Tinea capitis: a growing headcount. Br J Dermatol Nurs 1998; 2(3):10–12.
Winsor A. Sampling techniques. Nurs Times Plus 2000; 96(27):12–13.

ACKNOWLEDGEMENT

The author would like to acknowledge the expertise of Dr Richard Meyrick Thomas, Consultant Dermatologist, Salisbury District Hospital, in the preparation of this section.

9.9 IMPETIGO

Sara Burr

INTRODUCTION

- Impetigo is a superficial, bacterial skin infection that is commonly seen in paediatric practice. It is characterised by blisters with a fragile roof that easily ruptures, leaking fluid that (when dried) forms the typical honey-coloured crusts of impetigo. The infection can involve almost any part of the body although, in children, it commonly affects the face, nares and extremities.
- Impetigo has two classic forms: non-bullous and bullous, both of which are caused by infection with *Staphylococcus aureus* and/or *Streptococcus pyogenes* (group A β-haemolytic streptococcus, GABHS).
- Non-bullous impetigo accounts for the majority (>70%) of cases, is more common in pre-school/school-aged children and uncommon in those less than 24 months of age. In contrast, bullous impetigo is seen more frequently among infants and young children. However, there is an increased incidence of both types of impetigo in the warm, muggy, summer months and among children living in poverty (it is associated with overcrowding).
- The lesions of non-bullous impetigo are caused by *S. aureus, S. pyogenes*, or a mixture of both pathogens. The lesions usually form on skin that has been injured (i.e. infection occurs after an episode of poison ivy, eczema, insect bites, minor abrasion, etc.).
- The lesions of bullous impetigo are caused by *S. aureus* (phage type II). A warm, humid environment favours their development and, therefore, bullous impetigo is often found on moist, intertriginous areas that were previously intact (although it can occur on the face or extremities).
- Characteristics of bullous and non-bullous impetigo are summarised in Table 9.18.

PATHOPHYSIOLOGY

- Impetigo is highly contagious and is easily spread through direct physical contact and fomites. The impetiginous lesions are often itchy and, when scratched, can spread the infection to surrounding areas, additional sites on the body and/or to children, family members and close contacts. Consequently, household outbreaks are common.
- In non-bullous impetigo, bacteria colonise the skin surface and then superficially invade any areas where the integrity of the skin has been compromised. Conversely, the lesions of bullous impetigo appear to develop on intact skin as a result of localised toxin production by *S. aureus.*
- The reservoir for staphylococci is the upper respiratory tract, from which asymptomatic carriers can spread the bacteria to themselves or others. The reservoir for streptococci is thought to be from the skin and not from the respiratory tree.
- Regional lymphadenopathy and leukocytosis are common findings in non-bullous impetigo (90% and 50% of cases, respectively), whereas bullous impetigo does not usually cause regional lymphadenopathy or other

Table 9.18   Characteristics of Bullous and Non-Bullous Impetigo

Impetigo form	Characteristic
Non-bullous	• Most common form of impetigo seen in paediatric practice • Caused by *Staphylococcus aureus*, *Streptococcus pyogenes* (group A β-haemolytic streptococcus, or GABHS) or a mixture of both organisms • More common in children >24 months of age • Lesions usually form on skin that has already been injured • Lesion(s) typically begin as small, erythematous, and fluid-filled (i.e. vesiculopustular) • Lesions subsequently burst and leak serous fluid, leaving a punched-out ulceration with honey-coloured crust/plaque • Plaque is generally <2 cm in diameter • Lesions may itch but minimal pain and erythema of surrounding tissue • Regional lymphadenopathy is common • Lesions of non-bullous impetigo that are caused by *S. aureus*, *S. pyogenes* or a combination of both organisms appear identical
Bullous	• Caused by *Staphylococcus aureus* • More common in young infants and children (<24 months) • Lesions appear to develop on intact skin as a result of localised toxin production by *S. aureus* • Single or clusters of lesions with larger, fluctuant, transparent bullae that progress to cloudy blisters • Bullae rupture easily, leaving a scalded skin appearance: erythematous, denuded skin with a rim of scale • Propensity for moist, intertriginous areas (although also seen on face and extremities) • Regional lymphadenopathy, systemic symptoms and erythema of surrounding tissue uncommon

systemic symptoms. Neither form of impetigo typically results in systemic symptoms and, therefore, if a child seems quite ill with impetigo, additional investigation is imperative.

- Altered host immunity—e.g. IgA deficiency and defect in cellular immunity—in addition to underlying skin diseases that compromise the barrier function of skin, such as eczema, and fungal skin infections, predispose a child to the subsequent development of impetigo.

- The lesions of impetigo can resolve without treatment, but this will take several weeks as there is likely autoinoculation and continued spread as older lesions heal; prompt treatment prevents spread and speeds healing. Extension of infection beyond impetigo to cellulitis or abscess formation is uncommon and requires prompt investigation and treatment.

- Complications of impetigo are rare but include deep ulcerations or abscesses, cellulitis (see Sec. 9.6), lymphadenitis (see Sec. 15.3), osteomyelitis, toxic shock syndrome, scarlet fever and acute glomerulonephritis. The risk of

acute post-streptococcal glomerulonephritis is related to the strain of *S. pyogenes* responsible for the impetigo; some strains are more nephritogenic than others. The risk of cellulitis developing post-impetigo is <10%; however, factors such as the invasiveness and toxigenicity of the organism, integrity of the skin and the immune and cellular defences of the host impact this likelihood.

⬅ HISTORY

- Pre-existing skin conditions (e.g. atopic eczema, seborrhoea, varicella, etc.), condition of skin prior to lesion development (e.g. cuts, abrasions, bites, etc.) and history of trauma.
- Onset, location and appearance of original lesion(s).
- Length of time lesions present.
- History of pruritus and/or spread.
- History of exposure, including other family members with symptoms or exposure of other family members to child with impetigo.
- Daily hygiene routine (sharing of towels, bed clothes, etc.).
- Systemic symptoms.

- Treatment(s) used and results.
- Coexisting disease (especially immunocompromise).

🩺 PHYSICAL EXAMINATION

- **Head and ENT:** Routine examination, noting any lesions on face or scalp.
- **Lymph:** assess for regional lymphadenopathy in nodes that drain affected areas.
- **Skin:** head-to-toe assessment of all skin is important. Note extent of lesion(s) and appearance (especially distinction of bullous from non-bullous and the presence of satellite lesions).
- If systemic symptoms present (unexpected in uncomplicated impetigo), further investigation required.

🔎 DIFFERENTIAL DIAGNOSES

- Consider other infections that present with vesiculobullous rashes: enteroviruses, varicella zoster, herpes simplex, staphylococcal scalded skin syndrome (uncommon) and Gram-negative sepsis (uncommon).
- Consider non-infectious conditions that present with vesicles or bullae: burns, insect bite hypersensitivity and eczema (uncommon).

✚ MANAGEMENT

- **Additional diagnostics:** consider a swab with microscopy, sensitivity and culture. A swab can be taken of bullae fluid (bullous impetigo) or purulent material underneath crust (non-bullous). If systemic symptoms are present, consider FBC and blood cultures.
- **Pharmacotherapeutics:** the decision to treat topically or systemically is based on the age of the child, number and extent of lesions, location of lesions, carer's preference and prior experience with this infection in the past. Note that infants under 6 months of age should be treated systemically. Impetigo is usually treated systemically with flucloxacillin or erythromycin.

Topical antibiotics (e.g. Fucidin) can also be used for milder cases with no involvement of face (5 days maximum).

- **Behavioural interventions:**
  - Infection control measures are very important in order to prevent spread to others (careful hand washing, use of antibacterial soap, no sharing of clothes or bedding, use clean gauze instead of flannels or sponges, etc.).
  - Trim fingernails and keep short.
  - Wash clothes in hot water.
  - Treat underlying skin disorders (e.g. eczema). Steroid must be avoided on the impetiginised areas.
  - Until lesions treated, close skin-to-skin contact with the child should be discouraged (especially play and sleeping) and always followed with careful hand washing.

- **Patient education:**
  - Review with parents, carers (and the child) the mechanism for impetigo spread and the infection control measures to help prevent this. Tell them it is not uncommon for impetigo to spread through the household, with children frequently reinfecting themselves and others. Careful attention to infection control measures is the only way to prevent this.
  - Inform parents that impetigo is a superficial bacterial skin infection that usually heals rapidly and does not commonly cause systemic symptoms (fever, malaise, vomiting, headache, etc.) or scarring. Remind them to seek care immediately if any of these symptoms develop and/or if lesions appear deeper or more severe. Encourage parents to inspect lesions periodically.
  - Discuss with parents the importance of early detection and management of any broken skin in order to prevent future episodes of impetigo.

⇨ FOLLOW-UP

- Usually not required if lesions heal promptly with treatment.

⇄ MEDICAL CONSULT/ SPECIALIST REFERRAL

- Any child in whom complications develop, including cellulitis and/or abscess formation.
- Any child in whom initial management was not sufficient to manage the infection.
- Any child in whom there is an immune deficiency.
- Any child with systemic symptoms or a gravely ill appearance.
- Any infant less than 1 month of age as intravenous antibiotics are likely to be required.

⚥ PAEDIATRIC PEARLS

- Some soap substitutes with antibacterial properties are available to use as washes. They contain ingredients such as chlorhexidine and benzalkonium chloride which may be useful for children suffering recurrent episodes.
- If culture reveals both staphylococci and streptococci, there is no way to determine which is causing the infection and antibiotic choice must be effective against both pathogens.
- If the initial infection clears completely but the child becomes infected again, consider examining household contacts.

- Impetigo that is very wet and weepy responds well to potassium permanganate soaks twice daily (hold gauze swab soaked in solution to affected area for approximately 10 min).
- Children with underlying skin disease (e.g. eczema) are difficult to treat because of heavy bacterial skin colonisation and chronic mechanical damage to skin (e.g. scratching). In addition, impetigo on previously diseased skin may be difficult to recognise as it may appear only as a slight flare-up of the skin condition.
- If impetigo develops around the nose, it is almost always *S. aureus*.
- Uncomplicated impetigo does not usually scar; however, post-inflammatory pigment changes may last for weeks to months.

⊟ BIBLIOGRAPHY

Darmstadt G. A guide to superficial strep and staph skin infections. Contemp Pediatr 1997; 14(5):95–116.

Darmstadt G. Oral antibiotic therapy of children with uncomplicated bacterial skin infections. Pediatr Infect Dis J 1997; 16:227–230.

Darmstadt G, Lane A. Impetigo: an overview. Pediatr Dermatol 1994; 11:293–295.

Hurwitz S. Clinical pediatric dermatology: a textbook of skin disorders of childhood and adolescence. St. Louis: WB Saunders; 1981.

Jain A, Daum R. Staphylococcal infections in children: part 1. Pediatr Rev 1999; 20(6):183–191.

Rook D, Wilkinson S, Ebling D. Textbook of dermatology, Vol. 2, 6th edn. London: Blackwell Science; 1998.

Ruiz-Maldonado R, Parish LC, Beare JM. Textbook of paediatric dermatology. London: Grune and Stratton; 1989.

9.10 INFANTILE SEBORRHOEIC DERMATITIS (ISD) OR INFANTILE ECZEMA (INCLUDING CRADLE CAP)

Stephen Gill

📖 INTRODUCTION

- Infantile seborrhoeic dermatitis (ISD) is a form of eczema that occurs commonly. It mainly affects the face, scalp and flexures of the newborn and infant.
- A thick yellow scale on the vertex of the scalp, sometimes extending onto the eyebrows and nape of the neck is often called 'cradle cap'. This may present as a singularity or in combination with other skin involvement to complete the dry, scaly picture of ISD.
- The disorder is a matter of contention, as experts disagree on how to classify it. Most authorities regard ISD as a unique skin problem, whereas others incorporate it into the category of atopic eczema as a variant on the same theme.
- One major difficulty is that the child diagnosed with ISD may proceed to develop atopic eczema in later childhood or it may be coexistent with ISD during infancy. This clinical overlap confuses the statistical accuracy for both disorders and renders prognosis difficult.
- ISD is a common, often self-limiting problem of infancy that usually resolves with simple treatment (though in extreme forms it can linger on and cause significant distress).

🔬 PATHOPHYSIOLOGY

- The name 'seborrhoeic' dermatitis denotes the site of the target skin cells and, like the adult form of eczema with the same name, it has little to do with overproduction of sebaceous glands as traditionally thought. Rather, the symptomatology is a function of the three main features of ISD: skin dryness, inflammation and a potential for fungal and/or bacterial infection.

- A potential hormonal aetiology has been postulated for ISD (as it most commonly presents during infancy) and, likewise, ISD's predilection for intertrigous areas suggests a potential aetiological role for yeast cells (especially *Pityrosporum ovale*). A genetic link has also been hypothesised, as seborrhoeic dermatitis tends to run in families. However, at present there is a lack of consensus with regard to a definitive cause.
- While ISD is not thought to originate from a bacterial component, secondary infection of the lesions can worsen the condition. The same is true for secondary fungal infection, which can also complicate the clinical picture.
- Histiopathic findings of ISD are non-specific and similar to atopic dermatitis and, therefore, are not helpful in diagnosis. However, they include evidence of low-grade inflammation, parakeratosis, acanthosis and intracellular oedema.

⬅ HISTORY

- General growth and development.
- Age of onset, distribution and characteristics of the cradle cap.
- Other areas on body that have scaling, erythema or dryness (e.g. axillae, antecubital fossae, creases in the nappy area, eyebrows, nasolacrimal folds, eyelashes, cheeks, post-auricular areas, nape of neck, etc.).
- Presence of pruritus (babies with ISD are often unperturbed by their non-pruritic rash).
- Hygiene habits and products used (frequency of bathing use of soaps, moisturisers, baby creams, wipes, etc.).
- Family history of atopic-associated conditions (asthma, allergies, hay fever and/or others with eczema or ISD).
- Details of treatments used (if any) and their effectiveness (including any

complementary therapies or special dietary regimen).

🩺 PHYSICAL EXAMINATION

Systematic head-to-toe examination of the skin with inspection of all areas of the body. Note general growth and development of the infant in addition to:

- Presence, severity and distribution of lesions/scale (thick, yellow, greasy scales with erythema of the scalp are characteristic of cradle cap). Likewise, there may be involvement of other areas (axillae, antecubital fossae, creases in the nappy area, eyebrows, nasolacrimal folds, eyelashes, cheeks, post-auricular areas, nape of neck, etc.). Note that some authorities regard involvement of the axillae as a significant diagnostic sign of ISD.
- Distribution and pattern of any skin dryness.
- Any signs of secondary bacterial or fungal infection.

🔍 DIFFERENTIAL DIAGNOSIS

- Rule out napkin dermatitis, scabies, tinea capitis/corporis, bacterial infection, contact dermatitis and psoriasis. In severe or recalcitrant cases (especially if infant has systemic signs of illness), diseases such as Leiner's disease, Letterer–Siwe disease, Omenn's syndrome and Wiskott–Aldrich syndrome (although these are very rare). In addition, HIV should be considered, as severe, generalised seborrhoeic dermatitis has been reported to occur in a large percentage of patients infected with HIV.

➕ MANAGEMENT

- **Additional diagnostics:** there are no specific tests for ISD; the diagnosis is based on the classical clinical presentation. If there is some ambiguity with regard to possible fungal or bacterial infection, these cultures can be considered. A skin biopsy will shed little light on the diagnosis, is overly invasive and is not recommended.

- **Pharmacotherapeutics:** The frequent and liberal use of moisturisers is the foundation of ISD treatment. If simple moisturisers do not control the condition, steroid ointment can be added to the skin care regime. Hydrocortisone 1% ointment, applied twice daily to affected areas, is the first-line drug for markedly inflamed areas if severe pruritus is present. It is important to use the steroid on rehydrated skin (e.g. 20 min after moisturiser application or an oily bath) and apply sparingly, only to affected areas (e.g. only until the skin appears 'shiny'). The steroid can be discontinued when the inflammation is gone (and restarted if a flare-up recurs). Note that if control is not obtained within 3–4 days then the role of bacterial or fungal elements needs to be considered. In this case the hydrocortisone can be replaced with Timodine or Nystaform-HC. Both of these ointments are hydrocortisone combined with antiseptic and antifungal components.

- **Behavioural interventions:**
  - The avoidance of soaps and detergents (baby bath bubbles, shampoos) and the introduction of moisturisers are the single, most effective first-line treatment. Most babies with ISD can be adequately controlled with these simple and side-effect-free measures. More severe cases may require the application of tubular bandages to increase the efficacy of the emollients (see Sec. 9.3 for description of moisturisers, soap substitutes and techniques).
  - The scalp scale (i.e. cradle cap) of ISD is essentially water-soluble, but it dries out and becomes hard, water-resistant and adherent to the scalp (especially if frequently washed with detergent shampoos). Consequently, it is often necessary to soften the scale with a greasy emollient before removal is attempted ('picking' of hardened scale usually results in a bleeding scalp). As a general rule, a gentle staged approach to cradle cap (that is guided by the severity of the scaling and dryness) is recommended.
  - *Mild scalp scaling:* moisturise scalp to soften scale (massage in mineral oil, white petroleum, olive oil, emulsifying ointment or, in mild cases, baby oil). This can then be washed out with baby shampoo and moisturiser and reapplied after towelling dry. Repeat as often as is necessary.
  - *Moderate scaling:* leave moisturiser on the scalp for a few hours, then wash the hair with cradle cap shampoo. After the baby's bath (when scale is softer and still damp from the bath water), gently tease out residual scale with adult comb (not rounded baby comb). Repeat as often as is necessary.
  - *Severe scaling:* as above, except be sure to use a generous amount of a greasy moisturiser and leave it to penetrate overnight. In the morning, bathe baby and follow with an adult comb to tease out scale. After scale is reduced, wash hair again and reapply a moisturiser. The scale often builds up again after removal, so it is likely further treatments will be necessary to keep cradle cap under control.
  - Note that baby oil is likely to be too light for the job (and if perfumed, may be unsuitable for sensitive skin). Alternative greasy moisturisers include 50/50 liquid paraffin in white soft paraffin or emulsifying ointment; other greasy emollients (without perfume), almond oil, mustard oil, coconut oil or a mixture of 25% emulsifying ointment in coconut oil (this can be made up by the chemist). If the coconut oil solidifies it should be warmed in hot water to aid application.

- **Patient education:**
  - Review medication and behavioural interventions with the family and provide written reinforcement whenever possible.
  - Families will require support and encouragement with regard to the chronicity of ISD during the first months (or year) of life. However, be sure to counsel them on the likelihood that the ISD will resolve completely and that very good control (even in marked cases) can be achieved with careful skin care. Note that for some families, ISD can be extremely stressful; the degree of family upset may or may not be proportional to the severity of the ISD. The thick scalp scales may embarrass mothers, especially if others perceive her child as being 'unclean', 'dirty' or with poor hygiene.
  - Leaflets on ISD can be obtained from the National Eczema Society: tel: 0870-241-3604. They are a helpful adjunct to the consultation process. In addition, the Internet can be a useful source of information. Families can type 'eczema' into a search engine to find useful sites such as the Skin Care Campaign and the British or American Eczema Societies.

⇨ FOLLOW-UP

- With concordance to the skin care regime there should be some improvement within 1 week. If the ISD settles, then no further follow-up is required except for repeat prescriptions. However, some families will require ongoing support and/or treatment adjustment.

⇄ MEDICAL CONSULT/ SPECIALIST REFERRAL

- Any infant whose initial management has been unsuccessful or those where there is suspicion of a systemic illness complicating the picture.
- Any child in whom it is likely that there is a fungal or bacterial secondary infection, especially if control has not been gained with topical therapies.

PAEDIATRIC PEARLS

- Don't underestimate the degree of emotional 'angst' for mothers that skin disorders in their children cause. *Psychological Approaches to Dermatology* (Papadopolous & Bor, 1999) is a good textbook that gives an insight into how people view and react to skin disease in themselves and others.
- Axillary involvement, lack of itching/irritation and thick, greasy scale on the scalp differentiates ISD from atopic eczema.
- Do make sure your parent is fully aware of the difference between topical steroid and simple moisturisers and work hard to overcome steroid phobia.
- Do consider how the eczema is affecting the general well-being of the child and family. A useful tool for this is the Paediatric Dermatology Quality of Life Index (Lewis-Jones & Finlay, 1995).

- Do prescribe a good-sized amount of moisturiser. A 500 g tub encourages more frequent application and a small tube of moisturiser inhibits it.
- The baby's delicate skin is often reddened and made sore by well-meaning 'deep' massage of oils and moisturisers; a gentle approach is always best.

BIBLIOGRAPHY

Atherton D. The neonate. In: Champion RH, Burton JL, Burns DA, Breathnach SM, eds, Textbook of dermatology, 6th edn. Oxford: Blackwell Sciences; 1998: 474–477.

Boerio M. Pediatric dermatology: that itchy scaly rash. Nurs Clin North Am 2000; 35(1):147–157.

David TJ. Atopic eczema. Prescrib J 1995; 35(4):199–205.

Gill SJ. Use of topical steroids in childhood eczema. Br J Dermatol Nurs 1998; 2(4):10–11.

Goodyear HM. Skin microflora of atopic eczema in first time hospital attenders. Clin Exp Dermatol 1993; 18:300–304a.

Lewis-Jones MS, Finlay AY. The children's dermatology quality of life index (CDQLI): initial validation and practical use. Br J Dermatol 1995; 132:942–949.

Long CC, Mills CM, Finlay AY. A practical guide to topical therapy in children. Br J Dermatol 2000; 138:293–296.

McDonald L, Smith M. Diagnostic dilemmas in pediatric/adolescent dermatology: scaly scalp. J Pediatr Health Care 1998; 12(2):80–84.

Papadopolous L, Bor R. Psychological approaches to dermatology. London: British Psychological Society; 1999.

Rajka G. Infantile seborrhoeic dermatitis. In: Harper J, ed., Textbook of pediatric dermatology. Edinburgh: Churchill Livingstone; 2000.

Singleton J. Pediatric dermatoses: three common skin disruptions in infancy. Nurse Pract 1997; 22(6):32–50.

9.11 NAPPY RASH

Rosemary Turnbull

INTRODUCTION

- Nappy rash is a relatively common condition, which will affect a majority of children at some point in their early years.
- Affected infants are often fretful, irritable and uncomfortable; however, in the majority of cases, nappy rash will be short-lived and easy to clear.

PATHOPHYSIOLOGY

- Infant skin is more fragile and prone to injury from chemical and/or physical trauma due to a thinner dermis with less collagen and elastin fibres. In addition, the blood and nerve supply is immature and while the normal pH is acidic, moistness (from the occlusive nature of nappies) increases pH with a subsequent increase in skin permeability.

- Nappy rash results when these characteristics are combined with processes such as friction from the nappy itself; irritation from urine or faeces; and/or fungal contamination (*Candida albicans*).

HISTORY

- The child's general health and well-being, as well as nutritional intake to date.
- Onset and initial appearance of rash.
- Changes/alterations from the initial appearance (spread, additional lesions, worsening/improving, increased/decreased redness, etc.).
- Duration of rash and association with any other symptoms (history of diarrhoea, areas of bleeding, recent weight loss and/or other illnesses, etc.).

- Treatments used (if any) and effect on rash.
- Frequency of wet nappies and stool.
- Types of nappy used and frequency of changes.
- Infant skin products and laundry detergents used.
- History of atopy/skin problems (eczema, seborrhoea, allergies or asthma/wheezing).
- History of recent medication use (especially antibiotics).

PHYSICAL EXAMINATION

- The infant should be examined naked to ensure that all areas of the body can be observed. Assess skin colour and turgor. Check the extent/location of the nappy rash and whether any skin is unaffected. Nappy rash is characterised by a red, moist appearance (skin folds usually spared) over the area covered by the nappy. There may be fine, peripheral scaling with erythematous macules or papules and, in marked cases, ulceration and bleeding.

- Note that fungi are opportunists and it is not uncommon for *Candida albicans* (thrush) to be present alongside general nappy rash as it thrives in warm and moist environments. It will have a fiery, erythematous appearance, generally involving the inguinal folds and often with satellite pustules at nappy margins.
- Nappy rash complicated by seborrhoea will have typical greasy, yellow/pink scaly plaques, which are often found elsewhere (scalp, axillary folds, behind ears and eyebrows).
- Bacterial infection of the nappy rash will have yellow/golden crusts and/or pustules.
- Inguinal lymph nodes may be markedly enlarged.
- Consider head, ENT, respiratory and abdominal assessments if suspicion of systemic illness.
- Check mouth for oral lesions of thrush.

DIFFERENTIAL DIAGNOSES

- As many conditions may start in the napkin area it is important to consider other potential aetiologies: napkin psoriasis, *Candida albicans*, bacterial infection, nutritional deficiency, systemic disease (e.g. zinc deficiency and congenital syphilis, although rare) and non-accidental injury (NAI). It is essential to note any lesions with an unusual appearance; it is important that they are consistent with the history given.

MANAGEMENT

- **Additional diagnostics:** straightforward nappy rash is usually recognisable, but if *Candida* is suspected it is important to initiate antifungal treatment promptly. If there is no improvement after 48 hours, it is advisable to consider bacterial infection. Swabs can be taken to check for sensitivities, but treatment should be initiated and not withheld until

swab results are available. If systemic disease or nutritional deficiency are suspected, diagnostic evaluations would be aetiology-specific.

- **Pharmacotherapeutics:**
  - Uncomplicated nappy rash is best treated with non-soap cleansers and a mild barrier cream (e.g. zinc/castor oil cream or petroleum jelly) can be used.
  - Nappy rash with *Candida* infection will require a topical antifungal preparation such as clotrimazole or nystatin (applied twice daily) with the usual barrier preparations at other nappy changes.
  - Nappy rash complicated by seborrhoeic dermatitis will require a combination steroid and antifungal preparation such as: clotrimazole 1% and hydrocortisone 1% (Canesten HC) or miconazole 2% and hydrocortisone 1% (Daktacort). These preparations should be applied twice daily to affected areas only (use barrier preparations for other nappy changes). Due to the occlusive nature of nappies, any combination creams containing steroids must be closely monitored. In addition, nothing stronger than 1% hydrocortisone is indicated and the preparation should be discontinued as soon as the area is clear. The length of use will depend on severity, but the rash should resolve within 5–7 days.

- **Behavioural intervention:**
  - Change soiled nappies as soon as possible. In addition to reducing hydration and friction damage in the nappy area, nappy changing reduces the amount of contact time between the skin and the chemical irritants found in urine and the bacteria in faeces.
  - Nappy-free periods in a warm, dry room should be encouraged for *all* babies; they allow air to the skin and aid the healing process if baby is already suffering from nappy rash.
  - The area should be thoroughly cleaned using cotton wool and water with a mild soap or soap substitute if necessary. It is important not to scrub; gentle cleansing is all that is required.

  - Any baby wipes with alcohol and fragrance should be avoided, as the additives will irritate already inflamed skin.
  - It is particularly important to protect a baby's skin at night when they are at a higher risk of developing nappy rash. If the baby already has a rash, change the nappy during the night, and the use of a barrier cream is recommended.

- **Patient education:**
  - Discuss and reinforce behavioural interventions (above).
  - Family support is essential, as parents may feel guilty about their infant developing the rash. Reassure them that they have done nothing to cause the nappy rash, but stress that your advice can minimise and reduce the risk of nappy rash reoccurring.
  - Modern-day disposable nappies are designed to keep urine away from babies' skin. If a cloth nappy is used, advise parents/carers to use nappy liners and encourage thorough rinsing of the cloth nappy after laundering.
  - Reassure parents that vigorous and frequent cleansing can actually exacerbate the condition: only gentle washing (as above).
  - The use of baby powder (which can be inhaled by both parent and infant) can worsen nappy rash; its use should be discouraged.
  - Inform parents of the importance of contacting you should the rash deteriorate in any way.

FOLLOW-UP

- Review in the clinic or home within 1 week; if clear, no further follow-up required. Consider telephone support, management and/or follow-up if appropriate.

MEDICAL CONSULT/ SPECIALIST REFERRAL

- If rash persists despite all active measures.
- If the child is generally unwell.
- Your intuition tells you the rash is not consistent with the usual nappy rash.

PAEDIATRIC PEARLS

- Shiny and erythematous: think *Candida*.
- Nappy rash not responding: think about differential diagnoses.
- Any unusual lesions that are unexplainable: think of child protection issues.
- Management cornerstones include (1) prevention of nappy rash with expedient nappy changes after soiling; (2) consistent use of barrier creams; and (3) occasional nappy-free periods.

BIBLIOGRAPHY

Amsmeier S, Paller A. Getting to the bottom of diaper dermatitis. Contemp Pediatr 1997; 14(11):115–126.

Garcia-Gonzalez E, Rivera-Rueda M. Neonatal dermatology: skin care guidelines. Dermatol Nurs 1998; 10(4):274–281.

Higgins E, Vivier A. Skin disease in childhood and adolescence. Oxford: Blackwell Scientific; 1996.

Holbrook K. A histological comparison of infant and adult skin. In: Maibach H, Boisits E, eds, Neonatal skin: structure and function. New York: Marcel Dekker; 1982: 3–31.

ICM Research. Nappy rash survey. London: ICM; 1999.

Turnbull R. Treatment approaches to some childhood skin conditions. Comm Nurse 2001; 6(12):15–16.

Van Onselon J. Rash advice. Nurs Times 1999; 95(12):S37, 95.

Verbov J. Nutritional deficiencies manifesting as skin disorders. Dermatol Pract 1998; 6(5):5–8.

9.12 PEDICULOSIS HUMANUS CAPITUS (HEAD LICE)

Jan Mitcheson

INTRODUCTION

- Head lice is a common problem amongst school-age children and although infestation rarely affects general health, it is often the cause of much anxiety for parents and carers.
- Transmission occurs through head-to-head contact, in addition to spread through infected fomites (hats, hair slides, combs, hairbrushes, etc.).
- Lice infection is usually asymptomatic, although approximately one-third of patients experience itching.
- Diagnosis is confirmed by detection of the living louse and treatment consists of insecticide application.
- Parent education and support is of paramount importance in the identification, treatment and control of head lice.

PATHOPHYSIOLOGY

- Head lice are spread when there is sustained, direct, head-to-head contact which allows movement of the lice from one head to another.
- *Head lice cannot jump, fly, crawl or swim.* However, they can be spread via direct contact with infected combs, brushes, hats, bedding and upholstery as lice can live for 1–2 days off their human host (although most lice on inanimate objects are dead or dying).
- The life cycle of the head louse is approximately 17–20 days; they survive by clinging to hair and sucking blood from the host scalp. In early infection, the lice are usually concentrated around the parietal and occipital regions (i.e. behind the ears and back of the head). Head lice cling to the hair shaft via a chitinous ring (cement-like substance) and release noxious saliva that can cause pruritus, irritation and dermatitis.
- The female louse lays about six to eight eggs per day (close to the scalp), which take from 7 to 10 days to hatch, leaving a shell (nit) on the hair shaft. Given that hair grows roughly ¼ inch per month nits, found further down the hair shaft, are likely to be empty shells. The emerging nymphs stay on the original host for a further 7 days until they reach adulthood. Only the adult lice are contagious, as nymphs cannot spread to another host.

HISTORY

- Detection of living louse or eggs on hair shaft (identification of live eggs is difficult).
- Complaints of itchy scalp (include onset).
- History of potential head lice exposures (especially family members or close contacts).
- History of outbreak in school or nursery.
- Previous management of symptoms and infestation control measures (i.e. family members treated and interventions to rid hats, combs, brushes, etc., of louse infestation).
- Any other symptoms (secondary skin lesions, dermatitis of skin and neck area, etc.).

PHYSICAL EXAMINATION

- Visual inspection, as traditionally performed by the school nurse, has been found to be unreliable in the detection of head lice, producing unacceptably high levels of false-positives and -negatives. Combing wet hair (especially close to the scalp) with a plastic detection comb (teeth 0.2–0.3 mm apart) is considered to be a reliable way in which to detect head lice infestation. Louse specimens (and/or nits) can then be attached to clear sticky tape for confirmation by a health care professional.
- Note any secondary skin lesions or dermatitis of neck and shoulder areas. It is sometimes possible to visualise bite marks where lice have fed on scalp but these are often obliterated by scratching (which can result in secondary bacterial infection).

- Examine eyelashes and eyebrows for infestation.
- Posterior occipital and/or cervical lymphadenopathy is not uncommon as a result of scalp infestation.
- Family members/close contacts should likewise be examined (using the detection comb on wet hair) for infestation once an initial case of pediculosis has been confirmed.

⚡ DIFFERENTIAL DIAGNOSES

- A definitive diagnosis of pediculosis is only confirmed when live lice have been detected and confirmed by a community health care professional.
- Consider foreign bodies, secretions from the hair follicle (hair muffs), seborrhoeic dermatitis, contact dermatitis, eczema and impetigo.

✚ MANAGEMENT

- **Additional diagnostics:** rarely necessary. Transfer of live louse to sticky tape for further inspection by a health care professional is helpful in diagnosis. In addition, live nits will fluoresce under a Wood light whereas examination of a louse or nit under a microscope can confirm characteristic appearance and rule out foreign bodies (i.e. dandruff).
- **Pharmacotherapeutics:** There are currently four insecticides—malathion, permethrin, phenothrin and carbaryl—in use in the UK. Note that a number of licensed products, that nurses with prescribing status may prescribe, are listed in the *Nurse Prescribers Formulary* at N17–18. However, the Cochrane Collaboration Review (1999) could find only limited evidence of the effectiveness of any of these four insecticides and, as a result, its current policy is to manage each proven case using a mosaic of treatments (i.e. retreatment with a different insecticide if one treatment has failed or reinfection has occurred).
  For each treatment:
  - Apply two applications of an insecticide 7 days apart.
  - Hair should be checked thoroughly with a fine plastic detector comb

2–3 days after the second application.
- If adult lice are still present, the treatment should be repeated with a different insecticide.
- Investigate the reasons for treatment failure. Consider initial misdiagnosis, inadequate or incorrect application of treatment, and/or reinfection (often due to inadequate contact tracing or inadequate treatment of fomites).
- Some products can cause skin irritation, and alcoholic formulations should be avoided in small children and in patients with asthma. Likewise, malathion should not be used in infants less than 6 months of age.
- Shampoo formulations are not recommended.
- Interest in the use of naturally occurring products to treat head lice (quassia, tea tree oil, other essential oils, herbal remedies, petrol) has increased in recent years. However, evidence with regard to efficacy, standards of use and safety is limited. In addition, some therapies (i.e. petrol) can be dangerous.

- **Behavioural interventions:**
  - Routine inspection for lice infestation: comb wet hair periodically (with a plastic fine-toothed comb) as a means of detecting early head lice infection. Demonstration of techniques and written information for parents/carers is vital (see Patient education).
  - Mechanical treatment (*Bug Busting*): combing of wet, conditioned hair using a fine detector comb until all the lice have been removed. The combing needs to be repeated every 3–4 days for a period of 2 weeks. It is important to note that while there is a lack of substantive evidence to suggest that mechanical treatment methods are effective, such methods are gaining in popularity in the treatment of head lice. Mechanical removal of head lice may be an option in families who decline to use an insecticide or in whom treatment has repeatedly failed. However, *mechanical treatment is generally not recommended for whole populations.*

- Disinfection of fomites: all items in contact with the scalp (combs, hairbrushes, slides, hats, etc.) should be washed in hot (60°C) water. Likewise, all bedding, clothes and washable toys should receive the same treatment. Objects unable to be washed can be treated with insecticide powders or sealed in plastic bags and left for 2 weeks.
- Treatment of infested eyelashes: apply a petroleum-based ocular ointment to eyelashes 3–4 times daily for a period of 10 days; remove nits mechanically from lashes.

- **Patient education:**
  - Review medication regimen, including application instructions, length of time for applications, etc.
  - Stress the importance of concordance with all aspects of treatment. Remind families that appropriate home management (including medication, treatment of infected contacts and behavioural interventions) is essential for effective eradication of head lice infection.
  - It is often helpful to explain to parents the rationale behind the head lice treatments, including information on the life cycle of head lice.
  - Warn parents that pruritus may persist for up to 2 weeks after treatment (related to chemical irritation from the medication and/or sensitivity to the bite of the louse); this does not mean that there has been a treatment failure.
  - Patient education materials:
    The Prevention and Treatment of Head Lice (DoH, 2000) is available free to schools and health professionals in the UK from Department of Health, PO Box 777, London SE1 6XH.
    Bug Buster help line: 020-8341-7167, www.nits.net/bugbusting.

⮕ FOLLOW-UP

- Ideally, follow-up is advisable to evaluate treatment success within 2–3 days of the second treatment.
- Signs of treatment failure are the same as for the original diagnosis (i.e. detection of live lice).

MEDICAL CONSULT/ SPECIALIST REFERRAL

- Usually not necessary, as head lice infestation is rarely associated with serious clinical consequences, although in rare cases inflammation of the scalp and secondary infection can occur. In these cases, referral to a general practitioner may be advisable.

PAEDIATRIC PEARLS

- Lice infection is confirmed through detection of live lice or eggs; treat only true infections.
- The minimum volume for a single application is usually a single small bottle (50–59 ml); however, this amount may have to be adjusted upwards for very thick or long hair.
- Prophylactic use of insecticides (or automatic treatment of family members) is not recommended, although close contacts should be carefully checked for infestation after a case has been confirmed.
- Use of a white cloth or tissue to wipe the detection comb with after each

pass through the hair can aid in detection of hair debris and/or lice.

- Treatment failures are most likely due to failure to administer second application of insecticide; failure to recognise and treat other infected contacts; incorrect insecticide use (especially failure to leave on the hair for the recommended length of time).
- Do not overtreat. Chemical irritation and/or sensitivity from louse bites can result in pruritus that persists for up to 2 weeks; this is not a treatment failure.
- Insecticides work by killing lice and eggs (ovicidal). Effectiveness depends on the insecticide itself (assuming correct application) and some preparations have greater ovicidal activity than others. Consequently, the second application of insecticide is important. Note that shampoo formulations have low ovicidal activity and may not kill lice, so they are not recommended.
- Although there had been reported resistance to commonly used insecticides, it is important to rule out other causes for treatment failure and the possibility of psychogenic or allergic itching before retreatment.

BIBLIOGRAPHY

Anonymous. Treating head louse infections. Drug Therap Bull 1998; 36(6):45–46.

Chesney P, Burgess I. Lice: resistance and treatment. Contemp Pediatr 1998; 15(11):160–192.

Chosidow O. Scabies and pediculosis. Lancet 2000; 355:819–823.

Department of Health. The prevention and treatment of head lice (Leaflet L09/001). London: DoH; 2000.

Dodd CS. Interventions for the treatment of head lice. In: Cochrane Data base of Systematic Reviews, The Cochrane Library, Cochrane Collaboration. Oxford: Update Software; 1999.

Ibarra J. Primary health care guide to common UK parasitic diseases. London: Community Hygiene Concern; 1998.

Ibarra J. Interim report: study comparing visual inspection at school with the use of the 1998 Bug Buster Kit at home for the detection of head infestation. Shared Wisdom 2000; 5:10–11.

Roberts RJ, Casey D, Morgan DA, et al. Comparison of wet combing with malathion for treatment of head lice in the UK: a pragmatic randomised controlled trial. Lancet 2000; 356:540–544.

COMMON PAEDIATRIC PROBLEMS

9.13 PSORIASIS

Sandra Lawton

INTRODUCTION

- Psoriasis is a chronic inflammatory skin disorder characterised by episodes of flare and remission; it is not infectious.
- Although less common in children, it is probably underdiagnosed. It has been estimated that 10% of patients with psoriasis present before the age of 10, with the average age of onset being 8 years.
- Psoriasis usually presents as red, scaly, thickened patches commonly affecting knees, elbows, lower back and scalp (chronic plaque psoriasis); this presentation is easily recognised

and accounts for 65% of cases in childhood. In contrast, guttate psoriasis is less prevalent and accounts for 25% of cases. Other forms of psoriasis are shown in (Table 9.19).

- Scalp involvement affects 80% of children with facial, intertrigenous and napkin psoriasis seen commonly. Attacks of pustular and erythrodermic psoriasis are rare in children, as are psoriatic arthropathy and nail changes.
- There is a strong genetic component to psoriasis, with a variety of potential triggers playing a role in disease expression (Table 9.20).

PATHOPHYSIOLOGY

- The skin consists of two layers: the epidermis and the dermis. In normal skin, cells reproduce, move from the dermis to the epidermis and are shed slowly. This process takes about 28 days and is called 'proliferation'.
- In psoriasis, the new skin cells (keratinocytes) are made too quickly and push up to the surface of the skin with a 4-day turnover. In addition, there is a 30-fold increase in production of new epidermal cells.
- These combined phenomena result in (1) the characteristic silvery scale of psoriasis; (2) a thickened epidermis;

Table 9.19 Types of Psoriasis

Type	Distinguishing features
Chronic plaque psoriasis	• Accounts for approximately 65% of cases in children • Easily recognised, red/pink, well-demarcated plaques with dry, silvery-white scale • Knees are commonly affected • Auspitz's sign commonly seen (pinpoint bleeding if scales are picked off)
Guttate psoriasis	• Accounts for approximately 25% of cases in children; especially children and adolescents • Characterised by small, round, red spots that appear suddenly on the trunk and become scaly • Lesions are typically small, extensive and superficial (often described as looking like 'raindrops') • Streptococcal sore throat can trigger and, as such, is often self-limiting (lasting 2–3 months) • Some individuals may have recurrent attacks and occasionally lesions coalesce to become plaque psoriasis
Scalp psoriasis	• Common site of psoriasis in children • Characterised by a scalp which is dry and flaky or red and inflamed with well-defined plaques • Scaling is thick and may form 'lumps' on head; areas often affected include behind the ears and just below hairline • Associated hair loss almost always resolves spontaneously after psoriasis clears
Napkin psoriasis	• Infants develop typical psoriasis plaques or a bright, red, weepy rash in the nappy area
Flexural psoriasis (uncommon in children)	• Most common in women and obese patients • Commonly affects submammary, axillary and anogenital folds • Glistening red plaques are clearly demarcated (no scaling); often there is cracking in the depths of the folds
Pustular psoriasis (rare in children): two types	• Palmoplantar pustular psoriasis: characterised by localised, painful yellow/white pustules (3–10 mm) appearing on inflamed, erythematous skin; may leave brown marks (areas of hyperpigmentation) after healing • Most resistant to treatment with increased prevalence in females and associated with smoking • Generalised pustular psoriasis: a medical emergency and requires immediate referral to specialist care • Can be a complication of long-standing psoriasis or related to the withdrawal of corticosteroid therapy, hypocalcaemia, infections and local irritants • The top layer of skin may come away in sheets and the patient can become acutely ill
Erythrodermic psoriasis (rare in children)	• Medical emergency and, as such, requires immediate referral • Characterised by erythema of whole body with patches of scaling that is fairly superficial and, as such, different from chronic plaque • Patients can develop oedema of the limbs, cardiac failure and impaired liver and renal function (as a result of vasodilation) • Triggers include severe sunburn, withdrawal of systemic steroids, irritation of the skin from coal tar and dithranol and systemic infections
Psoriatic arthropathy (rare in children)	• Many types, may present before or after rash; indication for referral • Blood tests for rheumatoid factors will be negative, despite arthropathy for several years prior to skin signs • The prognosis in psoriatic arthropathy appears to be better than in rheumatoid arthritis, often with less pain and disability
Nail psoriasis (rare in children)	• Thimble pitting is the most common, followed by onycholysis (separation of the distal edge of the nail from the bed) • Treatment is often difficult

Table 9.20 Potential Psoriasis Triggers

Potential trigger	Association
Infection	• Throat infection with group A β-haemolytic streptococcus can often precipitate an outbreak of guttate psoriasis in children and young adults
Skin trauma	• Psoriatic lesion can appear at site of trauma (scratches, surgical wound, sunburn, skin infection); known as Koebner phenomenon lesions often take 7–14 days to develop
Medications	• Use of lithium, beta-blockers, antimalarials and some non-steroidal anti-inflammatory drugs have been known to exacerbate psoriasis
Alcohol	• An association between high alcohol intake and psoriasis has been reported
Climate	• In general, psoriatic symptoms improve in warm climates but may be exacerbated in cold ones
Sunlight	• While beneficial in 90% of cases, for some patients sunlight may exacerbate symptoms
Stress	• Anecdotal evidence suggests emotional upset and/or stress triggers flare
Smoking	• Smoking aggravates psoriasis and it is associated with palmoplantar pustular psoriasis

(3) activation of local immune processes (WBC infiltrates); and (4) an increased blood supply to the skin (capillary dilatation causes the erythematous, raised patches).

HISTORY

- Family history of psoriasis.
- Potential triggers.
- Date/child's age when lesion(s) appeared, including their location at onset, appearance and areas which are currently involved.
- Appearance of lesions and degree of associated pain, pruritus and discomfort.
- Recent illness prior to onset (particularly sore throat).

- Recent medications (particularly systemic steroids use).
- Recent trauma prior to onset and/or relationship of lesion to trauma.
- Joint pain.
- Current medication (topical and systemic): any known allergies.
- Previous treatment(s) and response.
- Improvement with sun exposure and/or seasonal variations.
- Knowledge about skin condition (psoriasis).

PHYSICAL EXAMINATION

- Systematic head-to-toe examination of the skin with special attention to the scalp, joint flexures, palms, soles and nails. Be sure to check in the retroauricular portion of the scalp and perianal region as these are sites of involvement that are commonly overlooked.
- Determine texture, temperature and perfusion of skin.
- Lesions should be examined in detail with meticulous description and documentation on a body plan.
- Determine the degree of pain, itching (pruritus) and soreness associated with the psoriasis. Auspitz's sign (pinpoint bleeding when scale removed) is found in plaque psoriasis while the Koebner phenomenon is the appearance of psoriasis lesions at the site of trauma (scratches, surgical wounds, sunburn or skin infections).
- Joints should be examined for signs of swelling or deformity (psoriatic arthropathy) as should palms and soles (to rule out pustular psoriasis).

DIFFERENTIAL DIAGNOSES

- The different patterns of psoriasis in childhood have different differential diagnoses; see Table 9.21.

MANAGEMENT

The goals of psoriasis management are centred on controlling symptoms, managing exacerbations, maintaining comfort and adapting regimens to individual children and their families. In addition, vital components of

Table 9.21   Differential Diagnoses of Psoriasis

Common clinical patterns in childhood	Consider
Chronic plaque	• Discoid eczema, tinea corporis, pityriasis versicolor
Guttate	• Drug eruption, pityriasis versicolor, pityriasis rosea, pityriasis rubra pilaris, tinea corporis, Gianotti–Crosti syndrome
Scalp	• Atopic eczema, scalp infestation, infantile seborrhoeic dermatitis
Napkin psoriasis	• *Candida* infection, irritant dermatitis, nappy rash, infantile seborrhoeic dermatitis, histiocytosis X

management include educating, supporting and empowering children (and their families) as well as improving their quality of life.

- **Additional diagnostics:** not routinely required, as the diagnosis of psoriasis is established from history and physical examination findings. However, the following can be considered: *throat culture* (useful if streptococcal infection is suspected, as group A β-haemolytic streptococcus is associated with acute onset of guttate psoriasis in children and adolescents); *further investigations* (skin biopsy, and bacterial, fungal and/or viral cultures are sometimes useful if there is diagnostic doubt); *haematological screening* (required if systemic medications are to be used as there are implications for the therapies prescribed).
- **Pharmacotherapeutics:** first-line interventions are topical treatments followed by phototherapy and systemic medications (specialist management only). Note that care needs to be taken with regard to topical medications in children (see Ch. 5). Table 9.22 summarises appropriate pharmacotherapeutics.
- **Patient education:**
  - Educate patients about their skin condition, its management and its chronicity. Stress the importance of controlling the disease through physical care, maintenance of skin integrity (avoiding trauma) and consistent use of medications (especially topical treatments).
  - Reinforce with families that following instructions as closely as possible is important; therapy that is too vigorous may worsen symptoms while non-adherence to treatment regimens will not result in improvements.
  - Discuss with families strategies to maintain comfort, such as tackling distressing symptoms (e.g. itch, soreness, dryness, bleeding and pain). Outline warning signs that require evaluation (appearance of pustules or increase in number; significant increase in symptom severity, especially if accompanied by fever or an ill-appearance).
  - Review lifestyle changes and trigger avoidance that help prevent recurrence (avoiding skin injury, streptococcal infection, sunburn, stress, insect bites, itching, tight clothes/shoes and occlusive skin dressings).
  - Teach patients and families about their medication uses, side-effects and potential problems. Reinforce instructions and monitor use frequently.
  - Inform families that skin care regimens can be adapted to suit their individual needs.
- **Behavioural interventions:** adherence to skin care regimen; keep home cool and central heating low; heat dries the skin; avoid perfumed products; find a hairstyle that avoids the need for grips and bands, which pull the hair; beware of the common triggers—how they affect the child and action to be taken.

FOLLOW-UP

- The majority of patients can be supported and treated in primary care if the skin care regimens, behavioural interventions and patient education points are followed. The support of secondary care would then be on an 'as required or indicated' basis. Therefore,

Table 9.22	**Pharmacological Management of Psoriasis**	
Treatment	Mechanism of action	Guidance
Emollients	• Soothe: relieve the irritation and itch (anti-pruritic) • Soften: lubricate and soften the plaques, keeping them more flexible and comfortable so they are less likely to crack • Hydrate: by keeping the plaque moist, scale removal is achieved, which in turn allows easier application and enhanced penetration of other topical therapies • Anti-inflammatory: emollients may slow down the rate of cell turnover (further research is required) • Potential steroid sparing effect: emollients may reduce the need to use topical corticosteroids as rate of cell turnover may be reduced (further research is required)	• Apply thinly, frequently, gently and in the direction of hair growth to prevent folliculitis (irritation and inflammation of hair follicles). Must be allowed to soak into the skin before active topical therapies are used (20 min); *it is no good putting therapies on scale* • Many types available: soap substitutes, bath oils, shower therapies and moisturisers, so it is important to be familiar with various options so that the patient can be involved in the choice • See Section 9.3
Coal tar	• Helps clear psoriasis by an antimitotic effect but the exact action is still unknown; used to treat psoriasis over many years	• Disadvantages include unpleasant odour and mess of application • Often used in conjunction with UVB (ultraviolet radiation) • Apply once or twice/day. Cover the whole plaque and wipe on rather than rub in • Most tars will stain bedding and clothing so patients should be advised to use old clothing and linen
Dithranol (anthralin)	• Inhibits mitosis and slows down the excessive rate of keratinocyte division. Has been used for over 100 years to treat psoriasis	• Stains skin, hair, linen, clothing and bath (a purple/brown colour) • In hospital, dithranol is applied and left on overnight • In primary care, short contact dithranol is applied once daily and removed after 30 min in the bath or shower • Treatment should continue daily for 3–4 weeks and the strength of the dithranol increased every few days • Apply to the plaque while sparing surrounding skin, as it will cause staining, irritation and burning
Topical steroids	• Use of topical steroids in the management of children with psoriasis occurs under specialist supervision	
Vitamin D analogues	• Vitamin D derivatives induce differentiation and suppress proliferation of keratinocytes	• Used in mild-to-moderate psoriasis • Easy to use and not messy • Two types: calcipotriol and tacalcitol (tacalcitol is not licensed for use in children)
Topical retinoids	• *Not to be used in children*	
Phototherapy	• Administered in specialist units only	• Often used in conjunction with other therapies • Short-term complications include erythema and 'sunburn' • Long-term complications include photoaging and possible (though slight) increased risk of skin cancers
Systemic drugs	• Administered in specialist units only	• Methotrexate, acitretin, ciclosporin • Not generally used in children: all have potential side-effects and complications. They require haematological monitoring and are used in recalcitrant forms only

it is important for primary providers to have a clear understanding of the indications for subsequent dermatology consultation/referral (see below).

✍ MEDICAL CONSULTATION/ SPECIALIST REFERRAL

• Any child with pustular or erythrodermic psoriasis requires immediate referral.
• Any child with acutely unstable psoriasis or widespread symptomatic guttate psoriasis that would likely benefit from phototherapy.

• Any child/family in whom the condition is causing severe social and psychological problems; prompts to referral should include sleeplessness, social exclusion and reduced quality of life or self-esteem.
• Any child in whom the rash is sufficiently extensive to make self-management impractical and/or the rash is in a sensitive area (such as face, hands, feet, genitalia) with the symptoms that are particularly troublesome.
• Any child in whom the rash is leading to time off school

sufficient enough to interfere with education.
• Any child who requires an assessment for the management of associated arthropathy.
• Any child that has (or develops) features that create diagnostic uncertainty and/or those children who fail to respond to management in general practice.

⊙ PAEDIATRIC PEARLS

• It is impossible to predict the prognosis for an individual. However, if treated properly, psoriasis will generally improve, with remissions sometimes lasting for years.

- Listen to the parents and child and consider their wishes; they will require a tremendous amount of support (both psychologically and practically). The chronic nature of the disease requires a high degree of care continuity and providers need to allow sufficient time for this.
- Strategies for supporting patients include use of support groups, coping techniques, stress management, counselling, listening and talking.
- Psoriasis is considered to be stable if there are no new plaques or, if plaques are present, the amount of scale is decreasing and the lesions are not increasing in size, distribution or redness.
- Useful addresses: *Psoriasis Association,* Milton House, Milton Street, Northampton NN2 7JG (tel: 01604-711-129) and the *Psoriatic Arthropathy Alliance,* PO Box 111, St. Albans, Herefordshire AL2 3JQ (tel: 01923-672-837 or http://www.paalliance.org/)

🖺 BIBLIOGRAPHY

Lawton S. Assessing the skin. Prof Nurse 1998; 13(4):S5–S9.
Lawton S. Psoriasis. Pract Nurs 1999; 10(20):29–34.
Lawton S. A quality of life for people with skin disease. London: Skin Care Campaign Directory; 2000. http://www.skincarecampaign.org/directory/slawton.htm
Mackie R. Topical coal tar. J Dermatol Treat 1997; 8(1):30–31.
Mitchell T, Penzer R. Psoriasis at your fingertips. London: Class Publishing; 2000.
National Institute for Clinical Excellence. GP referral practice: a guide to appropriate referral from general to specialist services: http://www.nice.org.uk/
Paige D. Psoriasis in children. Dermatol Pract 1998; 6(5):10–12.
Van Onselen J. Psoriasis in practice. London: Haymarket Publishing; 1998.
Williams HC. Dermatology. In: Stevens A, Raferty J, eds, Health care needs assessment: series 2. Oxford: Radcliffe Medical Press; 1997.

9.14 SCABIES

Rosemary Turnbull

📖 INTRODUCTION

- Scabies is a highly contagious condition caused by the parasite *Sarcoptes scabiei*; humans are the only known reservoir.
- It affects all age groups and is not gender-specific. Epidemics are reported to occur in 15-year cycles.
- Scabies is not particular to socioeconomic class and is not a result of poor hygiene. Close personal contact with an infected human (with or without symptoms) is necessary for transmission. The scabies mite can live 36 hours isolated from a human host, but the extent of fomite transmission is unclear.
- The scabies rash is characterised by cutaneous eruptions and an intense pruritus, this being particularly bad at night (especially in bed, as mite activity increases due to a rise in body temperature).

🔬 PATHOPHYSIOLOGY

- The female scabies mite burrows in the stratum corneum (rarely penetrating through the epidermis) for 15–30 days after the initial infestation.
- She lays her eggs in the burrow (travelling 2–4 mm/day) and can lay up to three eggs daily for 4–5 weeks (after which she dies within the burrow). The eggs take 3 days to hatch into larvae and subsequently undergo a further three nymph stages before the mites are capable of reproduction. After mating, the male will die and the gravid female begins the cycle again.
- As such, there may be no pruritus until 4–6 weeks after the initial infestation.
- The actual skin eruption is a consequence of an immune response to the scabies mite.

⬅ HISTORY

- Onset and duration of the rash.
- Degree of itching and temporal factors (i.e. Is the itch worse at night?).
- Progression/distribution of the rash (i.e. From where does it seem to spread?).
- Potential exposures to scabies (e.g. close contacts with scabies, outbreaks in nursery/school, etc.).
- Anyone else in the family itching or have evidence of a rash?
- Measures taken thus far to relieve itching (with results).

👁 PHYSICAL EXAMINATION

- The child should be examined closely (see Sec. 9.1), paying particular attention to the finger and toe webs.
- Carefully check the inner aspect of the wrists, the axilla, waistline and gluteal cleft.
- In infants, carefully inspect the soles of the feet as well as scalp and face.
- Examine the skin closely for burrows, which are characterised by grey-white scaly lines (typically an elongated 'S' shape with a broad base). In addition, punctate brown-black dots may be seen at the leading edge.
- There may also be evidence of excoriated areas of skin, nodules and vesiculopustular lesions.

- Secondary infection of the lesions and/or eczematous changes as a result of chronic scratching is not uncommon.

DIFFERENTIAL DIAGNOSES

- Diagnosis is crucial, as treatment may complicate pre-existing skin diseases such as eczema. Consider contact dermatitis, drug reaction, eczema, insect bites, infantile acropustulosis and papular viral exanthems.

MANAGEMENT

- **Additional diagnostics:** examination of the contents of the burrow under the microscope will reveal the scabies mite, eggs, larvae and/or mite faeces. Use a needle to extract the contents from the burrow. Visualisation of the mite or byproducts is the definitive diagnosis.
- **Pharmacotherapeutics:** Regular administration of chlorpheniramine (Piriton) suspension may offer some relief of pruritus. The current scabicide treatment of choice varies, as products are generally rotated to avoid resistance. *It is important to check the products currently being used in specific areas.* Commonly used scabicides include:
  - Derbac-M (malathion 0.5% aqueous solution). Applied to whole body from neck down. Leave on for 24 hours. In cases of reinfestation use only once weekly.
  - Lyclear Dermal Cream (permethrin 5% cream) 30 g tubes. Apply to entire body, including scalp and face, avoiding the eyes. Leave *in situ* for 8 hours.
- **Behavioural interventions:**
  - Follow administration instructions exactly. Written information should supplement verbal instructions. The medication will need to be applied over the entire body, including the scalp and face. Ensure that toe and finger webs are covered. Note that if the hands are washed before the appropriate length of time has elapsed, then more solution must be applied.
  - After desired time, bath/shower in warm water to remove all the solution. A normal bath/shower can then be taken.
  - Treat all close contacts (whether symptomatic or not) at the same time. Ensure enough lotion/cream is issued to treat all contacts. Do not rely on carer buying additional lotion.
  - All clothing and bed linen should be laundered in hot wash and dried at a high heat.
  - Use clean clothes and bed linens after treatment.
- **Patient education:**
  - Discuss with parents/carers the exact cause of the rash. Reassure them that it is quite a common problem and is not an indication of family hygiene.
  - Review the behavioural interventions above and stress the importance of treating all contacts at the same time. Explain to parents that the most common causes of ineffective treatment are misapplication of medication and failure to treat all contacts simultaneously. This is true whether family members are symptomatic or not (contacts may be infested and yet still asymptomatic).
  - Inform parents that until treatment is completed, the child must be kept away from nursery/school.
  - Warn families that the itching may persist for up to 6 weeks after treatment and it is not indicative of failed treatment. However, the appearance of new burrows suggests reinfestation and parents should return for re-evaluation/examination.

FOLLOW-UP

- None is usually required.
- Issue telephone number for parent to contact you if they see new papules after treatment.

MEDICAL CONSULT/ SPECIALIST REFERRAL

- Any child in whom the diagnosis is unclear.
- Any child who is immunocompromised.
- Any child with recurring infestation despite adequate treatment.

PAEDIATRIC PEARLS

- Suspect scabies in any sudden onset of itching and excoriations.
- Lyclear cream is best for children, as it can be used on the scalp and face.
- If there is a rash on the soles of an infant's feet, think scabies.
- Scabies is not particular to a socio-economic class.
- If reinfestation occurs, think a carrier has not been properly treated.

BIBLIOGRAPHY

Anonmyous. The management of scabies. Drug Therap Bull 2002; 40(6):43–46.
Hughes E, Van Onselen J. Dermatology nursing: a practical approach. Edinburgh: Churchill Livingstone; 2001.
Morgan-Glenn PD. Scabies: in brief. Pediatr Rev 2001; 22(9):322–323.
Prendiville J. Scabies and lice. In: Harper J, Oranje A, Prose N, eds, Textbook of paediatric dermatology, Vol. 1. Oxford: Blackwell Science; 2001.
Rasmussen JE. Scabies. Pediatr Rev 1994; 15(3):110–114.

9.15 VIRAL SKIN INFECTIONS (WARTS AND MOLLUSCUM CONTAGIOSUM)

Karen Spowart

📦 INTRODUCTION

- *Warts* are benign, proliferative, intraepithelial tumours caused by the human papilloma virus (HPV) of which there are more than 100 different types identified to date. Those responsible for skin warts are types 1–4.
- Warts commonly occur in children; approximately 10% of children between 5 and 10 years of age have warts. Those with atopic eczema are particularly at risk, as warts can develop at sites of trauma (Koebner phenomenon). Likewise, immunocompromised children are at increased risk of wart and molluscum infection, with those on long-term chemotherapy tending to develop large and very persistent lesions.
- Commonly encountered warts in children are outlined in Table 9.23. Although most HPV sites have preferred sites of infectivity, note that there is significant overlap between the various HPV types.
- In young children, perianal and genital warts are often acquired non-sexually (autoinoculation or heteroinoculation from carer's warts); *however, the possibility of sexual abuse must be considered and/or ruled out.*
- *Molluscum contagiosum* are discrete, smooth, pearly papules caused by a pox virus. They are commonly referred to as 'water warts'.

🧩 PATHOPHYSIOLOGY

- The incubation period for HPV ranges from 1 to 6 months, although a latency period of 3 or more years has been suggested. Humans are thought to be the only reservoir of HPV.
- The mechanisms of transmission are not well understood. However, transmission is thought to occur via direct physical contact (although fomite spread has been postulated). After infection, the child is able to spread the virus to themselves (autoinoculation). This is commonly related to the manipulation of the warts (i.e. picking, scratching, shaving). Transmission can also occur from the warts of a carer or parent (heteroinoculation).
- Vertical transmission (e.g. transmission from the birth canal) can result in anogenital and laryngeal warts.
- The dermal papillae of the wart are thin and contain abundant blood vessels. These vessels correlate with the 'black dots' and pinpoint bleeding seen after trauma to the wart.
- The incubation period for molluscum contagiosum is thought to be 2–7 weeks, but it may be as long as 6 months. Humans are the only known source of the causative virus.
- It is spread through direct contact, fomites and autoinoculation. The period of communicability is unknown, but infectivity is considered to be low (although outbreaks have occurred).

⬅ HISTORY

- Length of time the warts/molluscum have been present.
- Location and any pattern of distribution or spread (i.e. increasing or decreasing numbers of lesions, where lesions started, etc.).
- Associated pain.
- Treatments used prior to consultation (with results).
- The degree to which the warts are bothering parent and child.
- Other family members affected.
- Expectations of the consultation.
- If perianal or genital warts are present (especially if children are >3 years of age), a careful history for sexual abuse

Table 9.23	Commonly Encountered Warts in Children
Type of wart	*Characteristics*
Common	• Easily identified as a firm papule with a hyperkeratotic surface • Most commonly found on the hands, although any site can be affected • Particularly common in children and may be painful, especially when periungual
Plane	• Small flesh-coloured warts, often multiple, occurring on the face and backs of hands
Plantar (verrucae)	• Occur on the sole of the feet • Body weight causes them to grow inwards; the associated pressure can result in considerable pain • Multiple individual lesions (particularly on the heel) are known as *mosaic* warts • Plantar warts tend to be persistent and difficult to treat
Genital and perianal (anogenital warts)	• Caused by human papilloma virus (HPV) types 6, 11, 16 and 18 • In young children genital and perianal warts are usually acquired non-sexually (vertical transmission, inoculation by carer). However, the possibility of child sexual abuse must be considered and/or ruled out
Molluscum contagiosum (water wart)	• Caused by pox virus • Characterised by pearly white or skin-coloured papules that are waxy with central punctum • Lesions are usually multiple and grouped in clusters; typically occur on the face, neck and trunk • Spread is by direct contact and autoinoculation is common (secondary to scratching). As a result, lesions typically occur on adjacent skin surfaces

is required. This should include maternal or paternal history of anogenital warts and history of warts in close contact of child.

PHYSICAL EXAMINATION

- Privacy during the examination (especially with perianal or genital warts) is key. Children may have experienced name-calling at school or may be generally embarrassed about their warts (especially if they are multiple); therefore, they may be reluctant to show them and extra sensitivity is required.
- Examine the entire patient for a potential source of infection (especially important for perianal or genital warts). In addition, it is wise to check parents/carers to rule out heteroinoculation.
- Document size, location and number of lesions with a diagram; careful documentation at presentation allows for comparison at subsequent consults.
- Typical appearances of different types of warts are outlined in Table 9.23.
- Warts are more likely in areas of trauma. In addition, with autoinoculation, they may appear in a linear pattern.
- *While less common than other routes of transmission among children <3 years of age, it is important to carefully check for signs of sexual abuse when any child presents with perianal and genital warts.*

DIFFERENTIAL DIAGNOSES

- Most warts (especially common warts) are distinguishable on clinical grounds and the diagnosis is straightforward. However, the following should be considered:
  - *Flat warts:* consider dermal nevi, molluscum contagiosum, milia, folliculitis and lichen planus.
  - *Plantar warts:* consider corns, calluses, and foreign bodies. Mosaic warts (multiple lesions particularly on the heel) can be confused with pitted keratolytis.
  - *Anogenital warts:* consider condyloma lata, molluscum contagiosum, skin tags and haemorrhoids.
- The possibility of sexual abuse requires consideration if anogenital warts are present.
- The differential list for molluscum contagiosum includes folliculitis, warts and condylomata accuminata.

MANAGEMENT

Spontaneous resolution of both common warts and molluscum is high (66% of common warts will resolve within 2 years and most molluscum lesions have resolved within 1 year). Consequently, the decision to treat both common warts and molluscum is based on the child's age, extent of involvement and the degree to which the lesions are causing distress. In addition, because resolution of common warts is associated with cell-mediated immunity, watchful waiting is reasonable (especially in young children).

- **Additional diagnostics:** none usually required. Scraping of molluscum lesions will show molluscum bodies under magnification and the diagnosis of warts is typically apparent from physical examination.
- **Pharmacotherapeutics:** see Table 9.24.
- **Behavioural interventions:**
  - Stress the importance of 'no picking, scratching or manipulating warts'; it is often useful to cover the warts with a plaster.
  - Paring of common and plantar warts to remove excess keratin formation (and enhance treatment effects) is best achieved by gentle rubbing with a manicure emery board until the lesion is flat. Alternatively, disposable scalpel blades (sizes 10 and 15) are effective at removing hard skin of plantar warts.
- **Patient education:**
  - Review pharmacotherapeutics and behavioural interventions with parent and child.
  - Discuss with parents the risk of infectivity. More specifically, explain that the mechanisms of transmission are not well understood and as such, it is difficult to predict infectivity. Children with impaired skin integrity and/or immunodeficiency are at greater risk of infection, but otherwise the risk of infection is fairly low. Infected children should not be prevented from attending school or nursery.
  - Explain to parents (and child) that good skin care and avoidance of 'picking' will also prevent infection.
  - Concordance with wart paints is generally not very good. Careful explanation about the necessity to persist with wart paint treatments over a significant period of time is essential.
  - Review with parents the importance of follow-up if lesions return. Explain that it is possible to have subclinical or latent infections despite clearing and with reappearance, treatment is best initiated early.

FOLLOW-UP

- Generally unnecessary in the majority of cases.
- 3-weekly appointments for cryotherapy if tolerated.

MEDICAL CONSULT/ SPECIALIST REFERRAL

- Any child with suspected sexual abuse.
- Any child with extensive lesions, painful plantar warts or warts that are refractory despite adequate management.

PAEDIATRIC PEARLS

- Due to a large proportion of warts and molluscum resolving spontaneously, *no treatment* is reasonable, especially in young children.
- Approaches to treatment must be relevant to the severity of the problem. However, warts can be

Table 9.24 Pharmacotherapeutic Treatment of Warts and Molluscum

Type of wart	Treatment
Common	• Watchful waiting (see discussion in Management) • Daily application of a keratolytic such as Salactol (salicylic acid 16.7%, lactic acid 16.7% in flexible collodion) • Prior to application, the surface of the wart should be gently rubbed with an emery board until flat • A drop of the paint should be applied to the centre of the wart and allowed to dry • The process should be repeated until the wart has completely disappeared • For persistent warts the use of cryotherapy with liquid nitrogen can be used; however, this procedure is painful and not well tolerated in young children • Warts should be frozen for sufficient time (5–10 s) to cause the surrounding skin to develop a white halo. This can be repeated at 3-weekly intervals until the warts have resolved
Plane	• A weak over-the-counter (OTC) keratolytic in gel form such as 12% salicylic acid (Salatac) or 26% Occlusal are beneficial
Plantar (verrucae)	• Best treated initially with salicylic acid plasters (40%) • As much of the hard, overlying skin should be pared away as is possible with application of a piece of the salicylic plaster to exactly cover the wart; hold the plaster in place with an adhesive bandage • The plaster should be left in place for 24–48 hours with the process repeated until the wart has disappeared • Cryotherapy can be used in the treatment of plantar warts but is extremely painful and not well tolerated by children (see above) • For multiple plantar warts (*mosaic* warts) the use of formalin soaks is more effective • The affected area should be soaked every night for 10–15 min (it is necessary to protect the surrounding skin with petroleum jelly) • After each soak the soft tissue can be gently pared away
Genital and perianal (anogenital warts)	• Effective treatment can be obtained with podophyllin (15%, 20% or 25% in benzoin compound tincture) • Podophyllin is an extract of plant root and highly irritant. The surrounding skin should be protected with petroleum jelly. Note that it is usually an outpatient procedure • Use a cotton bud to paint the podophyllin onto the individual lesions. The paint should be allowed to dry • The treated area should be washed 4 hours after podophyllin application using soap and water • This treatment programme has to be repeated weekly for the next 4–6 weeks • Cryotherapy is also an effective form of treatment, but it has limitations with young children (see above) • In young children genital and perianal warts are usually acquired non-sexually (vertical transmission, inoculation by carer). However, the possibility of child sexual abuse must be considered and/or ruled out
Molluscum contagiosum (water wart)	• Watch and wait (6–12 months) for spontaneous resolution; family will require reassurance during this time. After 1 year without resolution, refer for dermatology evaluation • Cryotherapy is an effective treatment, but it has limitations with young children (see above) • Additional treatment available in specialist care (i.e. paediatric dermatology)

upsetting for both parents and children; name-calling and bullying are not uncommon (especially among children with extensive lesions). Consequently, it is important to negotiate a treatment plan that is acceptable to both parent and child and considers the degree of distress the lesions are causing.
• Whereas it is generally accepted that anogenital warts in young children (those under 3 years or age) are acquired through non-sexual contact, the possibility of sexual abuse must always be considered.
• Black pinpoint dots are often on the surface of warts; they are a function of thromboses capillaries.
• Plantar warts interrupt natural skin lines, calluses do not.
• Consider the possibility of underlying immunodeficiency in children with extensive, treatment refractory HPV infection.

☰ BIBLIOGRAPHY

Harper J. Handbook of paediatric dermatology. Oxford: Butterworth-Heinemann; 1990.

MacKie RM. Clinical dermatology: an illustrated textbook. Oxford: Oxford University Press; 1991.

Stewart K. How to perform cryosurgery for warts. Br J Dermatol Nurs 1998; 2(3):8–9.

Turnbull R. Paediatrics: skin infections in children. Br J Dermatol Nurs 1999; 3(1):12–14.

CHAPTER 10

Problems Related to the Head, Eyes, Ears, Nose, Throat or Mouth

10.1 CONGENITAL BLOCKED NASOLACRIMAL DUCT

Anna Hunter

📖 INTRODUCTION

- Blockage of the nasolacrimal duct is defined as an obstruction in the portion of the tear drainage system that extends from the lacrimal sac to the nose.
- Congenital blockage of the nasal lacrimal duct is a common complaint in the newborn period, as at birth the lower end of the nasolacrimal duct is frequently non-canalised (usually near the inferior meatus of the nose).
- Canaliculisation of the nasolacrimal duct occurs spontaneously or by conservative medical management during the infant's first year of life.

🔖 PATHOPHYSIOLOGY

- In fetal development, the nasolacrimal duct is the last part of the lacrimal drainage system to canaliculise.
- The lacrimal system has two parts (Fig. 10.1): the tear-secreting system (e.g. the lacrimal gland and its accessory lacrimal glands) and the plumbing system (e.g. the upper and lower lacrimal puncti, canaliculi and nasolacrimal ducts).
- Canaliculisation of the lacrimal apparatus begins at the end of the first trimester of pregnancy and is usually completed by the seventh month *in utero*. Occlusion of the nasolacrimal

duct is due to failure of complete canaliculisation of the lacrimal system at birth.
- Tears are composed of three layers: a lipid layer, an aqueous layer and a mucin layer. The lipid layer is the outermost layer and is produced by the meibomian glands of the eyelids; its function is to retard the evaporation of the aqueous layer.
- The middle, aqueous layer of the tear film is produced by the lacrimal gland and the accessory lacrimal glands (situated in the upper and outer orbital margins). The inner, mucin layer is produced by the goblet cells in the conjunctiva. This innermost layer has direct contact with the conjunctiva of the eye and provides a wettable surface for the aqueous layer to adhere to.
- Normal tears contain several antimicrobial substances such as lysozyme, betalysin, lactoferrin and immunoglobulins (IgA, IgG).
- Opening and closing of the eyelids (e.g. normal blinking) acts as a pumping mechanism. When the eyes are closed, tears (along with the micro debris) are collected and drawn into the lacrimal punctum; when the eyes are open, this mixture is expressed into the nose.
- In the baby with the congenital blocked tear duct, tears cannot drain and the stagnant tear film accumulates debris and exudate from the tarsal glands that becomes a focus for infection.

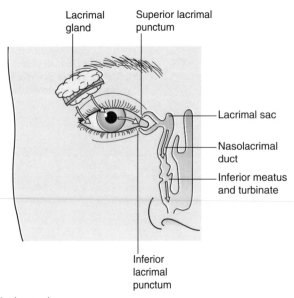

Figure 10.1 The lacrimal system.

HISTORY

- Onset of symptoms and when the watery discharge was first noticed: typically an infant presents to the surgery or clinic at about 2 months of age (the time when full tear flow is established) with a complaint of 'watery eye', or 'cold in the eye with matter'.
- Presence of discharge and if so, type amount, consistency, degree of inflammation, etc.
- Involvement of one or both eyes.
- Other eye infections or eye symptoms (especially at birth or soon after).
- General state of health and well-being (growth, developmental milestones, etc.).
- Other systemic complaints: fever, cough, irritability, upper respiratory tract infection (URTI) symptoms, etc.
- Treatments tried thus far with effectiveness.

PHYSICAL EXAMINATION

- Observe the general appearance, alertness and engagability of the infant. Pay attention to mother's level of anxiousness and confidence in handling/interacting with her infant. Outline the plan for the physical examination and describe your findings.
- **Head and ear, nose and throat (ENT):** inspect the eyelids (maceration, swelling, inflammation), especially the lower eyelid towards the nasal aspect. Note any crusted discharge around the lids and lashes; always compare the affected side with the unaffected. The lower lid margin may be macerated (as a function of the increased discharge). Inspect the conjunctiva (palpebral and bulbar); mild conjunctivitis of the palpebral membranes may be seen, but the bulbar conjunctiva is usually clear and white. Palpate gently around the nasal aspect of the lower lid (pressing gently on lacrimal sac); note any tenderness and/or expression of material from the puncta.

DIFFERENTIAL DIAGNOSES

- Additional causes of *increased tear production* include (all ages):

congenital glaucoma (rare), reflex tearing secondary to dry eye, seventh nerve palsies (rare), trichiasis, entropion.
- Additional causes of *decreased eye drainage* include (rare): imperforate puncta or canaliculi, ectropion, lateral canthus dystropia, traumatic injury to the nasolacrimal duct.
- The possibility of bacterial or viral conjunctivitis should be ruled out (see Sec. 10.3), as well as the possibility of nasolacrimal abscess and/or dacryocystitis (acute infection of the nasolacrimal sac).

MANAGEMENT

- **Additional diagnostics:** usually none are required unless the possibility of acute infection is under consideration and then a swab would be indicated. Some clinicians advocate the use of a dye disappearance test; fluorescein is applied to the conjunctival sac and after 5–10 min the patient is observed. If normal (i.e. negative test) the tear meniscus will have minimal staining after 10 min; in an abnormal (i.e. positive test) the height of the stain will either increase or fail to decrease.
- **Pharmacotherapeutics:** use a broad-spectrum antibiotic ophthalmic ointment such as chloramphenicol ointment (1%) applied three times daily to the affected eye or Fucithalmic 1% applied twice daily for a week. Ointment is preferable so the medication stays around the target area (e.g. the conjunctiva and lacrimal duct). Note that antibiotics should only be used if drainage is present with inflammation.
- **Behavioural interventions:**
  - *Remind carers to wash their hands before and after attempting nasolacrimal duct massage.*
  - Massage of nasolacrimal duct area (Creiger's manoeuvre) several times a day; the goal is to increase hydrostatic pressure on the walls of the blocked nasolacrimal canal in order to rupture the membranous obstruction. Place the index finger over the common canaliculus area to block the exit of the material

through the puncta and apply downward pressure. Alternatively, in order to promote canaliculisation of the duct, the carer can apply gentle pressure to the skin over the medial eyelids and lacrimal sac with 10 straight downward motions (towards the nose) 4 times daily.
- **Patient education:**
  - Review massage technique with carer and have him/her demonstrate this.
  - Discuss signs and symptoms of an acute eye infection, as it is not uncommon for the blocked duct to become infected (dacryocystitis).

FOLLOW-UP

- If spontaneous resolution (95% of infants by 12 months of age), none required. Consider re-evaluation at 6 months of age (if no resolution), as referral will need to be considered (see Referral).
- Consider follow-up phone contact if carer especially anxious.

MEDICAL CONSULT/ SPECIALIST REFERRAL

- Any infant in whom there is no resolution within 6 months, as it is likely that there will need to be probing of the canaliculus under a general anaesthetic. Note that the success rate for correction of the persistently blocked duct (dacryostenosis) is age-sensitive: 96% if probing and irrigation are performed before 13 months of age; 77% if the procedure is performed between 13 and 18 months of age; and 54% success rate if performed between 18 and 24 months of age. As such, consider the length of time between referral, initial consultation and likely waiting time for correction.
- Any infant in whom there is ambiguity with regard to the diagnosis.

PAEDIATRIC PEARLS

- The diagnosis of a blocked nasolacrimal duct can be confirmed if the contents of the nasolacrimal duct are expelled when gentle pressure is applied *underneath* the lacrimal duct on the nasal aspect.

- Nasolacrimal massage and instillation of ophthalmic medication are usually easier while the infant is feeding. Alternatively, if the carer sings a nursery song that involves 'beeping' the nose or stroking the cheek, nasolacrimal massage can be incorporated into the song's routine ('rub, rub, rub your little nose').

📇 BIBLIOGRAPHY

Crawford JA. Lacrimal duct disorders. Int J Ophthal 1984; 24:39–53.

Kanski J. Clinical ophthalmology, 2nd edn. Oxford: Butterworth-Heinemann; 1989.

Kushner B. Congenital nasolacrimal system obstruction. Arch Ophthal 1982; 100:597–600.

Nelson LB, Calhoun JH, Hartey RD. Pediatric ophthalmology, 3rd edn. Philadelphia: WB Saunders; 1991.

10.2 EYE TRAUMA

Rebecca C. Robert and Janet Marsden

📖 INTRODUCTION

- Eye trauma is a common reason for primary care or Accident and Emergency (A&E) visits. The reported incidence of traumatic ocular injuries depends on country, type of injury and treatment centre. Nonetheless, several common features appear in the paediatric population: (1) higher frequency of injuries occur in school-age children and adolescents; (2) the male-to-female predominance; (3) injuries are commonly sustained during sports and recreational activities (especially those that involve the use of a ball); and (4) injuries are more likely to occur during unsupervised play.
- Eye trauma ranges from relatively benign corneal abrasions to serious and potential sight-blinding globe ruptures. The decision to manage and/or refer depends on the extent of ocular trauma and its potential consequences.
- Nurse practitioners (NPs) must systematically and skilfully evaluate the eye trauma patient and make decisions with regard to appropriate management, referral and/or emergency treatment.
- The most common ocular injuries covered in this section are outlined in Table 10.1.

🔬 PATHOPHYSIOLOGY

- The clear, transparent cornea overlying the iris and pupil is composed of five

Table 10.1	Common Cause of Ocular Injury
Type of injury	Common causes
Corneal abrasion	• Scratching eye with finger, branch, paper, metal, hairbrush, mascara wand, foreign body, contact lens (foreign body between lens and eye, improper fit, trauma on entry/removal, overwear), sunlamp, welding or carbon arc
Chemical burn	• Alkali agents (lye, cements, plaster), acids, solvents, detergents, tear gas, mace, sparklers, flares that contain magnesium hydroxide
Ultraviolet light injury	• Ultraviolet rays from sunlight or tanning machine (inappropriate use without safety goggles)
Foreign body	• Commonly: dirt, glass, rust, hair. Think intraocular foreign body for potential penetrating foreign bodies such as metal striking metal, or objects that enter while hammering
Traumatic iritis and hyphaema	• Blunt trauma (e.g. fist, balls)
Ruptured globe/perforation	• Severe direct blunt trauma (e.g. fist, balls, stone), projectile injuries (e.g. pellet guns, sling shots), sharp instrument entering the orbit (can lids, toys), foreign bodies which strike the eye during hammering. Posterior rupture may occur after blunt trauma and may not be obvious
Intraocular haemorrhages	• Normal birth process (rarely present after 3–4 weeks) • Child abuse: shaking of baby (shaken baby syndrome)
Orbital (blow-out) fractures	• Blunt trauma to the front of the eye

layers, the outermost being the epithelium. Partial or complete removal of a focal area of this epithelial layer (e.g. scratching eye with a hairbrush) exposes nerve endings with resultant ocular pain. This type of injury is classified as a *corneal abrasion*. Healing of the outermost epithelial layer does not result in scarring; however, if the corneal trauma interrupts deeper layers, scarring may occur. Small foreign bodies are a frequent cause of *corneal abrasion*, but if there is deeper penetration of the cornea, scarring may occur. Injury with larger objects, such as pieces of glass or metal, may result in *corneal laceration*. In addition, corneal lacerations may perforate the cornea, as may very-high-speed foreign bodies.

- A penetrating or lacerating injury through the full thickness of the cornea or sclera is a severe injury and can lead to damage to underlying structures or even loss of ocular contents.
- *Chemical trauma* due to alkali or acid substances may also damage/disrupt the cornea and other tissues. Of these substances, alkalis are more damaging

due to their ability to lyse cell membranes and penetrate the cornea progressively. Acids precipitate proteins and therefore are not progressive; however, they may likewise cause devastating damage.

- Behind the cornea (and in front of the lens) lies the anterior chamber, a space normally filled with clear, aqueous fluid. Blunt trauma to the eye may cause rupture of iris vessels with subsequent haemorrhage into the anterior chamber, termed *hyphaema*. The ciliary body, lying at the base of the iris and just behind it, contains ciliary muscles whose function is to contract and relax. This, in turn, enables the lens to change shape, resulting in visual accommodation. Inflammation of the ciliary body with ciliary muscle spasm produces ocular discomfort. Cycloplegic agents (e.g. cyclopentolate, tropicamide and homatropine) help to relieve the spasm and therefore a component of the pain. They are often used in the treatment of corneal abrasions or in the case of uveitis to keep the iris away from the lens where it may adhere.
- Of the orbital structures, the medial wall and orbital floor are the most fragile and, as such, more susceptible to *fracture* from blunt trauma.
- A *ruptured globe* results from severe trauma that causes disruption and disorganisation of the integrity of the globe, possibly with loss of ocular contents. Posterior rupture occurs after a high-speed blunt trauma and may not be obvious.
- Ocular trauma may also cause an inflammatory response of the iris and ciliary body tissue with release of white blood cells and protein. This is known as *traumatic uveitis*.
- Figures 10.2 and 10.3 outline the important anatomy of the eye.

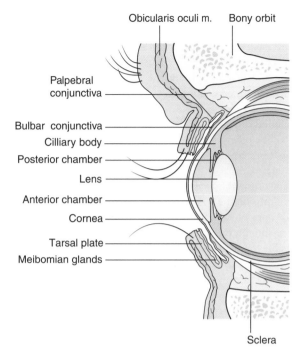

Figure 10.2 Anatomy of the eye (cross-sectional view).

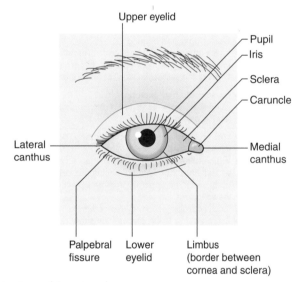

Figure 10.3 Anatomy of the external eye.

⇦ HISTORY

- Injury situation: how and when injury occurred (activity engaged in when trauma occurred); type of object, speed and direction (if known); and use of safety glasses.
- Vision-related symptoms: onset, course and severity or any visual changes (binocular vision, blurred or decreased vision, photophobia and/or tearing); and characteristics of any ocular pain (dull, sharp, foreign body sensation, burning).
- Previous history of eye problems: prior injuries, surgeries, amblyopia, congenital abnormalities and any medical conditions that increase susceptibility to infection (immunocompromise, diabetes, etc.).
- Visual acuity (prior to injury), if known, in addition to use of glasses or contact lenses.
- Date of most recent tetanus immunisation.
- Table 10.2 outlines historical information commonly associated with traumatic ocular injuries.

⊙ PHYSICAL EXAMINATION

- A systematic approach to the paediatric eye examination ensures a complete and accurate assessment of the eye. Move from external to internal—this approach is the least threatening to children and helps gain their confidence (especially among younger children who are especially fearful of eye examinations/drops).

- Note that a drop of ocular anaesthestic often greatly facilitates the examination and may aide in the diagnosis of corneal/conjunctival disruption (as symptoms will be relieved). Proxymetacaine is preferred in children as it does not sting.
- To open swollen (or forcibly shut) eyelids, place thumbs on the infraorbital and supraorbital rims (thus avoiding any pressure on the globe in the case of possible traumatic globe rupture). Likewise, take care if there is any possibility of fracture.

- Always examine both eyes. After completing the basic examination, proceed with fluorescein staining if indicated. Table 10.2 outlines physical examination findings characteristic of various ocular injuries.
- *Note that a history of an ocular chemical burn is an eye emergency and, therefore, the injured eye should be irrigated before completing a complete eye examination.*
- Assess visual acuity, peripheral vision and ocular movements: be sure to measure acuity in each eye individually (cover each eye well) and both eyes together. Note if there is an eye preference or if the child objects to the covering of one eye over the other.

Toys/bright objects can be used ('look for the toy') as an aid to the assessment of ocular movements and peripheral vision.

- Examine external eye structures, including the lid and orbital area. Note any swelling, lacerations, discoloration, crepitus, debris and/or discharge. Remove debris, discharge, etc., using warm water or saline irrigation.
- Examine conjunctival and corneal surfaces: note clarity, injection, haemorrhages, size, shape and response of pupils to light. If pupils demonstrate anisocoria, check under dim illumination to note whether the size difference of the pupil changes (change = abnormal, no change = normal variant). Check for irregularities in the *shape* of the pupil and iris. An irregularly shaped pupil may indicate damage to the iris or perforation of the globe.
- Assess the fundus and ocular components (including documentation of red reflex).
- Fluorescein staining is used to highlight any damaged corneal epithelial cells, such as in corneal abrasion. It also outlines any abrasions of the conjunctiva. To perform, use a single use Minim to instill a drop or a fluorescein-impregnated paper strip touched to the inferior canthus while the patient looks upward; then have the patient blink once. Any damage to the corneal epithelium will 'light up' a bright yellow colour. The colour is intensified by using the cobalt blue light on the ophthalmoscope (a slit lamp can also be use if available). Document the location and size of the epithelial defect (extremely helpful for future assessment of healing).

Table 10.2	Common Findings in Ocular Injuries
Type of ocular injury	*Findings*
Corneal abrasion	• Mild to sharp/severe pain with foreign body sensation, photophobia, tearing and redness • Fluorescein stain 'lights up' in the traumatised area, conjunctival injection, eyelid oedema
Chemical burn Conjunctival ischaemia Conjunctival blanching Vessel attenuation	• Ocular pain and burning • Epithelial defects 'light up' on fluorescein stain (may range from mild defects to corneal opacity), hyperaemia, mild eyelid oedema, burns of the periocular skin, abnormal pH
Ultraviolet light injury	• Ocular pain and photophobia • Fluorescein stain 'lights up' a diffuse punctate stain, injected eye, tearing and discomfort
Foreign body/perforation	• Foreign body sensation, pain, tearing, decreased vision (with intraocular foreign body) • Visualisation of foreign body on cornea or conjunctiva, may have vertical lines that 'light up' with fluorescein, differentiate a foreign body under the upper lid from an object dragged across cornea by the lid • Conjunctival injection, eyelid oedema • Sharp trauma to the cornea may show drainage of aqueous fluid (illuminated with fluorescein) or an irregular pupil
Conjunctival laceration	• Mild pain, foreign body sensation, red eye • Under white light and fluorescein staining, conjunctiva may appear to be rolled up on itself
Traumatic uveitis (iritis)	• Dull aching/throbbing pain, photophobia, tearing • Perilimbal injection, pain in traumatised eye when light is shone in either the non-traumatised or traumatised eye, small or large pupil sometimes decreased vision
Hyphaema	• Pain, blurred vision • Loss of red reflex, presence of haemorrhage in front of iris
Ruptured globe (sclera or cornea is disrupted)	• Pain, decreased vision • Dark spot on the sclera (may indicate uveal prolapse), oval-shaped pupil
Intraocular haemorrhages	• If retinal haemorrhages only, no symptoms • Retinal haemorrhages on fundoscopy
Orbital fracture	• Pain (especially on attempted vertical eye movement), local tenderness, binocular double vision, eyelid swelling, crepitus after nose blowing • Inability to look upward or lateral direction, point tenderness, crepitus, orbital oedema • Enophthalmos

DIFFERENTIAL DIAGNOSES

- The cause of the ocular injury is often apparent from the patient's history. However, infection should be ruled out (see Sec. 10.3) and non-accidental injury (NAI) should be considered as a possibility in children and adolescents presenting with traumatic eye injuries. In addition consider trauma complicated by infection, hordeolum, chalazion, dacryocystitis, herpes simplex keratitis (fluorescein stain illuminates lesion with a dendritic pattern), refractive error, orbital tumour, referred pain (e.g. sinusitis, tooth abscess) and glaucoma.

⊕ MANAGEMENT

- **Additional diagnostics:** with the exception of tests of visual acuity and fluorescein staining, any other tests require referral to ophthalmology.

- **Pharmacotherapeutics:** dependent on the specific ocular injury (Table 10.3). However, for the majority of eye trauma managed by NPs, pain can be controlled with oral analgesics and non-steroidal anti-inflammatory drug (NSAID) ophthalmic drops. Note that anaesthetic eye drops should only be used to facilitate the initial eye examination (and never for pain relief post-injury) as they will inhibit re-epithelialisation of the cornea. If their use is prolonged, further damage will result to the cornea. Any loss of corneal epithelium gives a route for pathogen ingress which may lead to corneal or intraocular infection. All corneal epithelial loss should be treated prophylactically with a broad-spectrum topical antibiotic.

- **Behavioural interventions:** aetiology-specific (see Table 10.3).

- **Patient education:** review with all families the medications to be

Table 10.3	Management of Ocular Trauma			
Type of injury	Behavioural interventions and pharmacotherapeutics	Follow-up	Ophthalmology referral	Comments
Corneal abrasion	• Fluorescein stain (with documentation of result) • Cycloplegic agent not typically used in young children; pain control can usually be achieved with ophthalmic non-steroidal anti-inflammatory (NSAID) such as diclofenac (Voltarol) or ketorolac (Acular). Note, however, these drugs are not licensed for use in children • Apply generous amount of broad-spectrum antibiotic ointment (chloramphenicol) • No patching required • Continue ointment four times daily for 5 days • Discontinue contact lens use until at least 1 week after completely healed	• Follow-up in 24 hours to assure abrasion has healed/decreased in size • Usually no further follow-up required if first 24 hours were uncomplicated; children usually heal quickly	• Abrasions not showing signs of healing within 24 hours • Increase or worsening of symptoms • Any abrasion due to contact lens use	• Antibiotic ointment generally preferred because it offers a better barrier function between eyelid and abrasion • Research has shown no benefit to patching and in young children may increase the risk of amblyopia development • Most corneal abrasions heal within 3 days • Use of cycloplegic agent among young children increases the possibility of amblyopia (even in 24 hours) Cycloplegic may be used in management of uveitis
Chemical burn	• Immediate irrigation with normal saline • Evert lid and irrigate underneath. Consider irrigating eye from medial to lateral aspect of eye • After 5–10 min of irrigation, check pH with litmus paper. Continue irrigation until pH reaches 6.8–7.5 (this may take 1–2 litres of fluid), then refer immediately • Do not delay referral to ophthalmology • Medication (antibiotics, steroids, cycloplegic, etc., as per ophthalmology) • Systemic pain medicine as needed	• As per ophthalmology	• Immediate referral	• Immediate (and copious) irrigation is vital • Bottled water or tap water may be used if no other fluids available • Helpful to set up intravenous (IV) tubing (without needle) and continuously irrigate with this apparatus
Ultraviolet light injury	• Fluorescein stain • If positive findings: apply drop of cycloplegic agent and provide systemic pain relief and ketorolac (Acular) NSAID ophthalmic drops. Note not licensed for use in children • Avoidance of sun, use of sunglasses, hat	• If symptoms settle, no further follow-up required	• If fluorescein stain reveals lesion → chloramphenicol ophthalmic drops or ointment • Ophthamology referral if no resolution within 24 hours	• Follow-up if no improvement in 24–48 hours • Importance of prevention (i.e. sun safety) reinforced, especially use of sunglasses when sun reflecting on snow or water; use of protective goggles with sun beds/lamps, etc. • If corneal injury, erosions will always be present

(continued)

Table 10.3 *continued*				
Type of injury	Behavioural interventions and pharmacotherapeutics	Follow-up	Ophthalmology referral	Comments
Foreign body of the cornea or conjunctiva	• Apply anaesthetic drop • If foreign body is visible, remove first then fluorescein stain • If foreign body is not visible, fluorescein stain first to help locate • Saline irrigation and/or gentle swabbing with a sterile swab dipped in saline • Irrigate with normal saline • If these two techniques do not work, refer to ophthalmology • Sweep conjunctival fornices with the sterile swab dipped in saline • Treat any corneal abrasions • If no corneal abrasion, apply antibiotic ointment single time • Artificial tears may be used every few hours for the irritated eye • Update tetanus vaccination as needed	• If symptoms settle, no further follow-up required • If corneal abrasion present, follow-up in 24 hours (as indicated for corneal abrasion)	• Refer if unable to remove superficial foreign body with techniques described	• Foreign body sensation expected for first 24 hours, if sensation continues for >24 hours, repeat examination and/or refer to ophthalmology • Eyelid eversion may be needed to remove foreign bodies—if vertical lines light up on fluorescein staining, look for foreign body under upper lid • If foreign body is metallic—a rust ring will often remain. Leave ring alone for 18 to 36 hours, refer to ophthalmology for removal (as it may require special instrumentation)
Corneal foreign body with penetrating trauma	• Do not irrigate • Guard eye and refer immediately • Update tetanus vaccination as needed	• As per ophthalmology	• Immediate referral for penetrating foreign bodies	• Importance of prevention reinforced
Lid laceration	• Control bleeding and refer immediately • Lid lacerations require meticulous repair to preserve anatomical and physiological function • Update tetanus vaccination as needed	• As per ophthalmology	• Immediate referral	• Importance of prevention reinforced
Traumatic uveitis (iritis)	• Refer immediately to ophthalmology (for dilated fundus exam); measurement of intraocular pressures (IOP); and treatment with cycloplegic agent plus steroid	• As per ophthalmology	• Immediate referral	• Importance of prevention reinforced
Hyphaema	• Keep patient calm and upright • Not usually admitted; discharged home to rest • Refer immediately to ophthalmology for treatment and/or evaluation of concurrent injuries	• As per ophthalmology	• Immediate referral	• Importance of prevention reinforced
Ruptured globe Penetrating injuries (treat as if ruptured globe)	• Place a rigid eye shield over eye (a trimmed Styrofoam cup or gallipot works well) • Maintain head of patient 45 degrees • Update tetanus vaccination as needed • Refer immediately	• As per ophthalmology	• Immediate referral	• Discuss prevention (if appropriate)
Intraocular haemorrhage	• If child abuse suspected, refer to ophthalmology for fundoscopic exam with eyes dilated. Note that retinal haemorrhages in infants should always trigger initiation of the child protection pathway; they are a child protection issue until proven otherwise • Initiate child protection pathways as appropriate	• As per ophthalmology	• Referral for fundoscopic examination	• Consider non-accidental injury (especially in young children and infants)
Orbital fracture	• Update tetanus vaccination as needed • Request that patient does not blow nose • Refer immediately	• As per ophthalmology	• Immediate referral	

used for home management, signs and symptoms of problems and the plan for follow-up care. In addition, promotion of eye safety and prevention of eye trauma should be reviewed. More specifically:

• Play should be supervised and sharp objects, pellet guns, air guns, etc., should not be used as toys.

• Extreme caution, avoidance or restricted use of fireworks such as sparklers.

• Use of protective eye wear in sports (or activities) where there is greater potential for injury. This includes use of safety glasses in classrooms such as woodworking and chemistry.

- Mandatory eye wear in sports for children with one functioning eye or recent ocular surgery.
- Familiarity with use of eyewash fountains in schools.
- Appropriate storage of strong alkalines such as caustic soda, oven cleaner, cement, mortar, plaster and household cleaners.
- Appropriate cleaning and wear of contacts lenses as well as annual eye examinations to check fit and condition of lenses.

⇨ FOLLOW-UP

- Dependent on the specific injury involved (Table 10.3) and at the discretion of ophthalmology. However, in general (and regardless of the aetiology of the injury), there should be improvement in pain and symptoms on a daily basis. If there is not (or if the symptoms become worse), an emergency re-assessment and/or ophthalmology referral are required.

⮂ MEDICAL CONSULT/ SPECIALIST REFERRAL

- Any child with significant symptomatology or traumatic injury.
- Any child with foreign body sensation for >24 hours.

- Any child without improvement in symptomatology within 24 hours.
- Any child with a corneal ulcer, chemical burn, penetrating trauma, orbital fracture, lid laceration, traumatic iritis, hyphaema or ruptured globe (Table 10.3).

⊙ PAEDIATRIC PEARLS

- Maintain an 'eye box' complete with anaesthetic ophthalmic drops, cycloplegic agents, antibiotic ointment and drops, indicator paper, fluorescein strips or drops, normal saline, eye shields, intravenous (IV) tubing, etc. This greatly facilitates an efficient, accurate eye examination and treatment.
- Patching is no longer the standard recommendation in the treatment of corneal abrasion (however, some cases may require patching by an ophthalmologist).
- Never prescribe anaesthetic drops— this will inhibit re-epithelialisation of the cornea.
- To instil ophthalmic drops in an uncooperative child, hold child tightly, pull lower lid down gently and instil drops into fornix or onto exposed globe. Alternatively, lie the child on his back and instil drops onto closed lids and ask him to blink (this will not work for ointment instillation).
- Consider an age-appropriate dose of chlorpheniramine, paracetamol or ibuprofen if child is unable to sleep.

- Retinal haemorrhages in infants should always trigger initiation of a child protection pathway; they are child protection-related until proven otherwise.

⊟ BIBLIOGRAPHY

Cheng H, Burdon MA, Buckley S, et al. Emergency ophthalmology. London: BMJ; 1997.

Coody D, Banks JM, Yetman RJ, Musgrove K. Eye trauma in children: epidemiology, management, and prevention. J Pediatr Health Care 1997; 11:182–188.

Flynn CA, D'Amico F, Smith G. Should we patch corneal abrasions? A meta-analysis. J Fam Practice 1998; 47(4):264–270.

Forbes B. The management of corneal abrasions and ocular trauma in children. Pediatr Ann 2001; 30(8):465–472.

Levin AV. Eye emergencies: acute management in the pediatric ambulatory care setting. Pediatr Emerg Care 1991; 7(6):367–377.

Marsden J. Ophthalmic emergencies. In: Dolan B, Holt L, eds, Accident and emergency: theory into practice. London: Ballière Tindall; 2000.

Marsden J. Treating corneal trauma. Emerg Nurse 2001; 9(8):17–20.

Rhee DJ, Pyfer MF. The Wills eye manual: office and emergency room diagnosis and treatment of eye disease, 3rd edn. Philadelphia: Lippincott, Williams & Wilkins; 1999.

Tingley DH. Eye trauma: corneal abrasions. Pediatr Rev 1999; 20(9):320–322.

Wingate S. Treating corneal abrasions. Nurse Pract 1999; 24(6):53–68.

10.3 THE 'RED EYE'

Judy Honig and Janet Marsden

▭ INTRODUCTION

- The 'red eye' refers to a variety of infectious and inflammatory ocular conditions. It is a very common ocular problem seen and treated in primary care. Although it is usually self-limiting and benign, it is important to identify

the likely aetiology of the red eye and determine if the condition warrants further evaluation and/or management.

- A diagnostic priority is to determine which ocular structure(s) are involved, as the differential diagnosis is largely determined by the sites involved (while

considering developmental influences such as age).

- As such, the objectives of the history, physical and management plan include (1) assessment of the acuity and severity of the problem; (2) appropriate (and timely) ophthamological referral (this is especially relevant among patients with prolonged symptoms of a non-emergent nature, as the referral of emergent conditions is usually readily apparent); and (3) maintenance of optimal visual functioning through adequate follow-up.

PATHOPHYSIOLOGY

- Pathophysiology is aetiology-specific. However, inflammation of the conjunctiva is by far the most common cause of red eyes. It is defined as hyperaemia of the bulbar and/or palpebral conjunctiva (mucous membranes covering the front part of the eyeball) and may be associated with inflammation of the episclera or sclera, the cornea, eyelid and (occasionally) deeper structures.
- Corneal ulceration, which also results in a red eye, affects the outer layers of the cornea and into the stroma (the third of the cornea's five layers). Corneal ulceration is commonly the result of pathogenic invasion (bacteria, virus or other) or may be the result of an autoimmune response.
- Note that the anatomy of the eye can be found in Figs 10.2 and 10.3 (see Sec. 10.2).

HISTORY

- Onset, duration and severity (including age at onset of problem).
- History of trauma (see Sec. 10.2).
- Detailed description of any discharge, including amount and appearance (profuse/scant, watery/mucopurulent, stringy/crusting, etc.).
- Systemic symptoms or recent history of infection (e.g. URTI, fever, chills, neck/joint pain, rashes, ear pain, sore throat, sneezing, etc.).
- Musculoskeletal complaints.
- Visual problems, including photophobia and blurry vision.
- Complaints of scratchiness or burning under the eyelids (especially common to have complaints of 'grittiness' with conjunctivitis).
- Foreign body sensation.
- Pain or tenderness in and around the eye.
- Use of contact lenses.

- Use of home treatments/self-management.
- Current medications.
- Exposure to chemicals, irritants and/or infections (e.g. herpes simplex).
- Exposure to others (family, classmates, daycare or nursery attendance) with the same symptoms.
- Is the red eye a recurring and/or seasonal condition.
- Family history of allergy or atopy.

PHYSICAL EXAMINATION

- **General appearance of the child:** this includes vital signs, activity level, allergic facies, obvious trauma, head lice, etc.

- **Head and ear, nose and throat (ENT):**
  - *Eyes:* careful examination to assess unilateral or bilateral involvement; oedema of the orbital/periorbital area, conjunctiva, eyelids or other structures (evert eyelid); redness/pinkness of conjunctiva (bulbar and palpebral), including the texture (e.g. 'bumpiness' of conjunctivae is associated with viral or allergic conjunctivitis); discharge (type, consistency, colour); pupillary function, ocular movements, visual acuity and fields of vision. Fluorescein staining can be used to assess the cornea (see Additional diagnostics). Be sure to note any pain; lesions/vesicles on the face, eyelids, and mucous membranes; tearing and/or foreign body sensations (evert eyelid). Note that subconjunctival haemorrhage is associated with *Haemophilus influenzae* and *Streptococcus pneumoniae* infections.
  - *Ears:* colour, opacity, landmarks, light reflex and mobility of the tympanic membrane. Note presence/absence of fluid behind drum.
  - *Nose:* colour and consistency of turbinates (grey, dull, swollen/boggy turbinates indicative of allergic disease); patency of nares and any nasal discharge.
  - *Throat/mouth:* hydration status, lesions, tonsils (colour, presence of

exudate, size) and condition of teeth. Also note cracked/peeling or bleeding lips and/or mucous membranes.

- **Lymph:** presence of cervical lymphadenopathy (especially preauricular and cervical adenopathy).

- **Routine cardiovascular, respiratory, abdominal and musculoskeletal examination.** Note any abnormalities, including painful joints.

DIFFERENTIAL DIAGNOSES

- The most common cause of a red eye is bacterial, viral, allergic or chemical/irritant conjunctivitis. However, given the non-specificity of the complaint 'my child's eye is red', it is important to think broadly with regard to potential aetiologies. Likewise, it is important to identify cases that require specialist intervention and/or immediate attention. An expanded list of conditions that can present with a red eye are outlined in Table 10.4.
- Note that it is important to consider the age of the child and associated epidemiology (season, exposures, temporal factors, etc.) when evaluating the complaint of a red eye.
- Always include Kawasaki's disease on the differential list especially when the red eye is accompanied by systemic symptoms (lymphadenopathy, desquamating or erythematous extremities, prolonged elevated temperature and mucous membrane involvement). Juvenile rheumatoid arthritis (JRA) may also present as intraocular inflammation. Early diagnosis has important implications for treatment, prognosis and morbidity.
- Likewise, consider the possibility of JRA if there has been prolonged ocular inflammation and complaints of achiness and/or painful joints (the chronic uveitis associated with JRA can easily be misdiagnosed as conjunctivitis).

MANAGEMENT

Largely aetiology-specific; however, general principles in management of the

Table 10.4 Differential Diagnosis of the Red Eye

Area of redness and/or involvement	Consider
Ocular adnexa	• *Infection:* hordeolum and chalazion, congenital blocked nasolacrimal duct, blepharitis, lice infestation, sinus infection, orbital/periorbital cellulitis, dental abscess, contact dermatitis, seborrhoea • *Trauma:* frequent eye rubbing, blunt trauma • *Tumours:* neuroblastoma, leukaemia, neurofibroma, orbital tumours • *Other:* prolonged crying, cavernous sinus thrombosis
Conjunctiva	• *Infection:* viral, bacterial or parasitic infection • *Tumours:* as above • *Toxic/environmental/drugs:* atropine, scopolamine, smoke/dust/pollen, make-up, contact lenses, chemical exposure • *Allergy/inflammatory:* allergic conjunctivitis, keratoconjunctivitis sicca (dry eye), nasal inflammation, collagen vascular diseases, Kawasaki syndrome, inflammatory bowel disease, Stevens–Johnson syndrome, juvenile rheumatoid arthritis (uveitis) • *Other:* subconjunctival haemorrhage (secondary to cough, vomiting, bacteraemia or blood dyscrasias)
Corneal involvement and conjunctival redness	• *Infection:* keratitis • *Trauma:* contact lenses, corneal ulcer/abrasion, chemical irritant
Pupil distortion with conjuctival redness	• *Trauma:* hyphaema or perforation • *Inflammation:* uveitis (will also have pupil miosis with reduced vision in one or both eyes)

red eye are outlined below and management of common causes of conjunctivitis in children are outlined in Table 10.5.

- **Additional diagnostics:** conjunctivitis in the neonate should be cultured (with appropriate technique and medium) to rule out gonorrhoea, chlamydia, herpes or other organisms acquired during birth. Note that a sticky eye in an infant less than 21 days old is a reportable disease and the appropriate notification forms should be completed and sent to the local public health medicine department. In older children, consider culture only if an unusual or serious pathogen is suspected (i.e. conjunctivitis in contact lens wearer). Purulent conjunctivitis in an infant with blocked nasolacrimal duct is unlikely to require culture, unless the infection does not clear with topical antibiotics (see Sec. 10.1). Use fluorescein staining with a slit lamp, pen torch with cobalt blue filter or ophthalmoscope if corneal involvement is suspected; this is especially important if there is associated ocular pain or foreign body sensation: see also Section 10.2. If preseptal or orbital cellulitis is suspected, blood cultures and a swab of the discharge should be obtained.

Computed tomography (CT) should be considered when orbital cellulitis or neoplasm are under consideration.

- **Pharmacotherapeutics:** Aetiology-specific; note, however, that if antibiotics are used they should be continued for 48 hours after the symptoms have resolved. Note that ophthalmic steroid preparations should not be used except under specialist care. Likewise, topical anaesthetics should never be used (except for the initial examination after corneal injury) as they delay healing time, can mask further damage and can lead to further corneal damage (see Sec. 10.2).

- **Behavioural interventions** (for conjunctivitis):
  - Careful handwashing before and after cleansing of eye area and administration of medication.
  - Cleanse crusted drainage on lids and lashes with cotton wool ball (or tissue) moistened with cooled, boiled water; wipe from the inside of the eyelid (by the nose) towards the outside; single cotton ball for each wipe on each eye.
  - Do not share pillowcases; wash clothes or towels.
  - Cool compresses to eye can provide symptomatic relief as can paracetamol

or ibuprofen if there is pain associated with the acute infection.
  - Be sure parents can get drops into the child's eyes. If struggling to get eye drops in, position child on his back with eyes closed; place eye drops on lid junction and then have him open his eyes. An opportunity for instillation of medication may be taken when the child is asleep by moving one of the lids gently and dropping the preparation onto the globe.
  - For eye ointment, run a ribbon of ointment along the inside of the lower lid and then have the child shut his eyes to spread the ointment over the globe.

- **Patient education:**
  - Review behavioural interventions (above) and stress with parent the importance of infection control (handwashing, no sharing of towels, etc.).
  - In general, the child can return to school or nursery 24–48 hours after antibiotic treatment is initiated (and if discharge has subsided).
  - Viral conjunctivitis often lasts up to 3 weeks, but secondary bacterial infection is common. Stress with parents the importance of returning or telephoning if there is no improvement or if things deteriorate.

⇨ FOLLOW-UP

- Generally none is necessary if the red eye resolves spontaneously or with treatment.
- Return for further evaluation/treatment if no improvement or deterioration of condition occurs.
- If, after initial improvement, the red eye returns, this may signal an adverse reaction to the medication. Discontinue medication and return to clinic. If no improvement after 7–10 days, refer.

⇄ MEDICAL CONSULT/ SPECIALIST REFERRAL

- Any child with a loss of, or a decrease in visual acuity.

Table 10.5	Common Causes of a Red Eye in Infants and Children			
Condition	Potential causes	Common findings	Treatment	Comments
Conjunctivitis (bacterial)	• *Haemophilus influenzae* • *Streptococcus pneumoniae* • *Neisseria gonorrhoeae* (uncommon but serious) • *Chlamydia trachomatis*	• Abrupt onset in one eye, often spreads to the other within 24–48 hours • Complaints of 'gritty' feeling in eyes • Mucopurulent drainage • Diffuse conjunctival erythema and oedema (chemosis) • Photophobia • Normal vision • Pupils are equal, round and reactive to light • Cornea is clear • Chlamydial infection in the newborn characteristically presents between 5 and 14 days after birth and has a sticky, watery and profuse discharge • Gonococcal conjunctivitis is characterised by marked oedema of the lids, with pain and copious purulent discharge; the swelling and discharge may be so significant that the eye is difficult to see	• Broad-spectrum ophthalmic antibiotic drops (chloramphenicol or fucidic acid) applied topically and frequently (e.g 2-hourly, especially during the first 24–48 hours; less often if fucidic acid as this is normally a twice a day formulation) • Continue treatment 24–48 hours after redness and discharge have resolved (usually 5–7 days) • Treat concurrent otitis media with systemic oral antibiotics • Suspected gonococcal infection requires immediate referral • Chlamydia infection will require systemic antibiotics and likely treatment of parents	• Can be accompanied by otitis media (conjunctivitis-otitis syndrome) • Careful handwashing and infection control measures • Symptoms in the newborn require referral, Department of Health reporting and (usually) treatment of parents • Reinforce with parents appropriate infection control measures (careful handwashing and no sharing of linens) • Discharge on lids and lashes can be removed with cooled, boiled water and cotton wool or tissues • Always treat both eyes with drops
Conjunctivitis (viral)	• Adenovirus is the most common • Herpes simplex • Varicella-zoster • Coxsackie virus	• Conjunctival hyperaemia and oedema with inflamed lymphoid tissue of membranes covering lids appearing as 'bumps' when eyelids everted • Complaints of 'gritty' feeling in eyes • Milky or watery drainage with less purulence (usually) than bacterial infections, but there may be more crusting (related to more serous drainage), especially in the morning • Often increased tearing but complaints of 'dryness'; the tears while profuse dry up quickly and, as such, the eye produces an increased quantity of watery discharge • May be punctate erosions of cornea when stained with fluorescein • Preauricular and submandibular lymphadenopathy is common (especially with pharyngoconjunctival fever) • Vision and pupils are normal • No photophobia (herpetic infection excepted)	• Treat as bacterial if uncertainty exists as to aetiology or if discharge is particularly sticky • If herpetic infection suspected, refer immediately • Adenoviral conjunctivitis is not responsive to treatment, and comfort should be maintained with the frequent use of artificial tears	• Difficult to distinguish adenovirus infection from bacterial infection • Adenoviral conjunctivitis may last 3–4 weeks and is highly contagious (frequent handwashing is imperative) • Concurrent pharyngitis or upper respiratory tract infection (URTI) (with negative group A β-haemolytic strep swab) is often diagnostic clue to viral aetiology (e.g. pharyngoconjunctival fever). Most commonly due to adenovirus infection and may be accompanied by systemic flu-like symptoms. Identification of adenovirus by polymerase chain reaction (PCR) test is very fast • Culture recovery of herpes virus is only successful in approx. 70% of cases
Conjunctivitis (allergic)	• Immunoglobulin E (IgE) mediated hypersensitivity • Exposure to seasonal (e.g. pollens) or other allergens (e.g. animal dander, smoke, moulds) • Contact lens allergy	• Conjunctival oedema with inflammation varying from pink to red • Often a 'bumpy' or 'cobblestone' appearance to palpebral conjunctivae • Can be unilateral or bilateral • Watery, stringy, mucoid drainage • Associated rhinitis, nasal congestion and pruritus • Seasonal • Vision and pupils normal	• Acute allergy with very oedematous conjunctiva; will settle quickly with supportive care • Cool compresses • Artificial tears/wetting solution • Remove offending allergen • Oral or topical antihistamine • Topical mast cell stabiliser • Topical steroid for specialist use only	• Consider season • Often history of atopy in family or child • Consider if just started with contact lens wear

(continued)

Table 10.5	continued			
Condition	Potential causes	Common findings	Treatment	Comments
Uveitis	• Inflammatory process often related to systemic disease	• Deep red inflammation • Dull iris colour • Pain in and around eye • Reduction in vision • Perhaps smaller, sluggish pupil in affected eye	• Immediate ophthalmology referral	• Usually treated with mydriatics and steroids • Systemic investigations will be commenced and appropriate referral made by ophthalmologists
Corneal ulcer	• Usually related to infectious process (viral or bacterial infection) • Three main types seen in ambulatory care: bacterial, marginal and dendritic	• Fluorescein stain will identify extent of lesion(s); however, often difficult to distinguish between the three main types • Cornea will have an area(s) of white or greyish opacity; it will not appear clear • Underlying corneal infiltrate will show up as a white spot, haze or opacity of the cornea. The borders of the affected area may look as if they are slightly heaped up • Complaints of pain, foreign body sensation tearing and (often) photophobia • Will likewise have concomitant conjunctivitis and possibly swollen lids	• Immediate ophthalmology referral • Antibiotics or antiviral treatment usually started after lesions scraped and Gram-stained • Follow-up as per ophthalmology	• Corneal ulcers with a lower threshold for ophthalmology referral than corneal abrasions • Delay in treatment of an infected ulcer can result in devastating intraocular infection • Discontinue contact lens use until ulcer completely healed (if applicable)

- Any child with an abnormal pupil and/or severe ocular pain.
- Any child with suspected herpetic (including varicella) or gonococcal conjunctivitis, periorbital/orbital cellulitis and/or foreign body.
- Any neonate with conjunctivitis or young child with marked conjunctivitis as they are at greater risk of orbital cellulitis due to their lack of a formed septum.
- Any contact lens wearer with marked pain and/or conjunctivitis (due to the unusual organisms that may be involved).
- Any child with corneal abrasion, corneal ulcer and/or pain for longer than 24 hours.
- Any child with a corneal opacity.
- Any child in whom the diagnosis is unclear or the red eye continues for a prolonged period (consider Kawasaki's disease, JRA or malignancy).

🔘 PAEDIATRIC PEARLS

- Straightforward conjunctivitis will not decrease visual acuity or result in pupillary involvement. If present on physical examination, these findings should prompt immediate consultation and/or referral.

- Thick, profuse and purulent discharge with foreign body sensation and eyes crusted shut with discharge is suggestive of bacterial conjunctivitis. Serous or lightly purulent discharge with profuse tearing is associated with viral infection. Bacterial conjunctivitis is, by far, the most common cause of a red eye in children. However, due to the increased risk of secondary bacterial infection in viral conjunctivitis, treatment of both infections is usually the same: broad-spectrum antibiotics with periodic removal of discharge. There should be improvement within 3–4 days with bacterial conjunctivitis and 2–3 weeks with a viral infection.
- Conjunctivitis in the neonate requires aggressive evaluation and treatment. Significant, sticky, watery conjunctivitis appearing in the newborn 5–14 days after birth is likely to be chlamydia infection. It will require systemic antibiotics, treatment of the parents and reporting to the public health department.
- Conjunctivitis accompanied by clusters of vesicles on face, eyelids and mucous membranes is indicative of herpetic infection (including varicella) and requires referral.
- Swelling of lids with erythema, diffuse conjunctival hyperaemia with a

'cobblestone' appearance, itchiness and rhinitis are often associated with allergic conjunctivitis. In addition, a cold compress over red eyes that results in resolution of erythema is a diagnostic clue indicative of allergic conjunctivitis. Large 'cobblestones' should be referred to an ophthalmologist, as control of symptoms may require the use of topical steroids.
- Corneal ulcers often present as a 'red eye' without a history of trauma and they are usually due to a viral or bacterial infection. As such, a low threshold for fluorescein staining will decrease the possibility of a missed diagnosis, which can result in a devasting intraocular infection.
- *Haemophilus influenzae* and *Streptococcus pneumoniae* infection are associated with subconjunctival haemorrhage.
- Consider Kawasaki's disease with bilateral red eyes, non-purulent drainage and systemic symptoms.
- Chronic uveitis is associated with pauciarticular JRA (involvement of less than five joints) and can be misdiagnosed as conjunctivitis. Although it is uncommon, it can lead to a loss of vision if not detected early. Note that uveitis is also known as iridocyclitis and iritis.

- Head lice that involve eyelashes can be treated by coating the eyelashes with petroleum jelly for a 12-hour period (see Sec. 9.12). In addition, consider the possibility of pubic lice in lashes (which will require referral).
- Children with recurrent styes (hordeola) can benefit from daily washing of eyelids with baby shampoo (diluted with water) to reduce bacterial growth. In addition, recurrent styes can be associated with increased glucose levels; consider checking urine.

📚 BIBLIOGRAPHY

Bertolini J, Pelucio M. The red eye. Emerg Med Clin N Am 1995; 13(3):561–579.

Dershewitz RA. Ambulatory pediatric care, 3rd edn. Philadelphia: Lippincott-Raven; 1998.

Gioliotti F. Acute conjunctivitis. Pediatr Rev 1995; 16(6):203–208.

Hoekelman RA, Friedman SB, Seidle HM, et al. Pediatric primary care. St. Louis: Mosby; 1997.

King R. Common ocular signs and symptoms in childhood. Pediatr Clin North Am 1993; 40:753–766.

Leibowitz HM. The red eye. New Engl J Med 2000; 343(5):345–351.

Marsden J. Identifying and managing non traumatic red eye in A&E. Emerg Nurse 1998; 5(9):34–40.

Marsden J. Systematic eye examination in A&E. Emerg Nurse 1998; 6(6):16–19.

Marsden J. Ophthalmic emergencies. In: Dolan B, Holt L, eds, Accident and emergency: theory into practice. London: Ballière Tindall; 2000.

Wagner RS. Eye infections and abnormalities: issues for the pediatrician. Contemp Pediatr 1997; 14(6):137–153.

10.4 COMMON ORAL LESIONS

Kelly A. Barnes and Thomas R. Ollerhead

📖 INTRODUCTION

- The NP may be the first health care professional to encounter an oral lesion in an infant, child or adolescent.
- Many of these lesions are benign, self-limiting and will not require treatment. However, it is important that the NP is familiar with the more common lesions and that she is able to determine the need for referral and follow-up of the less common (or less benign lesions).
- The incidence of individual lesions varies. Some lesions are so common that they are considered a normal developmental variant (e.g. geographic tongue or palatal cysts), whereas others will require specialist intervention and management (e.g. parulis).
- A glossary of dental definitions can be found in Table 10.6 and commonly encountered oral lesions are outlined in Table 10.7. Important anatomy of the tooth is illustrated in Figure 10.4.

🦷 PATHOPHYSIOLOGY

- Lesion specific (see Table 10.6).

Table 10.6	Glossary of Dental Terms
Term	Definition
Alveolar bone	• The bone of the maxilla and mandible which contains the teeth
Alveolar process	• If you were speaking about one arch, it would be the alveolar process of the maxilla or mandible
Alveolar mucosa	• The lining epithelium of the oral cavity
Alveolar ridge	• The ridge of bone where the teeth sit
Alveolar socket	• The socket is where the root of a tooth is housed within the alveolar bone
Alveolus	• A general term for alveolar bone
Ankylosis	• The cementum of the root is fused with alveolar bone, as such, the periodontal ligament space is absent in this condition
Anterior tongue	• The most forward aspect of the tongue
Apices	• The end of the root
Avulsion	• When a tooth is knocked completely out of the mouth
Buccal mucosa	• The lining mucosa of the oral mucosa on the side of the cheek
Carious	• Decay of the tooth's enamel and/or dentin
Carious communication	• Decay has progressed through the outer enamel into the dentin and entered the pulp chamber of the tooth. The pulp is normally a sterile environment, and when bacteria that cause decay enters this tissue, the stage is set for infection and abscess formation, be it acute or chronic

(continued)

Table 10.6 *continued*	
Crown	• That portion of the tooth which is seen in the oral cavity
Dorsal tongue	• The keratinised surface of the tongue (the taste buds are located on the dorsal aspect)
Eruption	• A tooth that emerges from the alveolar process to erupt through the soft tissue into the oral cavity
Exfoliation	• Primary (baby) teeth are lost when the permanent successors cause the resorption of the primary tooth roots
Intrusion	• A tooth that is forced inward into the alveolar process. This type of injury forces the periodontal ligament space to be compressed
Floor of the mouth	• The area under the tongue
Lateral luxation	• An injury to a tooth, whereby the tooth is moved in a lateral direction within the socket
Lingual	• Towards the tongue or having to do with the tongue
Lower anterior teeth	• The four incisors make up the four teeth in the anterior part of the mouth
Masticatory trauma	• Trauma sustained during mastication (eating)
Mucobuccal fold	• The fold of tissue within the oral cavity that makes up the vestible towards the lips or cheeks
Mucogingival junction	• The area where the keratinised gingiva (that surrounds the teeth) meets the soft, freely moveable, non-keratinised mucosa of the oral cavity
Occlude	• The action of bringing the teeth together into maximum contact (i.e. biting together)
Occlusal surface	• The chewing surface of the teeth, where the cusps and fossa are located
Periodontal structure	• The periodontium consists of the alveolar bone, cementum and the periodontal ligament. It is a general term for the collective support of the teeth
Primary dentition	• Baby teeth (milk teeth)
Pulp	• The nerve and blood supply of the tooth. It is this tissue which gives a tooth its vitality
Replantation	• When a tooth is avulsed (knocked out of the mouth) it can be replanted if it meets replantation criteria (see Sec. 10.5)
Root	• That area of the tooth that can usually only be visualised by a radiograph in a healthy dentition
Secondary dentition	• Permanent teeth
Subluxation	• An injury to a tooth whereby abnormal loosening occurs
Tooth germ	• The embryological structure where a tooth develops from
Upper anterior teeth	• The four upper incisors (laterals and centrals) make up the upper anteriors
Ventral tongue	• The underside of the tongue. Covered by vascular non-keratinised lining epithelium
Vermillion border	• Where the skin of the lips meets the skin of the face. It marks the transitional zone between internal mucous membrane and external skin

Table 10.7 **Common Oral Lesions**		
Lesion	Definition and appearance	Comments
Congenital lesions		
Palatal cysts	• Small keratin-filled developmental cysts • 1–3 mm in diameter and white or yellowish in colour • Usually occur in clusters of 2–6, although they can be singular • Appear most often along the midline of the palate near the junction of the hard and soft palates • May also occur more anteriorly along the midline or on the posterior palate, lateral to the midline	• Common in newborns • No treatment necessary (cysts are self-limiting and often resolve several weeks after birth)
Leukoedema	• Diffuse, greyish-white coloration of the buccal mucosa • Surface texture may appear wrinkled or thickened • Lesions are usually bilateral and will not 'rub off' • Stretching of the cheek skin greatly diminishes the appearance of the lesion (or causes it to disappear); this is diagnostic for the lesion	• Variation of normal oral mucosa • Increased prevalence in the black population • Does not require treatment
Natal teeth	• Natal teeth are present in the oral cavity at birth, whereas neonatal teeth erupt in the first 30 days of life • Often erupt in pairs and 85% occur in the mandibular incisor area • Thought to be caused by the superficial position of the tooth germ above the alveolar bone, which can result in insufficient root formation, mobility and premature exfoliation	• 1–10% of natal or neonatal teeth are supernumerary • Treatment dependent on maintenance of a normal complement of primary dentition to allow for normal arch development • Extraction recommended if extreme mobility or poor crown formation

(continued)

Table 10.7 continued		
Lesion	Definition and appearance	Comments
Commissural lip pits	• 1–4 mm invaginations that present as blind fistulas at the corners of the mouth on the vermillion border • May be unilateral or bilateral	• Seen more commonly in males than females • Tendency to run in families suggests autosomal dominant trait • No treatment required
Developmental lesions		
Geographic tongue	• Singular (or multiple) area(s) of irregular erythematous patches with thickened or elevated white borders • Seen on dorsal and/or lateral borders of the tongue • Erythema is caused by the atrophy of the filiform papillae of the tongue (aetiology unknown) • The lesions may change shape or coalesce over short periods of time (weeks to months) and will spontaneously regress and reappear	• Common, benign condition often detected in routine examination • Females affected more commonly than males (2:1) • Also called benign migratory glossitis or erythema migrans • Usually asymptomatic but can be sensitive to spicy foods • No treatment necessary
Fordyce granules	• Ectopic sebaceous glands found within the oral cavity • Present as yellow or yellowish-white papular lesions, usually occurring in clusters • Found most frequently on the buccal mucosa, on the cheeks and the inner surface of the lips, but may also be found in the retromolar area distal to the last molar and the anterior tonsillar pillar	• Represent normal anatomical variation of the oral mucosa • Very common; more than 80% of the population have Fordyce granules • First appear at approx. 10 years of age; increase in number during puberty • No treatment necessary
Retrocuspid papillae	• Appear as tissue enlargements of the mucosa that are lingual to the mandibular canine teeth at the mucogingival junction • Usually bilateral, 2–3 mm in diameter, soft, sessile nodules • Composed of normal mucosal connective tissue	• Have been reported in 72% of children less than 10 years of age • More common in females • No treatment necessary, most will regress with age
Benign tumours		
Mucocele	• Fluid-filled bulla-type lesion that may range from a few millimetres to a centimetre or more in diameter • Results from a traumatic rupture (e.g. lip biting or lip trauma) of a salivary gland duct that allow spillage of mucin into the surrounding soft tissue • 75% are found on the lower lip but can also affect buccal mucosa, anterior or ventral side of the tongue and floor of the mouth (termed a ranula) • If palpated, the lesion feels fluctuant but firm • Colour may be bluish grey (due to mucin in the tissues), although superficial lesions appear normal in colour	• 75% of cases found on lower lip • Duration may vary from a few days to several years • Most will rupture and subsequently heal on their own but long-standing ones may require surgical excision
Fibroma	• Represents a reactive hyperplasia of fibrous connective tissue in response to local trauma • Appears as an elevated, smooth surface nodule of normal mucosal colour • Most commonly found on the buccal labial mucosa, but may be anywhere in the oral cavity • Presents as either sessile or pedunculated and will usually feel firm to palpation • Can range from a few millimetres to several centimetres in diameter	• Most common benign tumour of the oral cavity • Usually asymptomatic, unless secondary trauma causes surface ulceration • If a known irritant is removed, the lesion may regress on its own • If fibroma is not associated with a known irritant, then surgical excision is indicated
Papilloma	• The papilloma appears as an exophytic growth with many cauliflower-like projections • The lesion is well-circumscribed, pedunculated, and of normal mucosal hue • Usually found on the tongue, hard/soft palate, buccal mucosa, gingivae, lips and/or uvula • The size ranges from a few millimetres to several centimetres in diameter	• Treatment consists of surgical removal • These lesions may or may not be associated with subtypes of the human papilloma virus (HPV)
Haemangioma	• Capillary haemangioma appears as flat area with reddish pigmentation which rapidly proliferates over first 6–12 months of life, producing an elevated lobulated mass that is red to purple in colour • See Section 9.4	• Most common benign tumour in infancy and childhood • Capillary haemangioma is the most common • If not an aesthetic issue or subject to masticatory trauma may be left untreated (will undergo spontaneous involution)
Congenital epulis of the newborn	• Soft tissue tumour that occurs on alveolar ridge of the newborn • Pink to red, smooth surface, pedunculated mass on alveolar ridge • Often presents just lateral to the midline on the maxillary anterior ridge, but can occur on the mandibular ridge	• 90% occur in females • Usually requires surgical excision, although complete regression has been reported in some cases

(continued)

Lesion	Definition and appearance	Comments
Odontogenic cysts		
Eruption cyst	• Soft, translucent swelling within the gingival mucosa overlying the crown of an unerupted deciduous or permanent tooth • Cyst is produced by the accumulation of fluid within the follicular space surrounding the developing tooth • Usually of normal mucosal colour but may be filled with blood, which will impart a purple to brown colour	• Usually found in children less than 10 years of age • Treatment is not usually required as the cyst often ruptures or regresses spontaneously, allowing tooth eruption • Alternatively, the cyst can be unroofed or if the tooth fails to erupt, excision of the roof of the cyst is indicated
Parulis	• Soft, fluctuant, gingival mass that can occur on either the facial or lingual gingival tissue of a non-vital tooth. It is commonly called a 'gum boil' • It is the result of the infectious process from necrotic pulpal tissue in a tooth with a carious communication or severe traumatic injury • In the acute stage of the infection, the gingival swelling will appear and is often accompanied by pain and tenderness to palpation and mastication • The tooth may be mobile and extrude from the socket	• The acute stage of the infection may be accompanied by systemic symptoms such as fever, malaise and lymphadenopathy • Accumulation of purulent material can lead to a sinus tract intraorally where drainage will occur • Patients that do not develop a sinus tract may develop a facial cellulitis as the infection spreads through the facial spaces (see Sec. 9.6) • Requires immediate referral to a dentist or oral surgeon • Treatment focuses on removal of the source of the infection. Options include endodontic therapy (e.g. root canal) or extraction of the tooth
Infectious lesions		
Herpes simples virus type 1 (HSV-1)	• Primary infection with HSV-1 in children is often subclinical, but if primary infection produces symptoms it is termed herpetic gingivostomatitis • Onset of gingivostomatitis is acute and accompanied by fever (39.4–40.5°C), cervical lymphadenopathy, irritability and multiple oral lesions • Lesions typically are small, pinpoint vesicles that rupture to form erythematous lesions that enlarge and develop focal areas of ulceration • Lesions can occur along gingival, anterior tongue, hard palate and buccal mucosa with concurrent gingival swelling, pain and erythema. Often there is foul odour to breath • Autoinoculation of eyes, face, chin, hands and genital area can occur (if ocular involvement, referral required see Sec. 10.3) • Recurrent infections occur in 30–40% of cases and represent a reactivation of latent HSV within the trigeminal ganglion. Most common site of recurrent infection is vermillion border of lips (termed herpes labialis) triggered by sunlight, stress, fatigue and trauma • Recurrent lesions characterised by multiple, small papules that develop into fluid-filled vesicles. The vesicle ruptures usually within 2 days and complete healing often occurs within 7–10 days	• HSV is a member of the human herpes virus family • HSV-1 is spread through infected saliva or active perioral lesions (highly infectious) • Most common cause of stomatitis in children <5 years of age; highest incidence occurs between 2 and 4 years of age • Treatment is supportive and palliative (analgesia, antipyretics, fluids, nutrition) • Cold ice lollies and/or fluids can be helpful in relieving pain and encouraging oral intake • Careful monitoring of food and fluid intake as dehydration can be a problem (secondary to oral pain and refusing fluids) • Mild cases resolve in 5–7 days but can extend to 2 weeks • Acyclovir can be used to ameliorate recurrent infections but it must be started very early • Highly communicable; newborns, children with eczema or burns and/or immunocompromised children must not be exposed
Herpangina	• Begins acutely with abrupt onset of fever up to 40.5°C, sore throat, dysphagia, malaise and sometimes headache, vomiting and abdominal pain • Oral lesions develop on the posterior oral cavity, usually on the tonsillar pillars, less frequently on the soft palate, tonsils or uvula • Lesions are small red papules that quickly evolve into small vesicles on an erythematous base that ulcerate rapidly, leaving shallow ulcers 2–4 mm in diameter	• Caused by Coxsackie A virus and less commonly by Coxsackie B (enteroviruses) • Highly infectious and can occur in epidemic form mainly in the summer • Treatment is palliative and supportive (analgesia, fluids, antipyretics) • Fever lasts 1–4 days, systemic symptoms improve in 4–5 days and recovery is usually complete in 1 week • Careful monitoring of food and fluid intake as dehydration can be a problem (secondary to oral pain and refusing fluids) • Ice lollies and/or cold fluids can be helpful in relieving pain and encouraging oral intake
Hand, foot and mouth (HFM)	• Enterovirus infection characterised by vesiculoulcerative stomatitis, papular or vesicular exanthema on the hands and/or feet and mild constitutional symptoms (low-grade fever to 38.5°C and malaise) • Lesions are almost always present and precede the appearance of the hand and foot lesions • The oral lesions are similar to those of herpangina but are not confined to the posterior oral cavity and may be more numerous	• Caused by Coxsackie A virus and less commonly by Coxsackie B (enteroviruses) • Highly infectious and can occur in epidemic form mainly in the summer • Treatment is palliative and supportive (analgesia, fluids, antipyretics)

(continued)

Table 10.7	continued	
Lesion	Definition and appearance	Comments
	• The labial and buccal mucosa as well as the tongue are the sites most commonly affected • Hand and foot lesions less consistently present (occur in 1/4 to 2/3 of patients). Maculopapular eruptions that progress to vesicles. Rarely tender or pruritic and most commonly on dorsal aspects of fingers and toes but may also appear on palms, soles, arms, legs, buttocks and face	• Cold ice lollies and/or fluids can be helpful in relieving pain and encouraging oral intake • Enlarged cervical nodes common
Recurrent aphthous ulcerations	• Ulcers arise on non-keratinised mucosa that is covered by a yellow-white fibrin purulent membrane surrounded by an erythematous halo • The buccal and labial mucosa, ventral surface of the tongue, floor of the mouth, mucobuccal fold and soft palate are all commonly affected sites • Minor aphthous ulcerations are usually between 3 and 10 mm in diameter and heal without scarring in 7–14 days. Pain is often proportional to the size of the ulceration • Major, recurrent aphthous ulcerations are commonly 1–3 cm in diameter, are deeper and more painful than the minor variant, take 2–6 weeks to heal and may cause scarring	• Painful ulcers that begin in childhood and often continue into adulthood • Onset of major aphthae is after puberty • Aetiology unknown, although an autoimmune or hypersensitivity reaction of the oral epithelium has been postulated • Contributing factors include local trauma, stress, food or drug allergies, nutritional deficiencies (folic acid, B12, and iron) and hormonal fluctuations • Treatment of minor aphthea is supportive (see HFM), wheras major aphthea may require topical steroids, and/or dexamethasone elixir in addition to analgesia, adequate fluids and good nutritional support
Candidiasis	• Characterised by adherent white plaques that resemble cottage cheese on the oral mucosa • The plaques can be removed by rubbing the area with gauze. The underlying mucosa will usually appear erythematous	• Opportunistic fungal infection caused by *Candida albicans* • Called 'oral thrush' • Commonly seen in infants and children • Predisposing factors include an immunocompromise (including premature birth), broad-spectrum antibiotic usage, and/or steroid therapy • Treatment includes debridement of mucous membranes with gauze prior to application of a topical antifungal (nystatin)

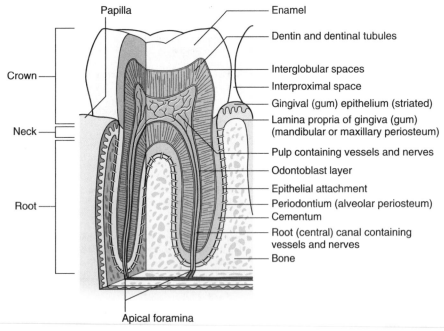

Figure 10.4   Anatomy of a tooth.

Labels: Papilla · Enamel · Dentin and dentinal tubules · Interglobular spaces · Interproximal space · Gingival (gum) epithelium (striated) · Lamina propria of gingiva (gum) (mandibular or maxillary periosteum) · Pulp containing vessels and nerves · Odontoblast layer · Epithelial attachment · Periodontium (alveolar periosteum) · Cementum · Root (central) canal containing vessels and nerves · Bone · Apical foramina · Crown · Neck · Root

⇦ HISTORY

• Age.
• Onset (acute or chronic), precipitating symptoms and duration of symptoms.
• Presence or absence of pain.
• Swelling, induration or fluctuance.
• Changes in the lesion(s) since onset.
• Treatments attempted (with results).
• History of trauma.

• Medication use (note that phenytoin, cyclosporin, and calcium channel blockers have been implicated in gingival hyperplasia).
• History of allergies.
• Other contacts/family members with similar lesions.
• Additional symptoms: fever, rash, malaise, systemic symptoms, inflammation.

🖐 PHYSICAL EXAMINATION

• **General appearance:** Note the general appearance of the child (ill, well, playful, etc.) with attention to vital signs and level of activity. If systemic symptoms are present (or suspected) a complete physical examination will be required (see Ch. 4).

• **Head and ENT:** careful assessment of the lesion(s) noting size, appearance, area(s) affected, presence of pain and/or inflammation, and distribution/location of the lesion(s).

• **Lymph:** thoroughly evaluate the lymph nodes of the head and neck as infected/infectious lesions in the mouth can inflame the head and neck lymph chains.

🔍 DIFFERENTIAL DIAGNOSES

- Dependent on the aetiology of the lesion; however, it is important to always consider oral pathology and systemic infection as part of the differential list.

➕ MANAGEMENT

The management of oral lesion is aetiology-specific (see Table 10.6). However, general principles of management of commonly encountered oral lesions are outlined below.

- **Additional diagnostics:** not usually indicated. Exfoliative cytology studies can be performed if the diagnosis is in question. If an oral infection (secondary to a carious lesion) is suspected, radiographic studies would be warranted. Likewise, if systemic illness is assumed, then consider a full blood count, C-reactive protein, cultures or other diagnostics that may assist in confirming the diagnosis.

- **Pharmacotherapeutics:** aetiology-specific; however (for the most part), medications used in the management of common oral lesions are limited to antipyretics, analgesics and, occasionally, antibiotics or antifungals.

- **Behavioural interventions:**
  - It is important to keep the mouth as clean as possible; if brushing is not an option (due to pain from the lesions), suggest rinsing the mouth after meals with warm water or brushing the teeth 30 min after an analgesic has been administered.
  - Other interventions are likely to be at the discretion of the dentist.

- **Patient education:**
  - Discuss with parents the aetiology of the lesion(s), home management, the expected course and unexpected events that should prompt a re-visit or follow-up phone call. It is very important that the parent understands when to seek care if the problem is not resolving as expected.

➡️ FOLLOW-UP

- If the lesion resolves as expected, then no further follow-up is required. However, if anxiety levels are running high, telephone follow-up can be effective in helping the family manage.
- Further follow-up is aetiology-specific, and is often at the discretion of the dentist or other health care professional.

⇄ MEDICAL CONSULT/ SPECIALIST REFERRAL

- Any child in whom the diagnosis is not clear.
- Any child with a gravely ill or toxic appearance.
- Any child with a suspected oral infection that will require specialist intervention (e.g. parulis).
- Any child in whom the oral lesion could present a safety hazard (e.g. loose natal teeth).

- Any child who is not able to maintain adequate food or fluid intake due to presence of the oral lesion(s).
- Any child with a long-standing, unresolved lesion (e.g. large mucocele, large fibroma, papilloma, congenital epulis).

🧒 PAEDIATRIC PEARLS

- Establish a good relationship with your local dentist; he can be an invaluable resource with regard to the identification and management of an oral lesion.
- Eruption cysts are much more common with the eruption of canine teeth and molars (30% of children will experience one) in contrast to a cyst associated with the eruption of an incisor (11%).

📑 BIBLIOGRAPHY

Dilley DC, Siegal MA, Budnick S. Diagnosing and treating common oral pathologies. Pediatr Clin North Am 1991; 38(5):1227–1264.

Dunlap CL, Barker BF, Lowe JW. 10 oral lesions you should know. Contemp Pediatr 1991; 8(12):16–28.

Flaitz CM, Coleman GC. Differential diagnosis of oral enlargements in children. Pediatr Dent 1995; 17(4):294–300.

Pinkham JR. Dental health examination and the pediatrician: an orientation to dental developmental age groups. Pediatrics 1989; 16(3–4):128–138.

Neville BW, Damm DD, Allen CM, et al. Oral and maxillofacial pathology. New York: WB Saunders; 1995.

10.5 COMMON ORAL TRAUMA

Kelly A. Barnes and Thomas R. Ollerhead

📖 INTRODUCTION

- Injuries to teeth in children are an increasingly common occurrence. It has been estimated that by 9 years of age approx. 35% of children will have experienced some degree of trauma to their teeth. By 14 years of age, this percentage has increased to approximately 50%.
- The aetiologies of the injuries vary, but include sport-related injuries, traffic accidents, bicycle accidents, falls, collisions with another person and dental injury secondary to seizure activity.
- Falls and child protection issues are responsible for the majority of dental

injuries in the 1 to 3-year-old age group while bicycle, skateboard and playground accidents account for most of the injuries in 7–10 year olds. Dental trauma amongst adolescents is often the result of fights, sports injuries and motor vehicle accidents.

- The most common injuries are tooth avulsion (the tooth is knocked completely out of the mouth); intrusion injuries (the tooth is pushed back into the gum) and fracture of the upper anterior teeth.
- The emphasis of this chapter will be directed towards (1) initial assessment of oral trauma; (2) description and classification of specific injuries; and (3) initial management of the most common oral injuries.
- The immediate post-trauma assessment and subsequent referral of oral injuries are critical in maximising the likelihood that a traumatised tooth can be saved. Consequently, it is important that nurse practitioners (NPs) (who may be the first point of contact post-injury) are familiar with emergency management and referral of traumatic injuries to the teeth.
- Note that a glossary of dental terminology can be found in Table 10.6 (see Sec. 10.4) and important dental anatomy is illustrated in Fig. 10.4 (see Sec. 10.4). Outlines of the primary and secondary (permanent) dentition are shown in Fig. 10.5. The illustration includes the average age of eruption for the teeth (both primary and secondary) and includes their anatomical names.

🔎 PATHOPHYSIOLOGY

- Aetiology-specific; however, the type and extent of injury to the oral cavity depends on the site, direction and force of the impact in addition to the ability of the periodontal structures to absorb the traumatic forces.
- Concussive, subluxation, lateral luxation and intrusive type injuries tend to occur if the lips cushion the

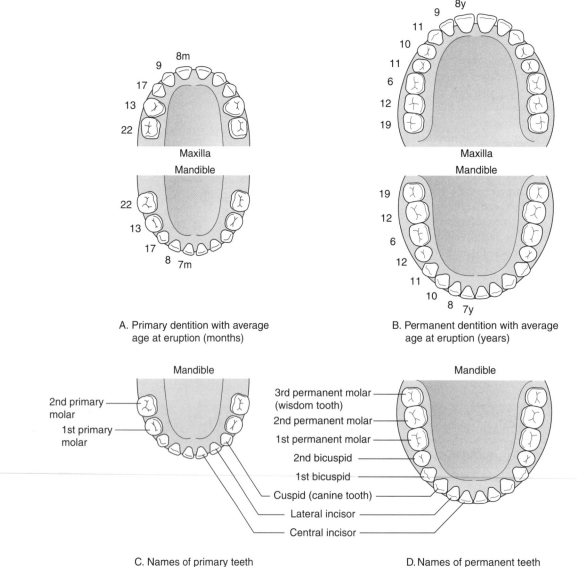

A. Primary dentition with average age at eruption (months)

B. Permanent dentition with average age at eruption (years)

C. Names of primary teeth

D. Names of permanent teeth

Figure 10.5 Primary and secondary dentition.

impact of the force. See Table 10.8 for definitions of these injuries.

- If a tooth sustains a direct force, the following are more likely to occur: fracture of the crown, displacement of a tooth and/or lip laceration(s).
- A force that is secondarily transmitted to the teeth by a blow to the chin is likely to produce a crown and/or root fracture, as well as the possibility of a mandibular fracture and dislocation of the temporomandibular joint (which is located just anterior to the external auditory meatus of the ear).

← HISTORY

- Cause of the trauma, including when and where.
- Description of the incident, including whether the injury was the result of a direct or indirect force.
- Treatment for the injury.
- Associated loss of consciousness, amnesia, vomiting or headache (e.g. rule out the possibility of associated head injury).
- Whether the teeth are sore to touch and/or chewing.
- Whether the teeth come together upon biting normally (i.e. occlude normally) or has there been a change in the bite.

Table 10.8 Differential Diagnosis of Trauma to the Teeth (World Health Organisation Classification of Traumatic Injuries to Teeth)

Type of injury	Definition	Comments and treatment
Injuries to the soft tissues of the perioral environment		
Abrasion	• The surface epithelium does not remain intact (i.e. it is 'abraded') as a result of the injury	• Abrasion injury can result in a contaminated wound • Treatment includes initial cleansing with an antibacterial solution followed by debridement to remove foreign material • A topical antibiotic cream can be applied with deeper wounds
Contusion	• Injury results when soft tissues are crushed between two surfaces • The underlying epithelium remains intact but the impact of the force injures capillaries and larger blood vessels, initiating an inflammatory response • Extravasated blood and fluid results in localised swelling and colour changes	• Minimal risk of infection as the epithelium remains intact and does not allow bacterial invasion • Treatment includes application of cold compress for initial 24-hour period, followed by application of warm, moist heat
Laceration	• Results from tearing of the soft tissue • These wounds can extend through all layers of the epidermis, dermis and muscle, and into the fascial planes of the head and neck	• These injuries should be evaluated for length and depth of the injury as well as structures affected • Treatment involves positive haemostasis, irrigation, debridement and preparation of wound margins for closure with sutures
Penetration	• Is most commonly the result of a fall when a child has an object (e.g. a toy) in the mouth. The most commonly involved areas include the lateral pharyngeal wall and posterior palatal areas	• The wound must be examined for extent of injury and presence of foreign body, as well as gag reflex and phonetic evaluation • Treatment involves wound irrigation, positive haemostasis and systemic prophylactic antibiotic administration
Injuries to secondary dentition		
Crown infraction	• An incomplete fracture of the enamel • A fracture or craze line may be present in the enamel	• *All of these injuries require immediate referral and follow-up by the dental professional* • These injuries are uncommon in children as the greater elasticity of their alveolar process (i.e. maxillary and mandibular bone), which is present with the primary and early mixed dentition, usually prevents fracture of the teeth (intrusive injuries or lateral luxation more common with primary teeth) • The incidence of these types of injuries increases with age and, as such, they are more likely to be seen in adolescents than in younger children
Uncomplicated crown fracture	• A fracture involving the enamel and dentin with no exposure of pulpal tissues	
Complicated crown fracture	• A fracture involving the enamel and dentin with exposure of pulpal tissues	
Uncomplicated crown–root fracture	• A fracture involving enamel, dentin and cementum with no exposure of pulpal tissues	
Complicated crown–root fracture	• A fracture involving enamel, dentin and cementum with exposure of pulpal tissues	
Horizontal root fracture	• A fracture involving the dentin, cementum and pulpal tissues. The tooth may appear elongated and displaced in a palatal direction	
Injuries to the tissues of the periodontum		
Concussion	• Injury has occurred to the structures supporting the tooth without displacement or loosening of the tooth	• The child will have an exaggerated response to biting pressure or percussion • Treatment includes relief of occlusion on opposing tooth, and analgesics for pain management
Subluxation	• Injury to the supporting structures of the teeth with loosening of the teeth in a horizontal direction	• Bleeding may be present in the gingival margin • Treatment includes relief of occlusion on opposing tooth, and splinting if necessary for patient comfort

(continued)

Table 10.8	*continued*	
Type of injury	Definition	Comments and treatment
Intrusion	• Displacement of a tooth into the alveolar socket • The tooth may or may not be visible upon examination of the oral cavity and, as such, may be mistakenly assumed to be avulsed	• Common injury of primary dentition (in addition to lateral luxation) • Note that among injuries occurring to the primary dentition, the quality of the bone (e.g. the alveolar process) has greater elasticity (as compared to the secondary dentition) and, as a result, tooth fracture is usually prevented • Treatment is dependent on stage of root development. In immature tooth (open apices) the tooth may be gently repositioned from a locked intrusive position. In mature tooth (closed apices), orthodontic extrusion is the preferred treatment modality
Lateral luxation	• Displacement of a tooth such that the crown portion is displaced either labially (towards the lips) or palatally (towards the palate)	• Comments are same as above • Treatment includes gentle repositioning of tooth, followed by splinting
Extrusion	• Partial displacement of a tooth out of the alveolar socket	• Treatment is dependent on stage of root development. In immature teeth (open apices) tooth should be gently repositioned, splinted for recommended period and followed closely for signs of pulpal necrosis. In mature teeth (closed apices), root canal therapy is almost certain, therefore may be instituted prior to splint removal
Avulsion	• Complete displacement of a tooth out of the socket • An avulsed tooth has ruptured the periodontal ligament fibres that attach the tooth to the alveolar socket, and severed the apical blood vessels and nerves	• Common injury in children and likely to be encountered by the nurse practitioner (NP) (accounts for 1–6% of all traumatic injuries to the secondary dentition with a much higher incidence in children) • *Do not replace avulsed primary teeth (increases the likelihood of damage to the underlying permanent (secondary) teeth)* • The prognosis is directly related to the stage of root development, length of time the tooth has been out of the mouth, the type of storage medium utilised and, most importantly, the *time lapse from avulsion to replantation* (1 h is the critical time frame) • Common sequelae of avulsion injuries include failure of reattachment of the periodontal ligament fibres; pulp necrosis; root resorption; and ankylosis. These can be minimised by proper handling and management immediately following avulsion • The most important factor for successful reattachment of the periodontal ligament fibres is speed of replantation • The parent should be instructed to replant the tooth in the socket immediately (with care taken to place the tooth in the proper orientation and to avoid touching the root surface) • If debris is present on the root surface, it should be gently rinsed with saline prior to replantation • *Do not rinse tooth with tap water* • If saline is not available and replantation by parent is not possible, store tooth in wet environment (milk or saline) with immediate referral to dental professional • Adjunctive drug therapy considerations include systemic antibiotics, tetanus consultation, chlorhexidine rinses and analgesics

• Whether there is spontaneous pain from the teeth.
• Whether there is a reaction to hot, cold and/or sweets and whether the sensation lingers after the stimulus has disappeared.
• Presence of any other injury in the mouth (e.g. lips, gums, tissue, etc.).
• Immunisation status (specifically tetanus).
• Past medical history.
• Note that the history and mechanism of injury should match, and that child protection issues need to be ruled out in all cases of oral trauma.

PHYSICAL EXAMINATION

• **Head and ENT:** examine the head and face for signs of swelling, facial asymmetry, extraoral signs of injury and any changes in skin colour. The bones of the skull, face and mandible should be gently palpated. Check the degree to which the child can open his mouth (i.e. degree of oral opening) and cranial nerve function. The presence of localised ecchymosis, crepitus, pain with palpation or dysaesthesia may indicate the presence of an underlying fracture. Displacement and mobility of a portion of the alveolar process that contains one or more teeth suggests fracture and will present as a noticeable discrepancy in the level or alignment of the teeth. The intraoral examination should include inspection and palpation of the buccal and alveolar mucosa, the teeth, alveolus, uvula, pharynx, tongue, palate and floor of the mouth.

• **Other examination:** Examination of the additional systems is dependent on the aetiology of the trauma and whether the possibility of further injury exists. For example, oral trauma secondary to a road traffic accident would warrant the assessment of all bodily systems.

⬚ DIFFERENTIAL DIAGNOSES

- See Table 10.8.

⊕ MANAGEMENT

- **Additional diagnostics:** aetiology-specific, although, in general, radiographs of the affected teeth are commonly performed. If any teeth or portions of teeth are missing (and unaccounted for) the possibility of aspiration must be ruled out, and therefore chest and abdominal radiographs should be considered. Consider radiographs, computed tomography (CT) or magnetic resonance imaging (MRI) of skull, face and mandible if suspicious examination findings are present or history suggests the possibility of severe trauma.
- **Pharmacotherapeutics:** aetiology-specific, but may include use of antibiotics (systemic or topical) and, commonly, analgesics for pain relief. Be sure dosages and choice of preparation is appropriate for the size and age of the patient.
- **Behavioural interventions:** aetiology-specific (see Table 10.8), but generally avoidance of mastication in affected areas is beneficial.
- **Patient education:**
  - Review the management plan, including a review of additional

diagnostics and behavioural interventions that will be necessary at home.
  - Discuss safety and the prevention of accidents/injuries through appropriate protective equipment, adequate supervision and suitable activities/play areas.
  - Outline the signs and symptoms of problems that would alert the family to seek additional advice and care.

⇨ FOLLOW-UP

- Aetiology-specific and often dictated by dental specialists.

⇄ MEDICAL CONSULT/ SPECIALIST REFERRAL

- Any child who has sustained severe trauma to the teeth.
- Any child in whom there is a suspicion of head injury or other severe injury.
- Any child with trauma to the 2° dentition.
- Any child with an avulsed tooth.
- Any child in whom there is suspicion of child protection issues.

⊙ PAEDIATRIC PEARLS

- In avulsion injuries, the single most important factor for successful reattachment of the periodontal ligament fibres is *the speed of replantation*. The prognosis for an avulsed tooth increases considerably if replantation occurs within 1 hour.

- If possible, do not rinse the avulsed tooth with tap water. Milk or normal saline are preferred storage media.
- Avulsed permanent teeth require a minimum follow-up evaluation period of 5 years.

▤ BIBLIOGRAPHY

Andreasen JO. Effect of extra-alveolar period and storage media upon periodontal and pulpal healing after replantation of mature permanent incisors in monkeys. Int J Oral Surg 1981; 10:43–53.

Andreasen JO, Hjorting-Hansen EI. Radiographic and clinical study of 110 human teeth replanted after accidental loss. Acta Odont Scand 1966; 24:263–286.

Andreasen JO, Hjorting-Hansen EI. Replantation of teeth II: histological study of 22 replanted anterior teeth in humans. Acta Odont Scand 1966; 24:287–306.

Andreasen JO, Andreasen FM, Bakland LK, et al. Traumatic dental injuries: a manual. New York: Blackwell Munksgaard; 2000.

Dewhurst SN, Mason C, Roberts GJ. Emergency treatment of orodental injuries: a review. Br J Oral Maxillofac Surg 1998; 36(3):165–175.

Dumsha TC. Management of avulsions. Dent Clin N Am 1992; 36:425–438.

Holt R, Roberts G, Scully C. ABC of oral health: dental damage, sequelae and prevention. BMJ 2000; 320(7251): 1717–1719.

Josell SD, Abrams RG. Managing common dental problems and emergencies. Pediatr Clin North Am 1991; 38(5):1325–1342.

Nelson LP. Pediatric emergencies in the office setting: oral trauma. Pediatr Emerg Care 1990; 6(1):62–64.

Nelson LP, Shusterman S. Emergency management of oral trauma in children. Curr Opin Pediatr 1997; 9(3):242–245.

Shusterman S. Pediatric dental update. Pediatr Rev 1994; 15(8):311–318.

10.6 ACUTE OTITIS MEDIA

Lee M. Ranstrom and Jo Williams

▭ INTRODUCTION

- Otitis media is a common diagnosis in paediatric practice. It is responsible for a significant number of primary

care visits and has substantial implications with regard to health care resources (e.g. management costs including medications and surgery).

- In the UK, about 30% of children under 3 years old visit their GP with acute otitis media (AOM) each year. About 1 in 10 children will have an episode of AOM by 3 months of age.

- White children are more commonly affected than black children, boys more than girls and children with craniofacial anomalies or Down's syndrome are likewise at greater risk. In addition, there is an increased incidence of otitis media among children from lower socioeconomic groups, those who suffer with enlarged tonsils, enlarged adenoids, asthma and those who attend group day-care/nurseries and/or use dummies. There is a lower incidence of otitis media among breast-fed infants.
- Episodes of otitis media occur more frequently during the winter months when there is a concomitant increase in upper respiratory tract infections (URTIs).
- Recurrent episodes of acute otitis media or chronic otitis media in young children increase the risk of hearing impairment.

PATHOPHYSIOLOGY

- The middle ear cavity is normally a sterile, air-filled space. During swallowing, air enters the middle ear through the eustachian tube.
- If there is eustachian tube malfunction (due to obstruction or abnormal mechanical factors), the middle ear cavity does not ventilate normally and negative pressure results as the air is absorbed. Consequently, an effusion occurs in the middle ear cavity, and bacteria from the nasopharynx may be drawn into the cavity. The proliferation and subsequent infection by microorganisms in the middle ear cavity results in the suppuration found in acute otitis media.
- Fluid obstruction of the eustachian tube can result from inflammation of the tube itself, or from hypertrophied nasopharyngeal lymphatic tissue. Viral illnesses and allergies are also thought to contribute to eustachian tube dysfunction. Mechanical factors associated with eustachian tube malfunction include reduced patency and poor muscular function.
- Otitis media among infants and young children has a developmental component. The eustachian tubes of this age group are more horizontal than

amongst older children and, therefore, they do not have the potential benefit of gravity to assist drainage.
- The most common offending bacterial organisms involved with otitis media are *Streptococcus pneumoniae*, *Haemophilus influenzae*, and *Moraxella catarrhalis*.

HISTORY

- Classic symptoms include a preceding URTI, fever, irritability, complaints of ear pain and diminished appetite. There may also be vomiting, diarrhoea, disturbed sleep and decreased hearing (older children). However, the overriding symptom in children with AOM is pain. The pain is acute, severe and deep in the ear. If the child is young, there may be ear pulling, crying and signs of infection (i.e. fever). If the ear drum perforates, the pain is suddenly relieved and a discharge will be observed.
- Note that up to one-third of children presenting with acute bacterial otitis media will not be febrile. Likewise, 'ear pulling or tugging' is not a reliable symptom.
- Onset, frequency and severity of symptoms.
- Rhinorrhoea, malaise, irritability, appetite and activity levels.
- Presence of fever, ear discharge and past history of ear infections.
- Additional symptoms (e.g. rashes, vomiting, diarrhoea, etc.).
- History of allergy to food or medication.

- Family history of allergies.
- Feeding techniques and practices (e.g. supine feeding, bottle to bed, bottle propping).

PHYSICAL EXAMINATION

- **General appearance and engagability of the child:** includes measurement of temperature (see Ch. 4).

- **Head and ENT:** visualisation of the tympanic membrane (TM) is the foundation upon which the diagnosis of otitis media is made. The normal TM is translucent with visible bony landmarks and a cone of reflected light that is easily identifiable (Fig. 10.6). If pneumatic otoscopy is performed on a normal TM, there will be resultant movement of the membrane (both laterally and medially) with negative and positive pressures. The diagnosis of acute otitis media is based on changes in the tympanic membrane with regard to colour, opacity, contour, the light reflex and mobility (if tested). Note that the colour of the tympanic membrane is the *least reliable indicator of middle ear pathology*. More specifically, a tympanic membrane that is red or yellow, swollen, with distorted bony landmarks and an absent or distorted light reflex is indicative of AOM. If pneumatic otoscopy is performed, the drum will not respond normally. In contrast, a TM that is red, but possessing good landmarks, a cone of light and good mobility, is not acutely infected. This is especially true

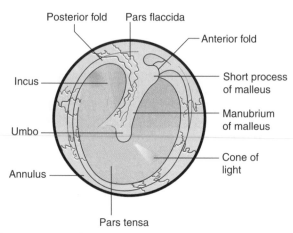

Figure 10.6 The tympanic membrane.

with the uncooperative child, as crying will flush the TM red. Careful assessment of eyes, nose and throat is required. Check for neck rigidity. Note that it is not uncommon for auricular and cervical nodes to be enlarged.

- **Cardiopulmonary:** routine assessment with special attention to the respiratory system.
- **Abdomen:** routine assessment.
- **Skin:** check for rashes.

DIFFERENTIAL DIAGNOSES

- Additional considerations in the infant/child who presents with upper respiratory tract symptoms, fever, irritability, decreased appetite and vomiting/diarrhoea include URTI, meningitis, acute gastroenteritis and viral illness.
- Ear pain with discharge can also be indicative of retained foreign body or otitis externa.
- Presence of a middle ear effusion without evidence of acute infection (i.e. a dull TM that is likely retracted with decreased mobility and fluid level/air bubbles visible behind the drum) should not be confused with acute otitis media and should not be treated with antibiotics.
- Eustachian tube dysfunction can cause transient ear pain but the tympanic membrane is normal.

MANAGEMENT

- **Additional diagnostics:** a tympanogram is helpful in diagnosis, but it can be normal in the early stages of an acute otitis media episode.
- **Pharmacotherapeutics:** The empirical treatment of acute otitis media is controversial. It has been demonstrated in placebo-controlled studies that 50% of *H. influenzae* and 20% of *S. pneumoniae* infections clear within 2–7 days without antibiotic treatment. However, in practice, suspected episodes of bacterial otitis media are usually treated with antimicrobials (this is especially true among infants and young children). More specifically, antimicrobial management is

dependent on the severity of the condition and whether the infection is bacterial. Mild viral otitis needs no treatment besides analgesia, whereas an episode of AOM (with bulging ear drum, etc.) warrants a broad-spectrum antibiotic such as amoxicillin or erythromycin. Younger children (i.e. those less than 2 years of age) require careful consideration if a 'watch and wait' approach is adopted (see Further Reading). Children meeting the criteria for recurrent acute otitis media (three episodes in 6 months or four episodes in 12 months with one in the preceding 6 months) complicate management, as antimicrobial prophylaxis needs to be considered.

- **Behavioural interventions:** practices to help prevent acute otitis media include (1) breast-feeding; (2) avoidance of passive smoking; (3) limited use of dummies; and (4) avoidance of bottle-feeding while in the prone position. Infants with more than one episode of acute otitis media should be encouraged to use a cup as soon as it is feasible.
- **Patient education:**
  - Review, with families, behavioural interventions to prevent episodes of acute otitis media (above).
  - Discuss the appropriate use of antibiotics, including the importance of not sharing antibiotics, completing the full course of antibiotics as prescribed and outlining potential adverse effects (e.g. allergic reactions, medication intolerance and vomiting/diarrhoea). Be sure to instruct parents on how to manage any adverse effects.
  - Show parents how to administer the medication to their infant/young child and warn them that symptoms will not improve immediately but that their child should be feeling better in 36–72 hours.
  - Review management of earache (e.g. paracetamol and ibuprofen).

FOLLOW-UP

- The tympanic membrane should be reassessed 3–4 weeks after completion of the antibiotic to ensure that symptoms have improved and that the

TM is returning to normal. Children who remain symptomatic despite 4–5 days of antibiotic therapy should be re-evaluated sooner.

MEDICAL CONSULT/ SPECIALIST REFERRAL

- Any child in whom the diagnosis is unclear.
- Any child with a gravely ill appearance or suspected serious bacterial illness.
- Any child who does not improve despite appropriate first-line antibiotic therapy.
- Any child who meets the criteria for recurrent acute otitis media.
- Any child in whom there is a hearing loss or documented effusion for >3 months.

PAEDIATRIC PEARLS

- An important goal of management is the judicious and appropriate use of antibiotics. They should be reserved for children with a documented acute otitis media determined through direct visualisation of the tympanic membrane.
- Remember that tympanic membrane colour is the least-reliable indicator of acute bacterial infection. Likewise, ear pulling (especially among infants) can be unreliable as both teething and seborrhoeic dermatitis (involving the area behind the pinna) can result in ear pulling.
- Pneumatic otoscopy, while not widely practiced, can be useful in the assessment of tympanic membrane mobility. This is especially true when the option of a tympanogram is not available. A bulb pump that fits into the head of the otoscope is available from otoscope manufacturers and medical suppliers.

BIBLIOGRAPHY

Bauchner H. Ear, ears, and more ears. Arch Dis Child 2001; 84(2):185–186.
Bluestone C. Management of otitis media in infants and children: current role of old and new antimicrobial agents. Pediatr Infect Dis J 1998; 7:S129–S136.

Damoiseaux RA, van Balen FA, Hoes AW, Verheij TJ, de Melker RA. Primary care based randomised, double blind trial of amoxicillin versus placebo for acute otitis media in children aged under 2 years. BMJ 2000; 320(7231):350–354.

Del Mar C, Glasziou P, Hayem M. Are antibiotics indicated as initial treatment for children with acute otitis media? a meta-analysis. BMJ 1997; 314(7093): 1526–1529.

Dowell S. Acute otitis media: management and surveillance in an era of pneumonococcal resistance: a report from the Drug-resistant *Streptococcus pneumoniae* Therapeutic Working Group. Pediatr Infect Dis J 1999; 18:1–9.

Dowell S, et al. Otitis media: principles of judicious use of antimicrobial agents. Pediatrics 1998; 101(Suppl 1): S7–S11.

Drake-Lee A. Clinical otorhinolaryngology. London: Churchill Livingstone; 1996.

Froom J. Antimicrobials for acute otitis media? a review from the International Primary Care Network. BMJ 1997; 315(7100):98–102.

Giebink G. Progress in understanding the pathophysiology of otitis media. Pediatr Rev 1989; 11(5):133–137.

Hogan SC, Stratford KJ, Moore DR. Duration and recurrence of otitis media with effusion in children from birth to 3 years: prospective study using monthly otoscopy and tympanometry. BMJ 1997; 314(7077):350–353.

Isaacson G. The natural history of a treated episode of acute otitis media. Pediatrics 1996; 98(5):968–971.

Klein J. Protecting the therapeutic advantage of antimicrobial agents used for otitis media. Pediatr Infect Dis J 1998; 17(6):571–575.

Linsk R. When amoxicillin fails. Contemp Pediatr 1999; 16(10):67–90.

Little P, Gould C, Williamson I, et al. Pragmatic randomised controlled trial of two prescribing strategies for childhood acute otitis media. BMJ 2001; 322(7282):336–342.

McCracken G. Treatment of acute otitis media in an era of increasing microbial resistance. Pediatr Infect Dis J 1998; 17(6):576–579.

O'Neill P. Acute otitis media. BMJ 1999; 319(7213):833–835.

10.7 AMBLYOPIA AND STRABISMUS

Andrea G. Abbott

📖 INTRODUCTION

- *Amblyopia* is diminished sense of visual form, which is not alleviated by the use of glasses. It is the most common cause of unilateral visual loss in childhood but can be overcome by appropriate treatment in early childhood (i.e. before the age of 7 or 8).
- *Strabismus* is manifest squint (i.e. a squint that is constant and noticeable) where one or other visual axis is not directed towards the fixation point (e.g. the eyes are misaligned). The misalignment can be horizontal, vertical or rotary.
- *Intermittent strabismus* is when the misalignment (e.g. squint) occurs from time to time or is present only when the child looks in a particular direction or at a certain distance. During the first 3 months of life, it is normal for a baby to show a slight strabismus. This intermittent squint should resolve by 3 months of age and, if it does not, intervention will be required.
- A child with a constant squint should be referred at once to a specialist (ophthalmologist or orthoptist), whatever the child's age. Most children that are seen and treated by an orthoptist will have a manifest strabismus and will suffer from poor vision (amblyopia). Amblyopia cannot be observed, but has to be detected by testing the child's vision. More specifically, accurate monocular and binocular visual acuities are the most sensitive indicators of amblyopia.
- Strabismus and amblyopia affect about 5% of the population. Consequently, it is likely that the nurse practitioner (NP) will, at some point, encounter strabismus or amblyopia in the clinical setting. Key to successful treatment is the NP's awareness of squint and amblyopia, so that early referral can be made (with all of the inherent implications for a positive outcome).

🔬 PATHOPHYSIOLOGY

- Factors necessary for the development of normal vision and eye alignment include:
  - normal anatomy of eye and orbit (see Sec. 10.2, Figs 10.2 and 10.3)
  - normal refractive systems (as tested by an optician)
  - normal sensory, psychomotor and motor pathway
  - normal mental development.
- Binocular single vision (i.e. the ability to use both eyes simultaneously so that each eye can contribute to a single common image) can be thought of in three stages:
  - *simultaneous perception* is the ability to perceive two images at the same time (one formed on each retina)
  - *fusion* is the ability to interpret the images (formed on each retina) as one
  - *stereopsis* is the perception of relative depth of objects.
- Abnormal synaptogenesis in the binocular cells of the visual cortex is responsible for *manifest squint*, whereas *intermittent strabismus* most often arises from one or more of the following (depending of the aetiology of the squint): neuronal degeneration, extraocular muscle atrophy, fibrosis or muscular infiltration.
- Amblyopia is unique to infancy and childhood and can be initiated by any condition that causes abnormal or unequal visual input between birth and

7 years of age. More specifically, amblyopia will result when the capability of one, or both, eyes to transmit normal and equal visual input is impaired (i.e. one of the two images that are transmitted from the eyes to the brain is ignored as the brain cannot cope with the two distinct images and therefore represses one image).

⬅ HISTORY

- **General medical history:** including past illnesses, head or facial trauma and developmental milestones (children with mental or physical disabilities are more likely to have a squint).

- **Birth history:** type of delivery, birth weight and gestational age. Note that some premature babies of low birth weight are more likely to develop refractive errors than babies of normal birth weight and gestation. In addition, forceps or ventouse extraction delivery can cause bruising of the soft tissue around the outer aspect of the eyes, leading to a convergent squint (this is less common than in the past).

- **Family history of squint and/or refractive errors:** squint is often familial and a history of squint in other family members is a useful confirmation of a true strabismus (as opposed to a pseudostrabismus). In addition, severe visual defects in early childhood are commonly due to hereditary disorders.

- **Squint history:**
  - The direction of squint or the limitation of eye movement.
  - The age at which it was first noticed.
  - Sudden or gradual onset (a history of sudden onset is usually reliable whereas gradual onset infers a longer duration than stated).
  - Who noticed the squint? (If the parents were first to observe the problem, it is likely to be more reliable than if the defect was seen by the family doctor, health visitor or school nurse).
  - Is the squint constant or intermittent? (The longer a squint has been constant, the greater the likelihood that there is a dense

amblyopia. If the deviation is intermittent, there is less chance of amblyopia. Note that a variable squint is often constant, but mistaken for an intermittent squint.)
  - Parental observations: does the child bump into things; fall over a lot (particularly on one side); or sit close to the TV?
  - Complaints of double or blurred vision.
  - Complaints of headache or blurred vision after a day at school.

- **Possibility of exposures:** contact with toxins, new climates, travel, nursery attendance or recent systemic medication (a recent onset of squint may be indicative of systemic illness).

👁 PHYSICAL EXAMINATION

- **Equipment:** a pen torch and small fixation target are vital pieces of equipment when assessing babies and small children. Most children are fascinated by lights and if the fixation target is colourful, it can attract and keep their attention. For tiny babies, a small squeaky toy can be used to attract their attention while assessing their eyes.

- **Eyes:** strabismus may be a presenting sign of ocular pathology, that can threaten sight or life. It is therefore paramount that babies have their red reflex checked wherever possible. The red reflex can be checked with an ophthalmoscope. Even a glimpse of the red reflex in either eye signifies that the retina is normal and that there is no obstacle to binocular vision. If a white or grey reflex can be seen on testing, the infant/child must be referred immediately to an Ophthalmic Casualty Department (rule out retinoblastoma, untreated cataracts or other pathology). In addition, physical examination of the eyes should include pupillary reactions, extraocular movements and tests of visual acuity. It is vital to observe where the corneal light reflections appear on the pupils; they should be in the same place in each eye. Normally, the corneal reflection is just nasal to the centre of

the pupil (Fig. 10.7). Unequal corneal light reflections are indicative of strabismus (Fig. 10.8). Note that pseudostrabismus is the appearance of strabismus most often caused by unequal epicanthal folds (excess folds of skin extending over the inner corner of the eye, partly or totally occluding the inner canthus). It is more common in children of eastern Asian heritage, although it can be present in 20% of white children. In pseudostrabismus the corneal light reflex is symmetrical in both eyes (Fig. 10.9). Other causes of pseudostrabismus are listed in Table 10.9.

- **ENT:** routine examination.

- **Neurological:** consider age-appropriate examination if history suggests possibility of neurological involvement (weakness, clumsiness, loss of gait, etc.).

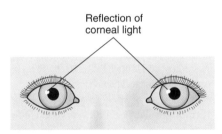

Figure 10.7 Symmetrical corneal light reflections.

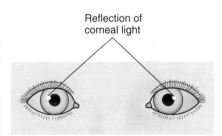

Figure 10.8 Asymmetrical corneal light reflections.

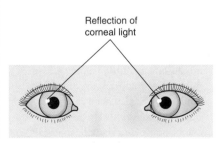

Figure 10.9 Pseudostrabismus.

Table 10.9   Aetiologies of Pseudostrabismus

Diagnosis	Characteristics
Epicanthus	• The eyes may appear to turn in (convergent squint) because the folds of skin are more prominent between the nose and the medial canthi. Therefore, less sclera is to be seen between the iris and the medial aspect of the eye, giving the impression of a squint • Careful inspection of the corneal light reflections can rule out strabismus (e.g. corneal reflection symmetrical in each eye) • Note it is possible to have a pseudostrabismus and squint coexisting in small children
Ptosis (droopy eyelid)	• Gives the appearance of a vertical squint because the eye under the drooping eyelid appears to be lower. Requires careful observation of the corneal light reflections
Facial asymmetry or misalignment of palpebral fissures	• Gives the appearance of a squint and is likely to require further investigation
Iris coloboma	• There is a keyhole appearance to the iris and, therefore, the eye appears to be darker and turn in. These patients should be seen by an ophthalmologist to exclude a retinal coloboma and investigate possible visual field loss
Anisocoria	• There is a difference in the pupil size in each eye, which can give an appearance of misalignment
Heterochromia	• There is a difference in colour between the two irises

❓ DIFFERENTIAL DIAGNOSES

- It is important to rule out pseudostrabismus (Table 10.9), the most common type of deviation seen in babies (Fig. 10.9). Note that symmetrical corneal reflections exclude the possibility of squint.
- Abnormal head postures can be due to visual or non-visual reasons and can be diagnosed easily through observation of the child's head position after giving him an occluder to wear over one eye (for about 10 min). If the child's head immediately straightens, it is likely that the posture has been adopted for visual reasons. If the child's head does not straighten after prolonged occlusion of one eye, then the posture may be due to structural changes in the neck and a referral to physiotherapy should be considered.
- Orbital deformities and tumours may result in abnormal globe position and orbital appearance without true strabismus.
- Children with facial asymmetry or misalignment of the palpebral fissures may give the appearance of a squint (and as such, may need referral). Likewise, children with an iris coloboma (e.g. a keyhole appearance to the iris that makes the eye appear darker and turn in) should be referred to ophthalmology to exclude retinal colobomata and/or visual field loss.
- Children with aniscoria (e.g. different pupil sizes) and/or heterochromia (e.g. colour difference between the two irises) may appear to have a misalignment (i.e. pseudostrabismus). They will require careful examination of their corneal light reflections to exclude strabismus.

➕ MANAGEMENT

- **Additional diagnostics:** rarely required; some additional testing may be considered by specialist care (ophthalmologist, optometrist or orthoptist) or if the strabismus is secondary to a systemic process (orbital cellulitis, tumour, etc.).

- **Pharmacotherapeutics:** eye examinations by ophthalmology and optometry are carried out under mydriasis—dilation of the pupil using 1% Mydrilate (cyclopentolate) to each eye; otherwise, there are no medications for treatment of strabismus.

- **Behavioural interventions:** The ophthalmologist, optometrist and orthoptist all examine patients who are referred for the evaluation of strabismus. The orthoptist initially performs a full orthoptic examination to check for squint and poor vision. This is followed by the ophthalmological examination to assess the fundus, media and development of the eye. Finally, the optometrist assesses the child for glasses. If treatment is required, interventions will include glasses for refractive error; occlusion therapy to overcome amblyopia (e.g. the covering of one eye to improve the vision of the uncovered eye); eye exercises to help control the squint; and/or surgery to likewise help control the squint or to improve the cosmetic appearance of the squint. Parents and children will require significant support and encouragement throughout their treatment.

- **Patient education:** Parents (and patient if appropriate) will need to know what the treatment will consist of and their role in it. This includes the likelihood that their child will need to be seen regularly, for an extended period of time (up to the age of 8 years). In addition, it is vital they understand that the eventual outcome of treatment is dependent on early intervention (i.e. starting at an early age) and good concordance. More specifically, the younger the child when treatment is instigated and the stricter the family is with the intervention, the better the outcome is likely to be.

➡ FOLLOW-UP

- Aetiology-dependent, but squint is typically followed with regular eye checks until the child is 8 years old.

⮂ MEDICAL CONSULT/ SPECIALIST REFERRAL

- Any child with a manifest or intermittent squint, asymmetrical corneal light reflections or unequal visual acuity between the eyes.
- Any child with a sudden onset of an eye turning inwards (who previously had normal alignment).
- Any child with an absent or abnormal red reflex.

- Any child with a suspected strabismus or amblyopia.
- Any child with a facial asymmetry or iris coloboma.

PAEDIATRIC PEARLS

- Pseudostrabismus is the most common referral of babies under 1 year to an ophthalmologist. However, be aware that a child can have epicanthus and a squint at the same time.
- Listen to parents: they are almost always the best observers of a child's eye because they are with them the majority of the time.
- If a red reflex is not present, an urgent referral to an ophthalmologist is necessary.
- A sudden onset of an eye turning inwards (in a child who previously had normal alignment) should always suggest the possibility of sixth cranial nerve palsy. *An immediate referral is indicated.*
- The importance of early identification and treatment of cataracts in young infants (less than 12 months of age) cannot be overemphasised. Untreated cataracts will cause dense amblyopia, whereas early diagnosis and treatment will aid in the recovery of vision (through the use of an intraocular lens and occlusion therapy). Always check for a red reflex in babies less than 12 months of age.
- 5–10% of the population suffer from amblyopia and strabismus. This is a significant number of patients and, therefore, it is likely that some will be seen by the nurse practitioner.
- The key to successful treatment is the NP's awareness of squint and amblyopia; early referral can dramatically improve the outcome.
- A worsening of squint in a child with a known squint may be indicative of a larger problem (e.g. a sudden increase in squint may indicate rising intracranial pressure in a child with hydrocephalus). Therefore, children with mental and/or physical disabilities (who often have a squint) need to be monitored regularly.
- Children who need glasses and occlusion need lots of support and encouragement.

BIBLIOGRAPHY

Bacal D, Wilson M. Strabismus: getting it straight. Contemp Pediatr 2000; 17(2):49–60.

Elkington AR, Khaw PT. ABC of eyes: squint. BMJ 1998; 297(6648):608–611.

Fielder AR. The management of squint. Arch Dis Child 1989; 64(3):413–418.

Joyce-Mein J, Trimble R. Diagnosis and management of ocular motility disorders. London: Blackwell Scientific; 1993.

Pratt-Johnson J, Tillson G. Management of strabismus and ambylopia: a practical guide. New York: Thieme; 1994.

Rowe F. Clinical orthoptics. London: Blackwell Science; 1997.

Sonksen PM. The assessment of vision in the preschool child. Arch Dis Child 1993; 68(4):513–516.

Stewart-Brown SL, Snowdon SK. Evidence-based dilemmas in pre-school vision screening. Arch Dis Child 1998; 78(5):406–407.

Von Noorden GK. Binocular vision and ocular motility, 4th edn. St. Louis: CV Mosby; 1990.

COMMON PAEDIATRIC PROBLEMS

CHAPTER 11

Respiratory and Cardiovascular Problems

11.1 ASTHMA AND WHEEZING

Michele Harrop

📖 INTRODUCTION

- During the last few decades, wheezing has become an increasingly common cause of consultation in paediatric practice. Recent epidemiological studies have suggested that up to 30% of all 3-year-old children have had at least one acute episode of wheezing.
- In the UK, 12–15% of children under 15 years of age have recurrent wheezing episodes; this represents a significant increase over the past 15 years and has been more noticeable in pre-school children. However, there is a recognised tendency to diagnose asthma more readily now than in the past; therefore, included in these data, may be children who have other reasons for their recurrent wheezing episodes.
- It is widely acknowledged that the diagnosis of asthma, especially in the very young, is extremely difficult: a distinction needs to be made between 'wheezing' and 'asthma'.
- *Wheezing* is a non-specific physical sign associated with restriction of airflow through narrowed airways. There are many causes as to why a child may present with wheeze (Table 11.1).
- *Asthma* is a chronic inflammatory disorder of the airways in which many cells and cellular elements play a role. The aetiology of asthma is multifactorial, although it is more common in children with personal or family history of atopy. Precipitating factors are known to include infection,

Table 11.1	Differential Causes of Wheezing
Aetiology	*Consider*
Allergic/ hypersensitivity	• Asthma
Congenital/ anatomical	• Cystic fibrosis • Bronchomalacia • Bronchopulmonary dysplasia • Undiagnosed congenital abnormality
Infectious	• Tuberculosis • Bronchiolitis • Pneumonia
Mechanical	• Foreign body • Obstructive mass (endotracheal tumour) • Recurrent aspiration • Pulmonary oedema • Cardiac failure • Inhalation injury
Miscellaneous	• Gastroesophageal reflux • Emotional/laryngeal wheeze • Factitious asthma

house dust mite, allergens from animals, exposure to tobacco smoke and anxiety.

- Wheeze in the first year of life may be primarily due to viral illness in predisposed infants rather than asthma (see Sec. 11.2), but the majority of wheeze that begins or persists into the second year of life is more likely to be part of the clinical entity recognised as asthma. Wheeze presenting in children under 2 years of age may be a mixture of viral respiratory illness and asthma. However, it is worthwhile remembering that 65% of children

with recurrent cough/wheeze in the first year of life will be symptom-free by 4 years of age.

🫁 PATHOPHYSIOLOGY

- Wheezing is thought to be generated by turbulent airflow which causes oscillation of the bronchial wall. The potential aetiologies of wheezing are numerous (Table 11.1).
- Asthma is a hyper-responsiveness of the airway triggered by inhalation of an array of environmental allergens and/or infectious antigens. The variable and reversible airflow obstruction is a result of airway invasion by inflammatory cells (mast cells, basophils, eosinophils, etc.) that respond to and produce various mediators (cytokines, lymphokines and leukotrienes). These processes result in (1) disruption of the airway epithelium with basal membrane thickening; (2) increased mucus production; and (3) hyper-responsiveness of airway smooth muscle and bronchospasm.
- Clinical manifestations of airway hyper-responsiveness in asthma include an acute wheezing episode and/or chronic respiratory symptoms (especially cough and wheeze).

← HISTORY

- *History of current wheeze:*
  - onset (acute or gradual) and potential triggers: upper respiratory

tract infection (URTI), animal dander, exercise, cold, etc.
- severity and duration of symptoms
- associated symptoms: cough, shortness of breath, chest tightness, fever, post-tussive vomiting, rhinorrhoea, diarrhoea, thick secretions, etc.
- medications/treatments used and effectiveness
- peak expiratory flow (PEF) measurements (if appropriate)
- possibility of foreign body aspiration or exposure to environmental toxins (fumes, smoke)
- history of atopy.

- *Past history and pattern of wheezing:*
  - age at first episode of wheeze, frequency, duration, severity and triggers (infection, cold, exercise, environmental stimulants) of past episodes
  - temporal characteristics (night vs day wheeze); year round or only wintertime
  - impact of asthma (hospitalisations, Accident and Emergency (A&E) visits, school absences, limitation of activity)
  - medications used with frequency (include frequency of systemic steroid use)
  - family history of atopy, asthma, allergy or infectious disease.

- *Environmental history:*
  - location of home (urban, rural, suburban)
  - heating system and/or fireplace
  - carpeting, stuffed animals and/or pets
  - exposure to cigarette smoke.

PHYSICAL EXAMINATION

- A calm and gentle approach should be adopted when assessing any child with respiratory difficulties.

- Astute observation of the child's general appearance (ill or well, alert, apathetic or lethargic), presence/absence of fever, work involved in breathing and the child's ability to speak in sentences, eat and drink.

- **Skin:** careful check for rashes/exanthems, perfusion, colour, skin turgor and presence of clubbing (sometimes seen in chronic asthma).

- **Head and ear, nose and throat (ENT):** note anterior fontanelle (if appropriate), nasal flaring/congestion, conjunctivitis, pharyngitis and state of tympanic membranes.

- **Cardiopulmonary:** assess for tachycardia, cyanosis, signs of poor perfusion and presence of heart murmurs. Check that the apical impulse is in the correct location for the child's age (i.e. congestive cardiac failure with cardiac hypertrophy is not responsible for the wheezing chest). Respiratory assessment includes rate, use of accessory muscles, presence of recessions (both intercostal and subcostal), chest deformities, adventitious sounds, end expiratory cough, degree of air movement and wheeze. Younger children will often bob their head when experiencing difficulty breathing. Inspiratory and expiratory ratios should be compared throughout lung fields. Note that children with severe attacks may not appear distressed and that assessment in very young children is difficult. Symptoms of *severe* respiratory compromise are outlined in Box 11.1.

- **Abdomen:** note use of accessory muscles, and palpable liver and/or spleen (can be displaced downwards if lungs are markedly hyperinflated).

DIFFERENTIAL DIAGNOSES

- Differential causes of wheezing are outlined in Table 11.1.
- Note that the correct diagnosis of asthma is based on the wheezing history (presenting complaints, signs/symptoms, frequency of episodes, etc.); clinical findings on physical examination; and assessment of lung function and respiratory symptoms (i.e. symptom diary kept for 4–8 weeks that monitors cough, wheeze, nocturnal symptoms, activity tolerance, school attendance, medication use and PEF).
- Diagnosis of asthma is particularly difficult in children less than 2 years of age. The characteristics of the wheeze (see Paediatric Pearls); and/or a 4–8 week treatment trial with symptom diary may both be of assistance in making a definitive diagnosis (see Management).

Box 11.1   Symptoms of severe respiratory compromise
Under 5 years of age
- Too breathless to talk - Too breathless to feed - Respirations >50 breaths/min - Pulse >140 beats/min - Use of accessory muscles
5–15 years of age
- Too breathless to talk - Too breathless to eat - Respirations >40 breaths/min - Pulse >120 beats/min - Peak expiratory flow (PEF) <50% of predicted (or best)
Life-threatening symptoms (all ages)
- Cyanosis - Fatigue or exhaustion - Agitation or reduced level of consciousness

MANAGEMENT

There is no single therapy that is effective for all causes of wheezing; specific management is based upon the aetiology of the wheeze:

- *Initial, acute episode of wheezing:* quickly determine the most likely cause and treat this expediently. However, a trial of β_2-agonists should be considered for a wheezing child in whom other causes have been excluded (e.g. foreign body, cardiac failure, allergic reaction, etc.) and where there is suspicion of reactive airway disease or bronchiolitis (Box 11.2).

- *Children less than 2 years of age with a history of wheeze only:* can attempt a 4–8 week trial of inhaled β_2-agonists, regular inhaled corticosteroids and a daily symptom diary as a basis for a definitive diagnosis. Treatment should be stopped if there is a poor response, and an alternative cause sought.

- *Asthma management is based upon a classification of asthma severity* (Table 11.2) *and the child's age.* Specific interventions are outlined in the British Thoracic Society (BTS) guidelines (Figs 11.1 and 11.2). Please refer to the full BTS guidelines (2003) for a comprehensive discussion of the management of acute and chronic asthma in children.

The additional interventions outlined below, for the most part, are applicable to both wheezing and asthma. They should

---

Box 11.2   Management of an acute wheezing episode

- Oxygen delivered via face mask to maintain SaO_2 >92%
- Nebulised β_2-agonists or high-dose metered dose inhaler (MDI) via appropriate spacer device
- Addition of nebulised ipratropium with β_2-agonist if respiratory distress is severe
- Oral (or parenteral) steroid administration
- Adequate hydration (oral or parenteral fluid administration)
- Frequent reassessment with treatment modification as required

---

Table 11.2   Classification of Severity of Asthma

Classification	Symptomatology
Mild persistent	• Symptoms at least once a week but less than once a day • Night-time symptoms more than twice a month • PEF[a] at least 80% predicted; variability 20–30%
Moderate persistent	• Daily symptoms affecting activity and treated with β_2-agonists • Night-time symptoms more than once a week • PEF 60–80% predicted; variability more than 30%
Severe persistent	• Continuous symptoms limiting physical activity • Frequent night-time symptoms • PEF less than 60% predicted; variability more than 30%

[a]PEF, peak expiratory flow.

be interpreted within the context of individual clinical discretion, local protocols and BTS guidelines. *The overall management aim (of both wheezing and asthma) is to give the minimum amount of therapy that will allow the child a lifestyle unrestricted by symptoms.*

- **Additional diagnostics:**
  - *Oxygen saturation (SaO_2):* should be performed routinely on all children with respiratory symptoms.
  - *Peak expiratory flow (PEF):* should be assessed in children >5 years of age. Note that PEF is height- and effort-dependent; use height-appropriate peak flow values (Fig. 11.3) but be cognisant that suboptimal PEF can overestimate the amount of bronchospasm present.
  - *Pulmonary function tests (PFTs):* suitable for most children >6 years of age. Lung function tests are not useful in an acute exacerbation but can be performed as part of follow-up.
  - *Chest X-ray:* required only if there is doubt about the diagnosis; the clinical examination suggests lung collapse/pneumothorax, acute infection (e.g. pneumonia, TB); and/or there is an unexpectedly slow response to prescribed treatment.
  - *IgE and RAST (immunoglobulin E and radioallergosorbent testing):* not performed as part of an urgent

investigation but if obtaining blood for analysis it may be helpful to check levels as it may aid in future management and prognosis.
  - *Additional bloodwork:* not routinely required, consider full blood count (FBC), C-reactive protein, urea, electrolytes, glucose and/or blood gases if clinical condition warrants.
  - *Microbiological studies:* consider if diagnosis is in doubt (e.g. sputum cultures, perinasal and/or cough swab, antigen detection, etc.); routine use is not advocated.
  - *Other:* further testing (HIV testing, Heaf test, pH probe, etc.) is dependent on aetiologies under consideration and would likely require referral.

- **Pharmacotherapeutics:**
  - Medication use for wheezing and asthma management is aetiology-dependent. However, pharmacotherapeutic mainstays of treatment include β_2-agonists (nebulised or inhaled and used with an appropriate spacer device), oxygen, corticosteroids, mast cell stabilisers (sodium cromoglicate), leukotriene receptor antagonists (montelukast) and theophylline.
  - The British Thoracic Society (BTS) guidelines (2003) for the management of asthma stress the importance of early intervention

with anti-inflammatory medications for the control of chronic asthma symptoms. They also note the importance of regular assessment and give clear guidance on how to step medication up or down depending on clinical findings. Although the BTS guidelines are presented as a series of steps, it is important that treatment is started at whatever level is appropriate to the severity of the disease at the time of consultation. Short courses of oral steroids may be needed at any step to gain control.

- **Behavioural interventions:**
  - avoidance of asthma/wheezing triggers (whenever possible)
  - daily PEF monitoring for children >5 years of age; accompanying symptom diary
  - concordance with medication regimes.

- **Patient education:**
  - Stress, with both carer and child, the importance of their active involvement in their own asthma management. The family should work with the health care provider(s) to develop a written management plan that is appropriate, practical and mutually agreeable.
  - Review the correct use of the child's inhaler device and check inhaler technique at each visit.
  - Discuss the difference between *'reliever,' 'preventer'* and *'protector'* medications and reinforce the appropriate dose and usage of each one.
  - Problem-solve with families the avoidance of trigger factors and household allergens.
  - Stress the importance of PEF monitoring and symptom diaries.
  - Review signs of worsening asthma (and or wheeze) and the actions to take if changes occur.
  - Outline the prevention and/or management of exercise-induced symptoms.
  - Reinforce the actions to take in an acute asthma attack and the indications for seeking medical assistance.

⇨ FOLLOW-UP

- *Aetiology- and severity-dependent: if there is spontaneous resolution of wheezing, no further follow-up is required. However,*

Age >5 years

ASSESS ASTHMA SEVERITY

Moderate exacerbation
- SpO_2 ≥92%
- PEF ≥50% best or predicted
- Able to talk
- Heart rate ≤120/min
- Respiratory rate ≤30/min

Severe exacerbation
- SpO_2 <92%
- PEF <50% best or predicted
- Too breathless to talk
- Heart rate >120/min
- Respiratory rate >30/min
- Use of accessory neck muscles

Life threatening asthma
- SpO_2 <92%
- PEF <33% best or predicted
- Silent chest
- Poor respiratory effort
- Agitation
- Altered consciousness
- Cyanosis

- $β_2$ agonist 2–4 puffs via spacer
- Consider soluble prednisolone 30–40 mg

- Oxygen via facemask
- $β_2$ agonist 10 puffs via spacer ± facemask or nebulised salbutamol 2.5–5 mg or terbutaline 5–10 mg
- Soluble prednisolone 30–40 mg

- Oxygen via facemask
- Nebulise:
  – salbutamol 5 mg or terbutaline 10 mg
  +
  – ipratropium 0.25 mg
- Soluble prednisolone 30–40 mg or IV hydrocortisone 100 mg

Increase $β_2$ agonist dose by 2 puffs every 2 minutes up to 10 puffs according to response

Assess response to treatment 15 mins after $β_2$ agonist

IF POOR RESPONSE ARRANGE ADMISSION

IF POOR RESPONSE REPEAT $β_2$ AGONIST AND ARRANGE ADMISSION

REPEAT $β_2$ AGONIST VIA OXYGEN-DRIVEN NEBULISER WHILST ARRANGING IMMEDIATE HOSPITAL ADMISSION

GOOD RESPONSE
- Continue up to 10 puffs of nebulised $β_2$ agonist as needed, not exceeding 4 hourly
- **If symptoms are not controlled repeat $β_2$ agonist and refer to hospital**
- Continue prednisolone for up to 3 days
- Arrange follow-up clinic visit

POOR RESPONSE
- Stay with patient until ambulance arrives
- Send written assessment and referral details
- Repeat $β_2$ agonist via oxygen-driven nebuliser in ambulance

LOWER THRESHOLD FOR ADMISSION IF:
- Attack in late afternoon or at night
- Recent hospital admission or previous severe attack
- Concern over social circumstances or ability to cope at home

NB: If a patient has signs and symptoms across categories, always treat according to their most severe features

Age 2–5 years

ASSESS ASTHMA SEVERITY

Moderate exacerbation
- SpO_2 ≥92%
- Able to talk
- Heart rate ≤130/min
- Respiratory rate ≤50/min

Severe exacerbation
- SpO_2 <92%
- Too breathless to talk
- Heart rate >130/min
- Respiratory rate >50/min
- Use of accessory neck muscles

Life threatening asthma
- SpO_2 <92%
- Silent chest
- Poor respiratory effort
- Agitation
- Altered consciousness
- Cyanosis

- $β_2$ agonist 2–4 puffs via spacer ± facemask
- Consider soluble prednisolone 20 mg

- Oxygen via facemask
- $β_2$ agonist 10 puffs via spacer ± facemask or nebulised salbutamol 2.5 mg or terbutaline 5 mg
- Soluble prednisolone 20 mg

- Oxygen via facemask
- Nebulise:
  – salbutamol 2.5 mg or terbutaline 5 mg
  +
  – ipratropium 0.25 mg
- Soluble prednisolone 20 mg or IV hydrocortisone 50 mg

Increase $β_2$ agonist dose by 2 puffs every 2 minutes up to 10 puffs according to response

Assess response to treatment 15 mins after $β_2$ agonist

IF POOR RESPONSE ARRANGE ADMISSION

IF POOR RESPONSE REPEAT $β_2$ AGONIST AND ARRANGE ADMISSION

REPEAT $β_2$ AGONIST VIA OXYGEN-DRIVEN NEBULISER WHILST ARRANGING IMMEDIATE HOSPITAL ADMISSION

GOOD RESPONSE
- Continue up to 10 puffs of nebulised $β_2$ agonist as needed, not exceeding 4 hourly
- **If symptoms are not controlled repeat $β_2$ agonist and refer to hospital**
- Continue prednisolone for up to 3 days
- Arrange follow-up clinic visit

POOR RESPONSE
- Stay with patient until ambulance arrives
- Send written assessment and referral details
- Repeat $β_2$ agonist via oxygen-driven nebuliser in ambulance

LOWER THRESHOLD FOR ADMISSION IF:
- Attack in late afternoon or at night
- Recent hospital admission or previous severe attack
- Concern over social circumstances or ability to cope at home

NB: If a patient has signs and symptoms across categories, always treat according to their most severe features

Figure 11.1 Management of acute asthma in children in general practice. Reprinted with permission from Thorax 2003; 58 (Suppl I).

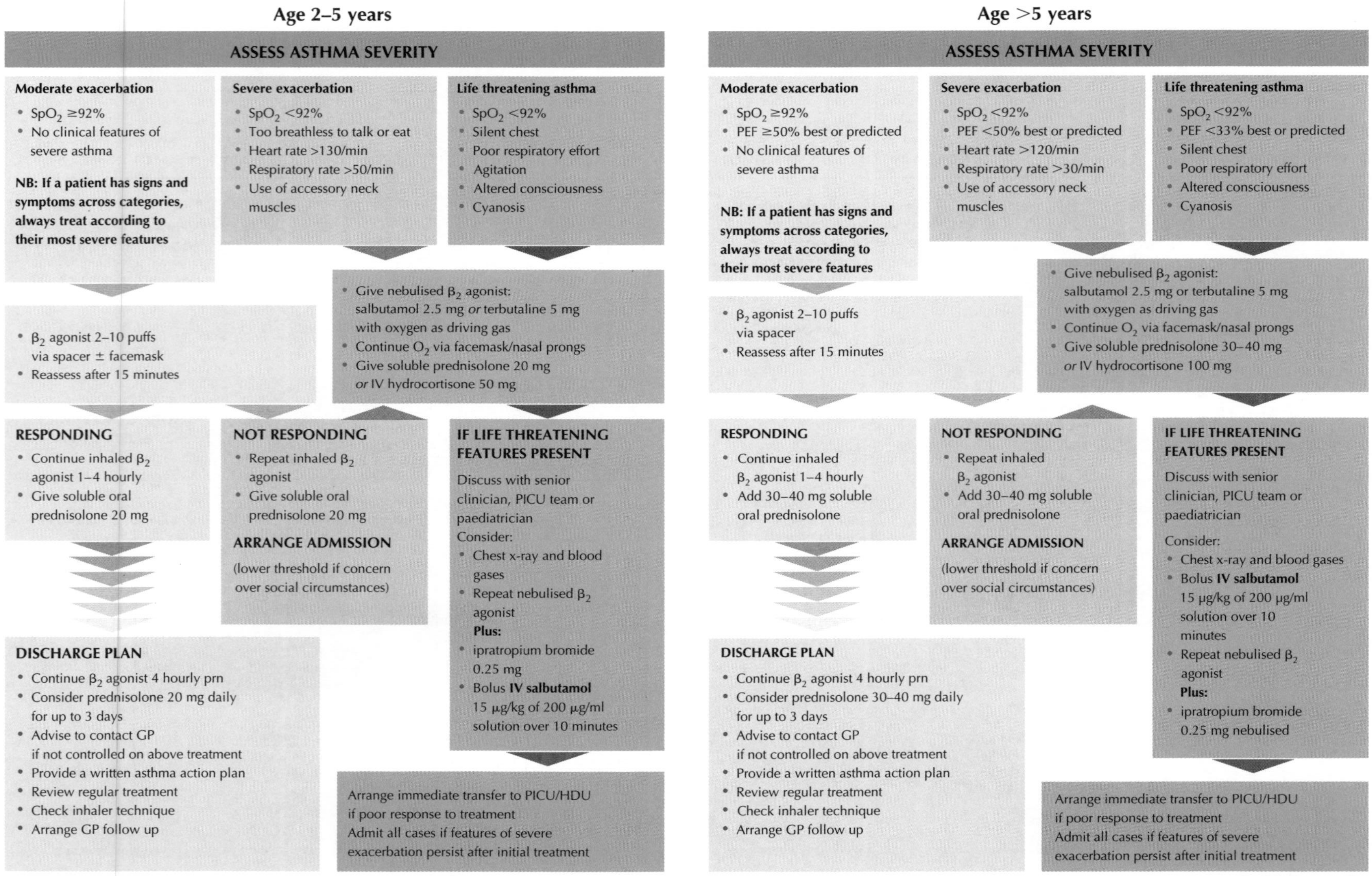

Age 2–5 years

ASSESS ASTHMA SEVERITY

Moderate exacerbation
- SpO$_2$ ≥92%
- No clinical features of severe asthma

NB: If a patient has signs and symptoms across categories, always treat according to their most severe features

Severe exacerbation
- SpO$_2$ <92%
- Too breathless to talk or eat
- Heart rate >130/min
- Respiratory rate >50/min
- Use of accessory neck muscles

Life threatening asthma
- SpO$_2$ <92%
- Silent chest
- Poor respiratory effort
- Agitation
- Altered consciousness
- Cyanosis

- β$_2$ agonist 2–10 puffs via spacer ± facemask
- Reassess after 15 minutes

- Give nebulised β$_2$ agonist: salbutamol 2.5 mg or terbutaline 5 mg with oxygen as driving gas
- Continue O$_2$ via facemask/nasal prongs
- Give soluble prednisolone 20 mg or IV hydrocortisone 50 mg

IF LIFE THREATENING FEATURES PRESENT

Discuss with senior clinician, PICU team or paediatrician

Consider:
- Chest x-ray and blood gases
- Repeat nebulised β$_2$ agonist

Plus:
- ipratropium bromide 0.25 mg
- Bolus IV salbutamol 15 µg/kg of 200 µg/ml solution over 10 minutes

---

RESPONDING
- Continue inhaled β$_2$ agonist 1–4 hourly
- Give soluble oral prednisolone 20 mg

NOT RESPONDING
- Repeat inhaled β$_2$ agonist
- Give soluble oral prednisolone 20 mg

ARRANGE ADMISSION
(lower threshold if concern over social circumstances)

Arrange immediate transfer to PICU/HDU if poor response to treatment

Admit all cases if features of severe exacerbation persist after initial treatment

---

DISCHARGE PLAN
- Continue β$_2$ agonist 4 hourly prn
- Consider prednisolone 20 mg daily for up to 3 days
- Advise to contact GP if not controlled on above treatment
- Provide a written asthma action plan
- Review regular treatment
- Check inhaler technique
- Arrange GP follow up

Age >5 years

ASSESS ASTHMA SEVERITY

Moderate exacerbation
- SpO$_2$ ≥92%
- PEF ≥50% best or predicted
- No clinical features of severe asthma

NB: If a patient has signs and symptoms across categories, always treat according to their most severe features

Severe exacerbation
- SpO$_2$ <92%
- PEF <50% best or predicted
- Heart rate >120/min
- Respiratory rate >30/min
- Use of accessory neck muscles

Life threatening asthma
- SpO$_2$ <92%
- PEF <33% best or predicted
- Silent chest
- Poor respiratory effort
- Altered consciousness
- Cyanosis

- β$_2$ agonist 2–10 puffs via spacer
- Reassess after 15 minutes

- Give nebulised β$_2$ agonist: salbutamol 2.5 mg or terbutaline 5 mg with oxygen as driving gas
- Continue O$_2$ via facemask/nasal prongs
- Give soluble prednisolone 30–40 mg or IV hydrocortisone 100 mg

IF LIFE THREATENING FEATURES PRESENT

Discuss with senior clinician, PICU team or paediatrician

Consider:
- Chest x-ray and blood gases
- Bolus IV salbutamol 15 µg/kg of 200 µg/ml solution over 10 minutes
- Repeat nebulised β$_2$ agonist

Plus:
- ipratropium bromide 0.25 mg nebulised

RESPONDING
- Continue inhaled β$_2$ agonist 1–4 hourly

NOT RESPONDING
- Repeat inhaled β$_2$ agonist
- Add 30–40 mg soluble oral prednisolone

ARRANGE ADMISSION
(lower threshold if concern over social circumstances)

Arrange immediate transfer to PICU/HDU if poor response to treatment

Admit all cases if features of severe exacerbation persist after initial treatment

---

DISCHARGE PLAN
- Continue β$_2$ agonist 4 hourly prn
- Consider prednisolone 30–40 mg daily for up to 3 days
- Advise to contact GP if not controlled on above treatment
- Provide a written asthma action plan
- Review regular treatment
- Check inhaler technique
- Arrange GP follow up

Figure 11.2 Management of acute asthma in children in A&E. Reproduced with permission from Thorax 2003; 58 (Suppl I)

telephone follow-up or a return visit is often helpful (especially with carers of young infants and children) to monitor resolution of symptoms and/or prognosis. All children with asthma require more frequent visits (both for monitoring and exacerbation management) as regular follow-up is required to enable good control of symptoms and reinforce knowledge.

- Children with mild-to-moderate asthma can be adequately cared for by their GP and asthma/practice nurse, and should be reviewed regularly every 3–6 months.
- Children with severe or brittle asthma should see a consultant paediatrician with a special interest in respiratory disease on a regular basis (every 3 months). Support by a paediatric respiratory nurse specialist is usually advisable/available.

⮂ MEDICAL CONSULT/ SPECIALIST REFERRAL

- Any child in whom the diagnosis and/ or aetiology of the wheeze is uncertain. This includes any child with a constant wheeze (e.g. no wheeze-free periods).
- Any child whose symptoms are not responding to conventional treatment, whose condition is deteriorating and/or whose clinical condition is indicative of moderate (or severe) respiratory distress.
- Any child who is a candidate for hospital admission.
- Any child requiring more than 400–800 µg of inhaled steroids in order to maintain adequate control of symptoms.
- Any child who is failing to thrive and/ or those less than 6 months of age.

- Any child with an abnormal chest X-ray, multiple A&E visits and/or hospital admissions.
- Any child in whom there is a high level of parental anxiety.

⚭ PAEDIATRIC PEARLS

- All that wheezes is not asthma.
- Beware the silent chest, as it is indicative of a lack of air movement and is considered a medical emergency.
- If a child in the community remains symptomatic (despite therapeutic doses of medication), check inhaler technique and concordance prior to stepping up treatment.
- The diagnosis of asthma is particularly difficult in children less than 2 years of age. Attention to the wheezing frequency and associated history often provide important clues.
- *Constant wheezing* (in children <2 years of age) with no wheeze-free periods indicates fixed airway narrowing and requires referral.
- *Episodic wheezing* (in children <2 years of age) that occurs in acute episodes only, is often due to viral infections and responds poorly to regular asthma treatment.
- *Interval wheezing* (in children <2 years of age) with symptoms between acute episodes is most likely to respond to asthma treatment.
- *Recurrent cough and wheezing* (in children <2 years of age) with a family history of atopy (especially in a first-degree relative) or eczema in the child would support the diagnosis of early asthma.
- *A dry cough* (either at night or with exertion) that may or may not be

associated with wheezing can be a typical presentation of mild asthma in the older child.

- *The importance of support in the community and consistent advice given by all professionals cannot be overemphasised. Paediatric asthma nurse specialists and practice nurses with training in management of childhood asthma hold the key to improving services for the increasing numbers of children affected by this disease.*

▤ BIBLIOGRAPHY

Asher MI. Worldwide variations in the prevalence of wheezing and asthma in children. Respir J 1999; 6(23S):410s.

British Thoracic Society. The BTS/SIGN British guidelines on the management of asthma. Thorax 2003; 58(Suppl 1). Available online: www.brit-thoracic.org.uk

Heaf D. How is recurrent wheezing managed in the under twos? In: National Asthma Training Centre, eds, Paediatric asthma: issues, diagnosis, treatment and management. London: Class Publishing; 1997:57–58.

Lenney W. Children's health: the management of asthma in childhood. Resp Dis Pract 1997; Autumn:10–13.

Lowhagen O. Asthma and asthma like disorders. Resp Med 1999; 93:851–855.

Martinez FD, Helms PJ. Asthma and wheezing in the first six years of life. New Engl J Med 1995; 332:133–138.

McKenzie S. Clinical features and their assessment. In: Silverman M, ed., Childhood asthma and other wheezing disorders. London: Chapman and Hall Medical; 1995:141–174.

Norton L. Asthma: support in the community. Paediatr Nurs 1995; 7(8):24–27.

Young S, Arnott J, O'Keeffe PT, et al. The association between early lung function and wheezing during the first two years of life. Eur Resp J 2000; 15:151–157.

11.2 BRONCHIOLITIS

Susan Peter

▢ INTRODUCTION

- Bronchiolitis is an acute, viral, respiratory infection affecting the small airways of infants and young children. It is the most common form of severe lower

respiratory tract infection during infancy, with respiratory syncytial virus (RSV) responsible for 75% of cases. Other pathogens implicated in bronchiolitis include influenza A, adenovirus, parainfluenza and *Mycoplasma*

pneumoniae. It is predominantly a disease of infancy, as most children (80%) have been infected by 12 months of age.

- Bronchiolitis accounts for significant morbidity in this age group, although mortality is low. Infants at greatest risk

> **Box 11.3 Clinical features of bronchiolitis**
>
> - Subcostal recession
> - Wheezing
> - Feeding difficulties
> - Apnoea
> - Tachycardia, tachypnoea
> - Fever in some infants (often low grade but can be as high as 39°C)
> - Cough that may initially be hoarse and dry for 3–5 days with progression to deep, wet and more frequent cough
> - Increasingly rapid distressed breathing
> - Coryza and snuffles often with thick purulent nasal discharge
> - Pallor, cyanosis (in severe cases)

for life-threatening episodes include those with pre-existing disease (those with neuromuscular disorders, immune deficiencies, congenital cardiac disease, chronic lung disease, infants less than 6 weeks of age or those born prematurely). Around 10% of babies develop bronchiolitis in their first year of life and one-fifth of these are admitted to hospital.

- In adults and older children bronchiolitis is manifested as a common cold (their larger airways tolerate the inflammation associated with infection much better), whereas in 40% of affected infants the infection progresses from the upper to the lower respiratory tract, giving rise to respiratory symptomology and feeding difficulties (Box 11.3).
- The main priority for the nurse practitioner (NP) is to accurately assess the severity of illness in order to differentiate infants with mild bronchiolitis (that can be safely cared for at home) from those with moderate-to-severe bronchiolitis (who require referral to hospital and/or admission).

PATHOPHYSIOLOGY

- RSV spreads easily from person to person through direct and indirect contact with respiratory secretions. Worldwide epidemics occur annually, peaking during the winter months in temperate climates and during the rainy season in warmer climates.
- After infection of a susceptible host, RSV replicates rapidly in the

bronchiolar epithelium, causing necrosis of the ciliated cells and subsequent destruction of cilia. The ciliary damage impairs clearance of secretions and, when combined with (1) increased mucous secretion, (2) submucosal oedema and (3) desquamation of cells, there is resultant bronchiolar obstruction, atelectasis and hyperinflation.

- The acute functional consequences of these changes are small airway obstruction, gas trapping and impaired gas exchange. The work of breathing and oxygen consumption are increased and manifest themselves in well-recognised clinical features (Box 11.3).
- In severely affected infants, impaired ventilation, combined with ventilation–perfusion imbalance and potential hypoventilation (due to apnoea or exhaustion) eventually lead to hypoxaemia and hypercarbia.

HISTORY

The possibility of bronchiolitis should be considered in any infant less than 1 year of age with a first presentation of wheeze or cough during the months of October to March. This is particularly true if associated with feeding difficulties or other clinical features outlined in Box 11.3. A higher index of suspicion must be incorporated into the history-taking process for neonates, in whom bronchiolitis often presents atypically, with minimal respiratory symptoms. Additional information to be collected:

- Age (infants less than 6 weeks of age and/or those who were born prematurely are at greater risk of respiratory compromise).
- Presence of pre-existing disease (children and infants with neuromuscular disorders, immune deficiencies, congenital cardiac disease, chronic lung disease are all considered to be at increased risk).
- Respiratory symptoms (presence/absence of cough and character, rhinorrhoea/nasal secretions) and severity of distress with temporal characteristics (condition improving or worsening).
- History of pallor or apnoea, or cyanosis (cyanosis is rare).

- Physical state and activity level (pallor, fatigue, exhaustion, restlessness/lethargy).
- Ability to feed, including amount taken per feed, frequency and reason for difficulties (e.g. blocked nose, cough, rapid respiration, exhaustion). Infants with bronchiolitis require an intake of 100 ml/kg/day.
- Presence of fever (elevations <39°C are common). *Note that only 1/3 to1/2 of patients diagnosed with bronchiolitis develop fever: absence of fever does not preclude a diagnosis of bronchiolitis.*
- Urinary output (last wet nappy, frequency and colour/strength of urine).
- Birth history (preterm, low birth weight, neonatal lung disease and infants weighing less than 5 kg are associated with increased risk of respiratory failure).
- Possibility of foreign body aspiration, gastro-oesophageal reflux (GOR) or inhalation of noxious agents (chemicals, fumes, toxins) should be eliminated. (These infants can present with wheezing.)

PHYSICAL EXAMINATION

- **General assessment:** assessment of the infant's general appearance, especially noting level of alertness and activity (extreme irritability or lethargy are worrying); degree of dyspnoea (including effort required to breath); ability to feed (assess hydration status) and temperature. It is helpful to observe the infant feeding and at rest. Table 11.3 outlines indicators of illness severity. *The infant's degree of respiratory effort and ability to feed are key observations to be noted.*

- **Skin:** observation of skin for exanthems, perfusion, colour (including absence/presence of cyanosis), and skin turgor (check on abdomen or midaxillary line).

- **Head and ENT examination:** note anterior fontanelle (may be slightly depressed with dehydration); nasal flaring and/or congestion/discharge (thick purulent secretions common). Include assessment of oral mucous membranes (slippery feel when hydrated) and state of tympanic membranes.

Table 11.3   Assessment of Illness Severity

Clinical parameter	Mild	Moderate to severe
Colour	Pink	Pallor, cyanosed or grey [a]
Physical state/activity level	Alert	Reduced conscious level [a] Exhausted or fatigued [a]
Heart rate	<140/min	>140/min
Respiratory rate	<60/min	>60/min
Oxygen saturation	SaO_2 >92%	SaO_2 <93%
Nasal flaring or grunting	None	Some—significant
Recession	Mild subcostal recession	Marked recession
Ability to feed	Able to take more than half of usual feeds	Taking less than half of usual feeds

[a] Indicates potentially life-threatening.

- **Cardiopulmonary:** note tachycardia and signs of poor perfusion (capillary refill >2 s); respiratory rate (may be decreased if fatigued/exhausted); accessory muscle use and recession (subcostal recession common). Note presence of cough, wheeze or grunting with careful auscultation of lungs (there may be widespread crackles, wheeze, prolonged expiratory phase and hyper-resonance to percussion).

- **Abdomen:** liver and spleen may be palpable as they are displaced downward from hyperinflated lungs.

🛈 DIFFERENTIAL DIAGNOSES

- Concurrent infection with other viruses or organisms such as *Chlamydia trachomatis* or *Mycoplasma pneumoniae* occurs in at least 5–10% of cases of RSV bronchiolitis. Differential diagnoses include asthma, pertussis, aspiration pneumonia, cystic fibrosis, congenital lung disease, congenital cardiac disease and immune deficiency. In addition, the possibility of GOR, foreign body aspiration and inhalation-related wheezing should be considered if history suggests.

✚ MANAGEMENT

Many infants with acute viral bronchiolitis can be managed at home; however, some require admission to hospital and a few need intensive care. Careful assessment at presentation is a priority in deciding where best to manage the infant (Box 11.4). Mild bronchiolitis without other risk

Box 11.4   Hospital admission criteria (consider admission if one or more of the criteria are met)

- Feeding: less than half of usual intake
- Marked recession, grunting
- Fatigue, exhaustion
- Infants from high-risk group: those with neuromuscular disorders, immune deficiencies, congenital cardiac disease, chronic lung disease and infants less than 6 weeks of age or those born prematurely
- Respiratory rate >60 breaths/minute
- Heart rate >140 beats/minute
- SaO_2 <93%
- History of apnoea

factors (see History) can usually be managed at home. Deterioration or more severe symptomatology (Table 11.3) will likely require hospital admission for monitoring, supplemental oxygen administration and hydration assistance.

- **Additional diagnostics:** RSV infection can be diagnosed rapidly from a nasopharyngeal aspirate using immunofluorescence techniques or enzyme-linked immunosorbent assay (ELISA). However, inability to detect RSV does not preclude a diagnosis of bronchiolitis or alter clinical outcome. *Oxygen saturation monitoring is invaluable and should be used whenever available.* Routine chest X-ray and blood work—full blood count (FBC), urea and electrolytes (U/E) and, C-reactive protein (CRP)—are rarely of value in mild cases but should be considered in severe cases or bronchiolitis, when there is suspicion

of additional pathology, or if a deterioration in clinical condition occurs.

- **Pharmacotherapeutics:** bronchodilators can produce modest, short-term improvement in clinical scores but there is no benefit on arterial oxygen saturation or the duration and rate of hospitalisation with their routine use. They are not recommended for routine management of bronchiolitis. *However, bronchodilators (ipratropium bromide or salbutamol) should be considered for those infants with previous episodes of wheezing for whom an initial dose should be administered and treatment continued only if improvement is noted.* There is no benefit from routine corticosteroid or antibiotic therapy. However, antibiotics should be considered when there are chest X-ray changes, raised white blood cell (WBC) count or CRP, clinical deterioration or suspicion of sepsis. Ribavirin (an antiviral agent) is occasionally used in hospital for infants with pre-existing disease early on in their illness.

- **Behavioural interventions:**
  - Careful handwashing (by family members and health professionals) is imperative. RSV sheds in respiratory secretions and is easily passed on via direct and indirect contact (the virus can stay on the hands for 30 min). Good handwashing routines and the use of gowns and gloves in hospitals have been proven to significantly reduce the risk of transmission. *Hospitalised patients (RSV positive) need to be isolated from uninfected patients.*
  - Adequate oral fluid intake (minimum = 100 ml/kg/day).
  - Antipyretics for fever and irritability.
  - Frequent observation of worsening of illness.
  - Sodium chloride (0.9%) nose drops can be helpful in clearing nose.
  - Supplemental oxygen, intravenous (IV) hydration and O_2 saturation (SaO_2) monitoring are likely additions for hospital care.

- **Patient education:**
  - Discuss and review behavioural interventions above (if hospitalised, discussion includes inpatient management and treatment).

Provide written information that outlines home management.

- Clear instructions regarding signs and symptoms that indicate a worsening condition (fast breathing, lethargy, poor feeding, dehydration, etc.). Reinforce these with written guidelines that include contact information for later questions/ concerns.
- Advise parents on feeding an infant with mild respiratory distress (total fluid needs, smaller frequent feeds, guarding against vomiting).
- Explain to parents that there should be improvement within 3–5 days, but a cough can continue for several weeks. Note that children can be reinfected with RSV during the same season. In addition, explain that an appreciable number of infants hospitalised with bronchiolitis will have recurrent wheezing episodes that tend to diminish after the first couple of years.

⮕ FOLLOW-UP

- Not required if symptomology resolves with supportive care.
- Return visit and/or phone call if parental anxiety or any deterioration in condition.

⮂ MEDICAL CONSULT/ SPECIALIST REFERRAL

- Infants that are classified as moderate to severe bronchiolitis.

- Infants considered to be at increased risk (see History).
- Infants who appear severely ill.

🐾 PAEDIATRIC PEARLS

- The two prominent clinical problems in bronchiolitis are respiratory problems and feeding difficulties. The main purpose for assessing severity at presentation is to decide where best to manage the infant.
- Hypoxia is common (and difficult to detect clinically), so it is vital to monitor arterial oxygen saturation with pulse oximetry.
- Be aware of apnoea, especially in young infants; likewise, respiratory failure may have sudden presentation.
- Mainstays of hospital treatment in bronchiolitis are careful monitoring, supplemental oxygen and hydration.
- Complicated bronchiolitis is more likely to occur in very young infants and those with pre-existing disease.
- Sudden deterioration suggesting atelectasis is due to mucus plugging.
- In cases of clinical bronchiolitis, common causes of false-positive ELISA tests include poor quality of sample; sample contamination; insufficient sample; and non-RSV bronchiolitis.
- For most infants, bronchiolitis is self-limiting with an excellent prognosis. However, 40–50% of infants hospitalised with bronchiolitis will have recurrent episodes of

wheezing until 2 or 3 years of age; some may eventually be diagnosed with asthma.

- Occasionally, some infants actually get slightly worse before they get better. This is due to atelectasis within the lung fields rather than worsening disease *per se*. However, this observation should be made carefully and it should not preclude follow-up evaluation to rule out secondary complications/worsening disease.

🗏 BIBLIOGRAPHY

Ackerman VL, Salva PS. Bronchiolitis. In: Loughlin GM, Elgen H, eds, Respiratory disease in children: diagnosis and management. New York: Williams & Wilkins; 1994:291–300.

Darville T, Yamauchi T. Respiratory syncytial virus. Pediatr Rev 1998; 19(2):55–61.

Kellner JD, Ohlsson A, Gadomski AM, et al. Bronchodilator therapy in bronchiolitis. In: The Cochrane Library, Issue 1. Oxford: Update Software; 1999.

Mulholland EK, Olindky A, Shann FA. Clinical findings and severity of acute bronchiolitis. Lancet 1990; 335:1259–1261.

Rakshi K, Couriel JM. Management of acute bronchiolitis. Arch Dis Child 1994; 71:463–469.

Schwartz R. Respiratory syncytial virus in infants and children. Nurse Pract 1995; 20(9):24–29.

Shaw KN, Bell LM, Sherman NH. Outpatient assessment of infants with bronchiolitis. Am J Dis Child 1991; 145:151–155.

11.3 PNEUMONIA

Elinor White

⬚ INTRODUCTION

- Pneumonia is an infection of the lower respiratory tract most commonly due to bacterial or viral pathogens and much less commonly the result of invasion by fungi, parasites or other organisms.

- Classification is usually by anatomical position (e.g. lobar, bilateral basal, interstitial or bronchial).
- Pneumonia is also classified by the infective pathogen (e.g. *Streptococcus pneumoniae* or *Mycoplasma pneumoniae*), both of which are the most common causes of bacterial

pneumonia in the UK. Respiratory syncytial virus (RSV) is the most common cause of viral pneumonia.

- The most frequent and consistent clinical presentations of pneumonia are tachypnoea, respiratory distress and increased work of breathing (recessions, nasal flaring, etc.). These signs indicate serious pneumonia in children and require careful evaluation.

- Bacterial pneumonia may develop secondary to a viral bronchitis associated with an upper respiratory tract infection (URTI). As such, recent upper tract infection is often part of the presenting history.
- The incidence of bacterial pneumonia is highest among children less than 2 years of age, with boys more commonly infected than girls (2 to 1 ratio). Children with pre-existing conditions are also at increased risk of bacterial pneumonia (e.g. cerebral palsy, severe learning disabilities, cystic fibrosis and other congenital syndromes).
- Viral infections of the lower respiratory tract are also more common in the under-2 age group. RSV is the most common cause of viral pneumonia, especially in infancy. It can produce large epidemics in infants and can be very serious among infants 6 weeks of age or less. Although RSV infection usually presents as bronchiolitis, RSV pneumonia may subsequently develop. It can be diagnosed following radiological evidence of consolidation and more focal clinical signs on examination.
- *M. pneumoniae* may cause an atypical presentation of pneumonia, usually in an older child (e.g. >4 years of age). The physical examination will be significant for moderate signs and symptoms of lower respiratory tract involvement; however, there will be marked patchy consolidation on chest X-ray. Focal findings of mycoplasma infection in the chest are often difficult to detect.
- Pneumonia caused by *Staphylococcus aureus* is not as common, but it can cause severe infection.

PATHOPHYSIOLOGY

- Pneumonia is usually spread by droplet infection, although less commonly it can be airborne; haematogenous spread is rare.
- Primary bacterial pneumonia is less common than secondary bacterial infection following a viral infection. The initial viral infection affects

the usual lung defences (e.g. altering normal secretions and flora, inhibiting phagocytosis and disrupting the epithelial layer). Subsequently, there is invasion of bacteria from the upper respiratory tree (commonly *S. pneumoniae*) and the development of a bacterial infection.

- In viral pneumonia, the invading pathogen often affects the conducting airways and the alveoli. The virus proceeds to disrupt normal lung function through the associated inflammatory response. Typically, the progression of symptoms in viral pneumonia is slower than occurs in bacterial illness.

HISTORY

- Age and duration of symptoms.
- Presence of fever, decreased activity and/or appetite, malaise, nausea, vomiting, chills and lethargy. Note that complaints of anorexia with decreased fluid intake are common.
- Cough, shortness of breath, trouble breathing or increased respiratory rate.
- Chest pain or abdominal pain (especially with right lower lobe pneumonia).
- Recent infections, especially a URTI.
- Exposure to others that are ill.
- Underlying medical conditions (including past history of pneumonia or respiratory problems).
- Travel abroad.
- Living conditions.
- Immunisation history.
- Drug allergies.

PHYSICAL EXAMINATION

- Thorough physical examination with careful attention to the respiratory system. Note the child's general appearance, colour, signs of respiratory distress and hydration status. Observe child undressed and in parent's arms to evaluate respiratory rate and work of breathing. A lot of information can be gained through careful observation; this is especially important in very young children as they can be difficult to examine. Note that colour and general appearance are key indicators.

- **Pulmonary:** note air movement throughout lung fields and any adventitious sounds (e.g. rales, crackles, friction rub, etc.). Wheezing is uncommon in bacterial pneumonia (mycoplasma excepted). In older children, the chest may be dull to percussion if an area of consolidation is present, whereas respiratory findings can be difficult to localise in younger children as sounds are easily transmitted from the upper airway and adjacent lung fields (due to the hyper-resonance of their chests).
- Note the degree to which child is struggling to breathe and presence of recession.
- Note any changes in chest shape that may indicate an underlying chronic respiratory condition (e.g. Harrison's sulcus or barrel chest).

DIFFERENTIAL DIAGNOSES

- Consider other causes of respiratory distress: foreign body aspiration, caustic ingestion, drug reaction, tuberculosis and asthma. Likewise rule out the possibility of metastatic disease, trauma, pulmonary or cardiac disease (cystic fibrosis, congenital heart disease) and sickle cell disease (acute chest syndrome).

MANAGEMENT

Hospital or community-based management of pneumonia is dictated by the degree of respiratory compromise and appearance of the child. Many older children with mild-to-moderate symptoms may be treated at home.

- **Additional diagnostics:** consider a chest X-ray, with posterior, anterior and lateral views, FBC, CRP, blood culture (considered the gold standard for diagnosis but only a small percentage will develop bacteraemia and many children will have already received antibiotics in the community), blood gases, mycoplasma serology and polymerase chain reaction (PCR). Note that sputum is often impossible to obtain in children, and throat swabs usually have no value in diagnosis.

Table 11.4 Antibiotic Therapy for Common Bacterial Pathogens

Pathogen	Antibiotic
Streptococcus pneumoniae	• Amoxicillin
Mycoplasma pneumoniae	• Erythromycin
Chlamydia trachomatis	• Erythromycin

Table 11.5 Age-Related Bacterial Pathogens

Age	Pathogen
Neonates	• Chlamydia trachomatis • Group B streptococcus • Gram-negative enteric bacilli (e.g. Escherichia coli, Klebsiella pneumoniae, Pseudomonas aeruginosa)
1–6 months	• Bordetella pertussis • Streptococcus pneumoniae
6 months to 5 years	• Streptococcus pneumoniae (most common) • Mycoplasma pneumoniae
>5 years	• Streptococcus pneumoniae • Mycoplasma pneumoniae (incidence increases with age)

However, a nasopharyngeal aspirate (NPA) is very useful in identifying viral pathogens.

- **Pharmacotherapeutics:**
  aetiology-specific (Table 11.4). Antibiotics are usually administered as it is extremely difficult to exclude a bacterial aetiology in case of suspected viral pneumonia. Antibiotic choice is usually based on the likely pathogen given the child's age (Table 11.5) and clinical findings.

- **Behavioural interventions:**
  - Temperature, pulse respiratory rate, effort and colour should be monitored.
  - Pulse oximetry with oxygen therapy administered to maintain an oxygen saturation level >90–92%.
  - Adequate rest, hydration and nutrition. Small frequent feeds should be given (if tolerated) so as not to overload the stomach and impair respiration.
  - If oral intake is not sufficient to maintain hydration, IV fluids will be required. Once dehydration is corrected, care should be taken not to overload.

- Children admitted to hospital should be nursed in the semirecumbent position supported with pillows, whereas infants should be nursed in a Derbyshire chair.

- **Patient education:**
  - review with families the aetiology of the pneumonia and the disease process
  - discuss with them the importance of concordance with the treatment plan, expected course the infection will take and signs and symptoms of a worsening clinical condition
  - outline for them the interventions involved in their child's care and negotiate their role in care delivery
  - talk about follow-up care, including other professionals that may be involved (children's community team, respiratory nurses, etc.).

➡ FOLLOW-UP

- Uncomplicated cases of pneumonia usually recover within 1–5 days and do not require follow-up or repeat X-ray.
- Follow-up is indicated if a child shows no improvement or has a recurrence.
- If the pneumonia is complicated by effusion or collapse, an 8-week post-infection chest X-ray should be obtained (it takes 6–8 weeks for the lung consolidation to resolve).

⇄ MEDICAL CONSULT/ SPECIALIST REFERRAL

- Any child less than 2 years of age.
- Any child with a toxic appearance, cyanosis, oxygen saturation <92% on room air and clinical signs of respiratory distress (e.g. tachypnoea, intercostal/subcostal recession, seesaw breathing, nodding respirations, nasal flaring and/or exhaustion).
- Any child who is unable to tolerate oral fluids sufficiently to maintain hydration.
- Any child with a deteriorating condition.
- Any child who does not improve after appropriate antibiotic therapy.
- Any child with parents who are unable to cope with the child's illness.

🔎 PAEDIATRIC PEARLS

- There is an increased risk of pneumonia in the first year of life if there is parental smoking, lower social status and residence in industrial communities.
- Radiographic findings may lag behind clinical presentation if the child is dehydrated and/or it is very early in the disease process.
- Right upper lobe (RUL) pneumonia can occur during the first year of life, which may be due to aspiration of feeds when lying down.
- Wheeze is rare in bacterial pneumonia (mycoplasma excepted). However, wheezing may be heard in pneumonia secondary to viral infection.
- Be aware of the possibility of aspiration of a foreign body, particularly with recurrence to the same lobe or if brief response to therapy.
- Remember the possibility of tuberculosis and/or HIV. Poor response to appropriate antimicrobials requires careful attention and re-evaluation.
- With recurrent episodes of pneumonia, consider compromised immunity and/or cystic fibrosis.
- Do not overlook the importance of nutrition and adequate hydration.
- Empyema (an infected pleural effusion) is more common in children with pneumonia caused by Streptococcus pneumoniae.

📖 BIBLIOGRAPHY

Anonymous. Managing childhood pneumonia. Drug Ther Bull 1997; 35(12):89.

Behrman RE, Kliegman RM, Jenson HB. Nelson text book of pediatrics, 16th edn. Philadephia: WB Saunders; 2000:1818.

Berman S, Simoes EA, Lanata C. Respiratory rate and pneumonia in infancy. Arch Dis Child 1991; 66(1):81–84.

Campbell JR. Neonatal pneumonia. Sem Resp Infect 1996; 11(3):155–162.

Choo S, Finn A. New pneumoccocal vaccines for children. Arch Dis Child 2001; 84(4):289–294.

Churgay CA. The diagnosis and management of bacterial pneumonias in infants and children. Prim Care 1996; 23(4):821–835.

Clements H, Stephenson T. Pneumonia: current challenges and treatment. Curr Paediatr 1999; 9:154–157.

Efron D. Royal Children's Hospital paediatric handbook, 6th edn. London: Blackwell Science; 2000.

Fete TJ, Noyes B. Common (but not always considered) viral infections of the lower respiratory tract. Pediatr Ann 1996; 25(10):577–584.

File TM. The epidemiology of respiratory tract infections. Sem Resp Infect 2000; 15(3):184–194.

Gordon RC. Community acquired pneumonia in adolescents. Adolesc Med 2000; 11(3):681–695.

Halpin D. Managing pneumonia in general practice. Practitioner 2001; 245(1619):108–113.

Hay W, Hayward AR, Levin MJ, et al. Current pediatric diagnosis and treatment, 14th edn. Hartford: Appleton and Lange; 1999.

McCracken GH Jr. Diagnosis and management of pneumonia in children. Pediatr Infect Dis J 2000; 19(9): 924–928.

Milner AD, Hull D. Hospital paediatrics. Edinburgh: Churchill Livingstone; 1992:102–105.

Overall JC Jr. Is it bacterial or viral: laboratory differentiation. Pediatr Rev 1993; 14(7):251–261.

Schmitt BD. Pediatric telephone advice, 2nd edn. Philadelphia: Lippincott Raven; 1999.

Schutz GE, Jacobs RF. Management of community-acquired bacterial pneumonia in hospitalised children. Pediatr Infect Dis J 1992; 11(2):160–164.

Schwartz MW. The 5 minute consult, 2nd edn. Philadelphia: Lippincott, Wliams & Wilkins; 2000.

11.4 STRIDOR AND CROUP (LARYNGOTRACHEOBRONCHITIS)

Joan Marshall

INTRODUCTION

- Stridor is a harsh, vibratory sound of variable pitch caused by partial obstruction of the upper airway. Although most stridor is caused by benign clinical conditions, it is a frightening respiratory problem for parents and children. Occasionally, it may be a sign of a serious or even life-threatening disorder and as such, requires careful evaluation.

- Acute inspiratory stridor is usually associated with obstruction of the laryngeal area and is most commonly observed in children with croup. Croup comes under the umbrella term 'croup syndrome', a non-specific term that refers to any condition producing inspiratory stridor and includes laryngotracheobronchitis (LTB), spasmodic croup, bacterial tracheitis and epiglottitis. *Note that the terms 'laryngotracheobronchitis' and 'croup' are often used synonymously.*

- *Viral croup* (acute laryngotracheo-bronchitis or LTB) is an acute illness that commonly occurs in children between 6 months and 3 years of age (peak incidence is during the second year of life with boys affected more commonly than girls). Most croup episodes are caused by parainfluenza viruses (types 1, 2 and 3), although numerous other pathogens can also be involved (RSV, adenovirus, enterovirus and rhinovirus).

- Children with viral croup present with acute inspiratory stridor, barking seal-like cough and hoarse voice. It is usually preceded by a cold for a few days, poor appetite, sore throat and low-grade fever; it differs from other types of croup as it is of gradual onset (12–48 hours). The child's symptoms may become more evident at night time and the stridor can become more severe when the child is upset and/or crying.

- *Spasmodic croup* (spasmodic laryngitis) is usually caused by allergic agents, gastroesophageal reflux (GOR) or psychological factors. The condition (which can be atopic) occurs in children aged between 1 and 3 years and is characterised by an *abrupt* night-time onset (awakening the child from sleep) of marked inspiratory stridor. It usually settles without any intervention after a few hours. Spasmodic croup may also be considered a variant of viral croup, especially when it recurs over several nights and is accompanied by a mild URTI. A small percentage of children with spasmodic croup may also have asthma.

- *Chronic inspiratory stridor* is most commonly caused by laryngomalacia. This condition results from a flaccid epiglottis combined with partial laryngeal collapse on inspiration; it is usually seen in infancy.

PATHOPHYSIOLOGY

- Acute infection (usually through respiratory droplet spread) provokes an inflammatory response that results in (1) mucosal oedema; (2) inflammation of the subglottic area; and (3) increased mucus production that can affect the entire respiratory tract.

- The localised inflammation of the subglottic region produces the barking cough and inspiratory stridor, but it is subglottic oedema (significantly narrowing the area) which can result in respiratory compromise. During inspiration, the walls of the subglottic space are drawn together. This can aggravate the localised inflammation and result in further oedema, more narrowing and significant respiratory distress.

- Because a child's airway is narrow, only a small amount of oedema is required to reduce the diameter and cause increased airflow resistance. It is therefore, extremely important that a child with croup is kept calm and quiet. A distressed and upset child will have more turbulent airflow, which compounds the problems of increased resistance and respiratory distress.

HISTORY

- Age, frequency and duration of symptoms.
- Activity and nature of symptoms at onset (playing, sleeping, gradual or abrupt).
- Quality of cry, cough and voice.
- Progression of symptoms since onset, home treatment and factors that have relieved or aggravated.
- Other associated symptoms (URTI, fever, vomiting, diarrhoea, abdominal pain, hoarse voice, rhinorrhoea, etc.).
- Difficulty with breathing, swallowing and/or intake of oral fluids.
- Previous history and treatment of croup.
- History of stridor at birth, airway malformation, intubations and cardiac or respiratory problems.
- History of allergies and/or atopy and immunisation status.
- Possibility of foreign body or chemical aspiration.

PHYSICAL EXAMINATION

- Astute observation is key and a 'hands off approach' should be adopted. Keep the child as calm as possible: it is important to leave the child with carer in an upright position.
- Focus observations on the degree of respiratory compromise: rate, grunting, recessions, colour, work associated with breathing, ability to take oral fluids, degree of stridor and positioning (leaning forward, drooling and ill-appearance suggest epiglottitis). Note signs of engagability with carer, tiredness, increased agitation, drowsiness, lethargy and altered mental status. A croup scoring system (Table 11.6) can be helpful in assessing the severity of symptoms. While there is subjectivity associated with the scoring, it can be a useful adjuvant to monitor a child over time. A score of 3 or more is likely to require more aggressive management.
- **Head and ENT:** examination of the oropharynx remains controversial as the risk of increased distress to the child must be balanced with the

information likely to be gained from direct visualisation. Likewise, inspection of the tympanic membranes needs to be considered with regard to the degree of distress this will cause the child. Neck masses or bruising suggest stridor that is related to bacterial infection or trauma.

- **Cardiopulmonary:** air entry is assessed as well as presence of cyanosis, wheezes/crackles, quality of voice and air entry into lungs. Note whether stethoscope is required to hear stridor and whether there is stridor at rest.

DIFFERENTIAL DIAGNOSES

- Diagnosis of croup is typically apparent from the history and physical examination; however, consider additional diagnoses as presented in Table 11.7.

MANAGEMENT

- **Additional diagnostics:** laboratory tests/procedures are not usually required for the diagnosis. However, the following procedures

Table 11.6 Croup Scoring System[a]

Observation	Score			
Level of consciousness	0 normal (alert, interactive)	1–4 minimal to moderate alteration	5 altered mental status (lethargic, disorientated)	
Air entry	0 normal	1 slightly decreased	2 very decreased	
Inspiratory stridor	0 none	1 at rest (with stethoscope)	2 at rest (without stethoscope)	
Retractions	0 none	1 slight	2 moderate	3 marked
Colour	0 without cyanosis	4 cyanotic when agitated	5 cyanotic at rest	

[a]Adapted from Super (1989) and Westley (1978).

Table 11.7 Differential Diagnosis of Croup

Potential aetiology	Characteristics
Congenital:	
• Tracheomalacia • Laryngomalacia	• Presents in first month of life, child is well, stridor increases with excitement
Infectious:	
• Epiglottis	• Stridor with toxic appearance, forward leaning, drooling (no Hib immunisation)
• Retropharyngeal or peritonsillar abscess	• Muffled voice, fever, ill appearance, stiff neck dysphagia
• Diphtheritic croup	• Missing/incomplete diphtheria vaccinations
• Bacterial tracheitis	• Ill/toxic appearance with fever and stridor that is rapidly progressing in severity; incomplete immunisations (Hib)
Toxins:	
• Foreign body aspiration	• Playing and well before sudden onset of stridor in a healthy child, may be accompanied by coughing/choking and history of play with small objects
• Caustic ingestion (smoke or heat irritation)	• History of exposure to heat, smoke or chemicals
Allergic/inflammatory:	
• Hypersensitivity or anaphylaxis	• Documented allergy, history of insect sting, new medication or food
• Asthma	• History of labile and severe asthma

may be of use in clinical decision making:

- Pulse oximetry should be documented at least once; note that it is not diagnostic for respiratory failure.
- FBC, CRP and blood cultures may be of help if bacterial infection is suspected. Note however, that venepuncture is likely to increase anxiety with a resultant increase in respiratory distress. *Invasive diagnostics are not routinely recommended and, if required, should be carried out in a controlled environment when the child's airway is deemed secure.*
- Neck/chest X-ray usually unnecessary; an anterior and posterior view may show subglottic narrowing and a lateral view may rule out epiglottitis, retropharyngeal abscess and foreign body.

- **Pharmacotherapeutics:**
  - Paracetamol: (10–15 mg/kg every 4 hours as required) to reduce pyrexia.
  - Steroids: the efficacy of systemic steroids in decreasing mucosal oedema and subglottic narrowing is well established. Choice of preparation (and administration route) are influenced by the setting and clinical judgement. Improvement is typically seen within 1 hour of steroid administration and, therefore, dexamethasone is a first-line treatment for moderate-to-severe croup. Note that oral dexamethasone is as effective as nebulised budesonide and the oral solution is readily available. In addition, both nebulisation and intramuscular (IM) injection can increase distress to the child and their use should be considered carefully: (1) dexamethasone, orally ($150\,\mu g$/kg) or IM injection ($0.6\,mg$/kg; max = $10\,mg$); (2) nebulised budesonide ($2\,mg$) in a single dose.
  - Nebulised epinephrine/adrenaline ($1/1000$) 5 ml with high-dose oxygen can be used with moderate-to-severe cases to reduce inflammation/oedema.

- Antibiotics: reserved for bacterial infections and are of no benefit in the treatment of viral croup.

- **Behavioural intervention:** the mainstay of treatment for mild croup is paracetamol, observation and adequate fluid intake. In some areas, humidity and/or use of mist tent therapy is still advised for the treatment for croup though recent research challenges the efficacy of this treatment. Caution should be exercised in using steam-generated humidity, as the risk of scalding the airway is more dangerous than the croup itself. In some instances, humidity can also induce bronchospasm.

- **Patient education:**
  - Clear and explicit discharge instructions (with contact phone number) should be given to the carer: this will include symptoms of worsening illness and/or increasing respiratory distress (breathing becomes more difficult, poor colour/pallor/cyanosis, drooling/difficulty swallowing, refusing liquids, increased heart rate and significant fever).
  - Reinforce with parents the importance of seeking care if any of those symptoms develop or if the child becomes restless, irritable, exhausted or confused. Likewise, parents should call if they are worried/concerned about their child's condition or home management.
  - Review home management of mild croup (fluids, fever control, comfort measures, observation) and let parents know that symptoms should gradually resolve over 3–4 days (although it is not uncommon for the stridor to last up to 1 week and the cough for longer).
  - Reassure parents that there will be no long-term damage to the respiratory system.

⇨ FOLLOW-UP

- Generally not indicated for uncomplicated viral croup, as the condition is self-limiting. Follow-up phone contact may be beneficial for anxious parents.

⇄ MEDICAL CONSULT/ SPECIALIST REFERRAL

- Any child with a toxic appearance or one who is cyanosed, dehydrated or exhausted.
- Any child in whom epiglottitis is suspected.
- Any child with tracheal, sternal or subcostal recessions at rest, other signs of respiratory compromise/distress (respiratory rate >50–60) and/or deteriorating condition.
- Any child under 1 year of age and/or any child in whom there is no improvement after initial treatment.
- Any child whose diagnosis is uncertain or who has a history of chronic, persistent or recurrent stridor which is likely to require further investigation/treatment.
- Any child in whom there is a suspicion of foreign body aspiration.
- Any child where there are family/social reasons to suggest the child cannot be cared for at home (including extreme carer anxiety).

◯ PAEDIATRIC PEARLS

- Clinical discretion must be used with regard to examination of the throat in a child with stridor. The likelihood of missed pathology needs to be balanced against the possibility of increased upset caused by examination of the oropharynx.
- Reduce anxiety levels by having a calm, confident and 'hands off' approach.
- Regular reassessment is required as a child can deteriorate quickly, developing a partial/complete airway obstruction.
- In young infants with recurrent croup, the following should be considered: congenital abnormalities, underlying anatomical problems and GOR.
- Bacterial infection of the lower respiratory system is a complication of croup. It can cause progressive airway obstruction that leads to a life-threatening event. Urgent intervention with hospital admission is required in these cases.

COMMON PAEDIATRIC PROBLEMS

2

- Always consider the possibility of foreign body aspiration or ingestion as a potential aetiology (especially in toddlers).
- Beware the toxic/ill appearing child: always consider epiglottitis. It is a medical emergency and will require an ENT/anaesthesia input.

BIBLIOGRAPHY

Couriel JM. Management of croup. Arch Dis Child 1988; 63(11):1305–1308.

Dawson K. The management of acute laryngo-tracheo-bronchitits (croup): a consensus view. J Paediatr Child Health 1992; 28(3):223–224.

Geelhoed G. Croup. Pediatr Pulmonol 1997; 23(5):370–374.

Kadas A, Wald E. Viral croup: current diagnosis and treatment. Contemp Pediatr 1999; 16(2):139–153.

Klassen TP. Croup: a current perspective. Pediatr Clin North Am 1999; 46(6):1167–1178.

Leung KC, Cho H. Diagnosis of stridor in children. Am Family Physic 1999; 60(8):2289–2296.

Madden V. Coughing associated with laryngitis in children: croup. Prof Care Mother Child 1997; 7(4):93–94.

Malhoutra A, Krilov L. Viral croup. Pediatr Rev 2001; 22(1):5–11.

Pappas D, Hayden G, Owen-Hendley J. Epiglottitis and croup: keys to therapy at home and in hospital. Consultant 1997; 4:857–867.

Super R. A prospective randomized double-blind study to evaluate the effect of dexamethasone in acute laryngotracheitis. J Pediatr 1989; 115:323–329.

Westley C. Nebulized racemic epinephrine by IPPB for the treatment of croup. Am J Dis Child 1978; 132:484–487.

11.5 SYNCOPE

Ritamarie John

INTRODUCTION

- Syncope is described as a sudden, transient, reversible loss of consciousness and muscle tone.
- Syncope is not a rare event in paediatrics; it has been estimated that 15% of children will have a syncopal episode at some point during childhood.
- Most syncope does not reflect cardiac disease but it is important to differentiate worrisome from benign syncope.
- Potential aetiologies for syncope include cardiac, neurocardiac, seizure migraine, breath-holding spells, hypoglycaemia, hysteria, orthostatic and situational. As there is a potential for life-threatening causes of syncope, a careful history and physical examination is key.
- Syncope causes significant anxiety for families, playmates and school personnel. In order to alleviate their fears, it is vital that the family's concerns are taken seriously. Likewise, it is imperative not to falsely reassure patients and families.

PATHOPHYSIOLOGY

- The specific pathophysiology of syncope is dependent on the aetiology of the episode.
- The most common mechanism of syncope is vasovagal (i.e. neurocardiac syncope). It is caused by autonomic dysfunction, in which a variety of external stimuli (pain, emotional upset, long periods standing, etc.) trigger increased vagal tone that subsequently causes a decrease in heart rate and peripheral vasodilatation. This primary vasodepressor response results in hypotension, decreased cerebral perfusion pressure and a syncopal episode.
- The child with breath-holding spells may involuntarily activate the Valsalva reflex, thereby increasing intrathoracic pressure, decreasing venous return and subsequently decreasing cardiac output. These processes lead to cerebral ischaemia, unconsciousness and decreased muscle tone (i.e. syncope). With the onset of cyanosis, generalised clonic jerks and bradycardia can occur.
- Hyperventilation causes syncope by producing cerebral vasoconstriction. If the patient simultaneously does a Valsalva manoeuvre the cerebral hypoperfusion is accentuated.
- Cough syncope occurs because of decreased venous return to the right heart, reduced left ventricular filling and decreased cardiac output, resulting in hypoperfusion to the brain.
- Functional problems associated with the heart (e.g. outflow obstruction, myocardial dysfunction or arrhythmias) may lead to syncope as a result of decreased cerebral perfusion and/or cardiac ischaemia. Cardiac syncope is potentially fatal and requires careful evaluation and treatment.

HISTORY

- Duration of the episode including what happened during the episode with regard to the child's colour, unusual eye and limb movements, loss of continence and length of time child was unresponsive.
- It is crucial to obtain information (from the child and observers) about what happened before the event (e.g. activity, environment, presence of seizure-like activity, and whether the child 'knew' or felt that she was going to pass out).

- Position prior to the episode, as standing-associated syncope suggest a vasovagal mechanism.
- 24-hour dietary recall and the association of the syncope to meals.
- Presence of associated symptoms: palpitations, chest pain, headache, sweating, nausea and/or auditory or visual auras.
- Medication history, including over-the-counter (OTC) medicines, herbal remedies and weight reduction medications, all of which can induce arrhythmias. Note that families may not consider herbal or homeopathic medications as part of the history, so use of these products needs to be explored.
- History of exposures (e.g. alcohol, carbon monoxide, drug use).
- Past medical history, including previous cardiac surgery and history of Kawasaki disease.
- Family history of syncope, sudden or early death, epilepsy, neurological disease, deafness (long QT syndrome may have familial deafness), endocrine disorders, long QT syndrome, cardiomyopathies, arrhythmias or myocardial infarction at a young age.
- A social history should include careful enquiry regarding stressors, sexual abuse or any secondary gain that might result from a syncopal episode.
- Note that a worrisome history in a child presenting with syncope includes an age <6 years, recumbent position, prolonged loss of consciousness of 5 min or longer, presence of cardiac disease or heart murmur, and syncope occurring with exercise.

👁 PHYSICAL EXAMINATION

- A complete physical examination with special attention to the cardiovascular and neurological systems.
- Check blood pressure sitting, standing and supine. An orthostatic change in heart rate or blood pressure should be noted (i.e. a drop of 20 mmHg when moving from a supine to a standing position). Compare blood pressure readings in each arm.
- Listen for murmurs in at least two positions (e.g. sitting and supine) and check peripheral and central pulses.

- If hyperventilation is being considered, the child should be hyperventilated to see if syncope occurs.
- Careful and thorough neurological examination.

❓ DIFFERENTIAL DIAGNOSES

- Syncope can be divided into cardiac, non-cardiac and neurocardiac aetiologies (Table 11.8).
- It is imperative that cardiac causes of syncope are differentiated from benign causes of syncope (e.g. breath-holding spells, vasovagal, hyperventilation and cough-induced syncope). A careful history and physical assessment is the basis upon which further clinical or laboratory testing is based.

✚ MANAGEMENT

The management of syncope is largely dependent upon the aetiology of the episodes.

- **Additional diagnostics:** Many children will have a clear history of vasovagal syncope and additional diagnostics are not necessary. Note that electrocardiography (ECG) is suggested for all cases of unexplained syncope, as ruling out life-threatening cardiac disease is a priority. In addition, consider a chest X-ray and FBC as initial tests (Table 11.8) with more extensive investigation coordinated by specialist care for children with recurrent or unexplained episodes.
- **Pharmacotherapeutics:** aetiology-specific. Note that among children with cough syncope and asthma, better control of their asthma will reduce the syncope. Scopolamine or other anticholinergics (e.g. atropine) can be used in frequent and severe cyanotic breath-holding spells as they will increase the heart rate by blocking the vagus nerve. Pseudo-ephedrine prevents venous pooling and blocks systemic hypotension when used as an adjunctive medication for vasovagal syncope. If iron-deficiency anaemia is present with breath-holding-induced syncope, correct anaemia as it has been reported to worsen the

frequency and severity of the breath-holding spells.
- **Behavioural interventions:**
  - For breath-holding spells, it is better to keep the child horizontal and wait (if loss of consciousness >2 min, activate emergency services).
  - Prevention of syncope by avoiding situations that have resulted in syncope (e.g. long periods standing in a warm room, maintaining adequate hydration and nutrition, etc.).
  - In hyperventilation syncope, reassurance and rebreathing into a bag can prevent the episodes.
  - Children with recurrent syncope should take precautions similar to those used among children of a similar age with epilepsy. More specifically, close monitoring when participating in water-related activities and restrictions on climbing. Note, however, that most children with recurrent syncope do not experience spells during vigorous activity.
- **Patient education:**
  - Parents (and children) will require significant reassurance, support and education regarding the syncopal episodes. Review behavioural interventions (above).
  - As most cases of syncope are vasovagal, breath-holding or hyperventilation-related, families will need to understand why these episodes happen and what can be done to prevent them. Note that most children outgrow their breath-holding episodes; however, they may be predisposed to vasovagal syncope as adults.
  - Parents should keep a record of the syncopal episodes if the child experiences more than two episodes within 6 months.
  - Reassure parents that pallid breath-holding spells do not result in brain damage.

➡ FOLLOW-UP

- Families need to return if the syncope reoccurs. Of particular concern is any syncope associated with exercise.

Table 11.8	Differential Diagnoses of Syncope in Children				
Aetiology	History	Physical examination	ECG	Chest X-ray	Comments
Neurocardiac					
Vasovagal	• Can be precipitated by prolonged time in a warm room, crowding, acute illness, anaemia, pain, fear, exhaustion, hunger • Prodromal symptoms: nausea/vomiting, pallor, lightheadedness/vertigo, visual disturbances, sweating and shortness of breath • Post-episode complaints of fatigue, lightheadedness, anxiety, nausea, and/or headache • Mental alert post-episode • Family history of syncope	• Normal examination	–	–	• Most common cause of syncope • Usually a clinical diagnosis based on history and lack of physical examination findings • Tilt table test can be used to confirm the diagnosis of neurocardiac syncope
Non-cardiac					
Breath-holding spells (BHS)	• Pain, anger, frustration or fear trigger BHS • Typical history: brief cry or forced expiration followed by apnoea (e.g. holding of breath) with cyanosis or pallor occurring, loss of consciousness and possible brief tonic or clonic jerking • Consciousness returns rapidly • Symptomatic between spells	• Normal examination	–	–	• If history is not typical of BHS, rule out epilepsy or cardiac syncope • Check haemoglobin as anaemia can cause/exacerbate • Propensity for vasovagal syncope in later childhood and adolescence
Hyperventilation	• Episode of hyperventilation precedes syncopal episode	• Normal examination	–	–	• Consider referral to psychology if behavioural aetiology and/or recurrent episodes
Cough syncope	• History of asthma • Recovery begins within seconds of loss of consciousness • Night-time occurrence with cough awakening child from sleep before syncopal episode	• Finding consistent with asthma	–	+/–	• Asthma management needs to be reviewed
Situational	• Defecation, neck stretching, venepuncture or other condition trigger episode • Consciousness returns rapidly	• Normal examination	–	–	• Diagnosis made on historical grounds
Seizures	• History of aura possible • Description of 'spell' more consistent with epilepsy than seizures (occurrence while at rest, unusual eye and limb movements, prolonged loss of consciousness, postictal stupor, etc.)	• Normal cardiac examination although tachycardia is a feature of the seizures	–	–	• Syncopal episode may trigger seizure in a susceptible child
Toxins/drugs	• History of exposure(s) and/or ingestion	• Findings dependent on toxin	+/–	+/–	• Safety counselling imperative
Migraines	• History of aura, severe headache, associated nausea, vomiting, photophobia and relief by sleep • Family history of migraines	• Normal examination	–	–	• Syncope related to pain of migraines • Positive family history of migraines in 75% of cases
Orthostatic hypotension	• Lightheadedness upon arising rapidly from sitting or recumbent position	• Drop of ≥20 mmHg within 2 min of standing upright	–	–	• Consider pregnancy in sexually active adolescent female • Dehydration and prolonged bedrest may predispose
Cardiac					
Outflow obstruction	• Syncope accompanies exercise • May be +ve family history of 'heart problems' • May have chest pain with exertion • No prior warning of syncope	• Abnormal cardiac examination (e.g. murmurs, rate abnormalities)	+/–	+/–	• Includes aortic stenosis and hypertrophic cardiomyopathy
Myocardial dysfunction	• As above	• As above	+/–	+/–	• Includes myocarditis, Kawasaki disease and Duchenne dystrophy
Arrhythmias	• As above • May complain of palpitations, 'funny beats' or dizziness with exertion	• As above, although murmur may not be heard • May have irregularities of rate	+	+/–	• Includes long QT syndrome, ventricular tachycardia, Wolff–Parkinson–White and sinus node dysfunction • Deafness may accompany long QT syndrome

⮂ MEDICAL CONSULT/ SPECIALIST REFERRAL

- Any child in whom the aetiology of the syncope is not readily apparent from the history or physical examination (e.g. those without classic vasovagal, breath-holding or hyperventilation-related syncope).
- Any child with recurring syncope or episodes associated with a recumbent position, prolonged loss of consciousness, presence of cardiac disease (or strong familial history of cardiac disease), exercise, cardiac symptoms or seizures.
- Any child less than 6 years of age with syncope that is not related to breath-holding spells.
- Any child in whom there is the possibility of a behavioural component to the episodes.

⌕ PAEDIATRIC PEARLS

- Vasovagal syncopal events are more common in pre-adolescents and adolescents and are induced while standing up in warm places.

- Children under 6 years of age with syncope not associated with breath-holding spells are more worrisome.
- There are rare causes of syncope such as familial dysautonomia, which is found in people who are of Ashkenazi Jewish descent. This will present early in childhood.
- Cough-induced syncope may be the sign that asthma is not in good control.
- Recurrent syncope related to prolonged QT interval may be missed on routine ECG, as it may only occur with exertion.
- Carbon monoxide may cause syncopal spells: enquire about exposures.
- Temporal lobe epilepsy may mimic a syncopal episode and/or syncope may trigger a convulsion in an epileptic child.
- Cardiac-related syncope is associated with little or no prodrome and occurs even when the child is lying down. There may be a prolonged loss of consciousness, history of palpitations, family history of sudden death and the episode may be associated with exercise.

- Consider pregnancy in a sexually active adolescent female with a vasovagal syncopal episode.

▤ BIBLIOGRAPHY

Ackerman M. The long QT syndrome. Pediatr Rev 1998; 9(7):3232–3238.

Benditt D, Lurie K, Fabian W. Clinical approach to diagnosis of syncope: an overview. Cardiol Clin 1997; 15: 165–176.

Braden D, Gaymes C. The diagnosis and management of syncope in children and adolescents. Pediatr Ann 1997; 26(7):422–426.

Feit L. Syncope in the pediatric patient: diagnosis, pathophysiology and treatment. Adv Pediatr 1994; 43: 469–494.

Lewis D, Dhala A. Syncope in the pediatric patient: the cardiologist's perspective. Pediatr Clin N Am 1999; 46:205–219.

Narchi H. The child who passes out. Pediatr Rev 2000; 21:384–388.

Prodinger R, Reisdorff EJ. Syncope in children. Emerg Med Clin N Am 1998; 16(3):617–626.

Willis J. Syncope. Pediatr Rev 2000; 21:201–204.

11.6 CHEST PAIN

Ritamarie John

▭ INTRODUCTION

- Chest pain is a common complaint in children and adolescents. It is found in children of all ages, with an average age at presentation of 12 years.
- The different aetiologies of chest pain in children have a developmental component. Young children are more likely to have a respiratory, gastrointestinal (GI) or cardiac source for their chest pain and they are more likely to have an organic cause for the pain. Older children and adolescents may still have a cardiac, GI or respiratory aetiology, but psychogenic, musculoskeletal or idiopathic causes increase in this age group. There is no racial or sexual predilection.

- The main objective in the evaluation of chest pain in children is to differentiate children that will require further work-up and referral from those in whom, analgesics, reassurance and follow-up are the mainstays of management.
- Remember that chest pain is significant for families as it tends to be associated with cardiac disease and death; these fears can add to the anxiety levels of both parents and children.

⯎ PATHOPHYSIOLOGY

- Chest pain can arise from several sources in children. The pain may come from the structures within the thorax or it can be referred from visceral organs.

- Cardiac disease will cause ischaemic chest pain, worsening with exercise and increased workload on the heart. This pain is from thoracic sympathetic nerves as well as the cardiac nerves. Pain from the pericardium can arise from the phrenic or the laryngeal-oesophageal plexus, causing substernal pressure or shoulder, neck or arm pain. Mitral valve prolapse can cause chest pain due to papillary muscle or endocardial ischaemia. Aortic pain will arise in the adventitia of the blood vessel and is produced from stimulation of the sympathetic chain.
- Pleural pain comes from irritation of the parietal pleura since the visceral pleura is insensitive to pain with signals transmitted via intercostal nerves.

- Central diaphragmatic pain comes from the phrenic nerve and, therefore, the child may present with shoulder pain on the affected side.
- Musculoskeletal causes of chest pain result from stimulation of the sensory nerves in the affected intercostal muscle or dermatome.
- Oesophageal pain is produced by stimulation of the nerves in the spinal segments and may present with anterior superior chest pain and/or pain around the neck.

⬅ HISTORY

- A careful history is imperative; allow the child and family to express their concerns. Explore the child's fears about the pain. Adolescents will worry that their heart is causing the chest pain.
- Onset, severity and frequency of the pain, including the length of time before the family sought care.
- Type of pain (burning, sharp, stabbing, etc.) and whether it interferes with everyday activities.
- Precipitating, aggravating and relieving factors.
- The association of pain to exercise and meals.
- Recent trauma or muscle overuse.
- Intake of spicy foods and medications (especially tetracycline or other 'tablets').
- Recent use of cocaine (and if positive, frequency and extent of use).

- Use of oral contraceptives and history of recent leg trauma (i.e. to rule out possibility of embolism).
- Recent or significant stress.
- Associated symptoms: fever, weight loss, syncope, palpitations, joint pain, rashes, attention-seeking behaviour.
- Past medical history, including asthma, Kawasaki disease, diabetes and sickle cell disease.
- Family history of cardiac problems (including sudden or early death, syncope or heart disease), asthma, sickle cell disease, cystic fibrosis and smoking.

👁 PHYSICAL EXAMINATION

- A thorough and complete physical examination is required, as the potential aetiologies of chest pain are numerous (Table 11.9). Pay particular attention to the cardiac, pulmonary and abdominal examinations.
- Worrying physical examination findings include severe distress, chronically or acutely ill appearance, cardiac involvement (e.g. murmurs, arrhythmias, tachycardia), pulmonary findings (e.g. rub, rales, wheezing), skin rashes/bruising, abdominal pathology, concomitant arthritis and acute anxiety.

🔎 DIFFERENTIAL DIAGNOSES

- The most common causes of chest pain in children and adolescents include musculoskeletal, trauma,

respiratory conditions, GI problems, cardiac pathology and various miscellaneous causes (breast mass, cocaine abuse, sickle cell crisis, thoracic tumour). The history and physical examination findings are the basis upon which further testing is considered and the differential list is narrowed (Table 11.9).

⊕ MANAGEMENT

- **Additional diagnostics:** aetiology-specific (see Table 11.9); however, if the history of physical examination suggests cardiac pathology consider electrocardiogram (ECG), chest X-ray, 24-hour cardiac monitoring and exercise stress testing. Likewise, if a pulmonary aetiology is suggested, consider a chest X-ray and pulmonary function tests.

- **Pharmacotherapeutics:** aetiology-specific; for many cases of benign chest pain, OTC analgesia (paracetamol, ibuprofen or antacids) are sufficient. Note, however, that serious aetiologies are not well correlated with frequency and severity of pain.

- **Behavioural interventions:** aetiology-specific; however, for the majority of benign chest pain, reassurance, relaxation (including stress management) and analgesia will suffice. A symptom diary that includes reference to activity or stress levels in addition to the pain often helps the child and family see the associations and triggers for the pain.

Table 11.9	Differential Diagnoses of Chest Pain in Children	
History	*Physical examination findings*	*Additional diagnostics, differential diagnoses and comments*
Musculoskeletal		
• Pain of acute onset • History of blunt trauma • Pain relieved by analgesics	• Pain in chest wall with area of localised tenderness possible • May have bruising • Breath sounds clear	• Consider soft tissue injury, rib fracture, muscle haematoma with possibility of cardiac or great vessel contusion if significant blunt trauma • Consider rib X-ray • Consider mechanism of injury, as rib fractures can be related to child protection issues • History and physical examination findings should match
• History of muscle strain, vigorous exercise or activity and/or lifting of heavy weights/objects • Pain relieved by analgesics	• Generalised tenderness over chest wall • Pain reproducible with same activity • Can have patient put hands together and push/pull apart (or push against examiner's hands) in order to reproduce pain • Breath sounds clear	• Consider chest wall strain • No other diagnostics indicated

(continued)

Table 11.9 continued		
History	*Physical examination findings*	*Additional diagnostics, differential diagnoses and comments*
Musculoskeletal		
• History of significant and forceful cough for an extended period of time (may complain of post-tussive vomiting) • Pain relieved by analgesics • Complaints of rib pain on inspiration	• Tenderness of chest wall with increased tenderness at costochondral junctions • May be swelling at costochondral junction • Breath sounds/lung fields clear • Significant cough	• Consider costochondritis • If cough related to asthma, improve asthma control • No other diagnostics indicated
Gastrointestinal		
• Pain worse on swallowing • Child may be drooling to avoid swallowing • Current medication (e.g. tetracyclines may cause oesophageal irritation) • History of 'choking' or ingestion • Complaints of burning pain • History of spicy food intake • History of eating disorders (bulimia)	• Normal examination • In bulimia there may be erosion of enamel on posterior upper teeth; salivary/parotid gland enlargement; calluses of knuckles or hands; muscle weakness and hypotension	• Consider oesophageal foreign body aspiration or caustic ingestion • Consider chest X-ray • Note that foreign body may not be radiopaque • If no resolution consider referral for evaluation and endoscopy • Consider gastro-oesophageal reflux (GOR), oesophagitis • Check stool for occult blood
Cardiac		
• Pain improves when child sits up and forward • Pain is acute, sharp and stabbing; increased on respiration • Ill-appearing child with fever	• May hear friction rub, distant sounding heart sounds, neck vein distension and pulsus paradoxus	• Consider ECG, chest X-ray, 24-hour cardiac monitoring • Consider pericarditis
• Complaints of 'funny beats' or 'heart beating very fast' • May have chest pain on exertion • May have history of syncope (see Sec. 11.5)	• Examination may be normal or arrhythmia (including tachycardia) may be heard	• Consider arrhythmias • Consider ECG, chest X-ray, 24-hour cardiac monitoring
• Ill-appearing child with/without fever • Pain on exertion • History of fatigue, dyspnoea	• Subtle findings on physical examination: tachycardia, ectopic beats and/or gallop rhythm • May have orthostatic changes in pulse (≥30 beats/min decrease) and blood pressure (≥20 mmHg drop) when changing position (supine to standing) • Check for an enlarged heart (point of maximal impulse to the left of the nipple line) • May have systolic murmur	• Consider ECG, chest X-ray, 24-hour cardiac monitoring • Consider myocarditis
Pulmonary		
• Complaints of cough, fever, ill-appearance	• Adventitious sounds • Increased respiratory rate	• Consider pneumonia • Consider chest X-ray
• Complaint of pain with exertion ('unable to catch breath') • History of asthma in family • Cough associated with exercise or night time	• Prolonged expiratory phase with or without wheeze • Use of accessory muscle	• Consider asthma
• Acute onset of sharp pain and complaints of respiratory distress	• Decreased breath sounds on one side, respiratory distress, hypotension	• Consider pneumothorax • Obtain chest X-ray
Other		
• History of cocaine use • Pain may be temporally linked to drug intake	• Tachycardia • Anxiety • Cocaine intoxication may present with pneumothorax, hypertension and arrhythmias	• Consider cocaine use • Obtain drug screen • Will require intervention around drug use/abuse
• Complaints of breast enlargement, breast tenderness or asymmetry	• Normal examination	• Consider physiological breast changes of puberty and/or pregnancy

- **Patient education:**
  - Reassure children and families (after acknowledging and addressing their fears) that most chest pain is benign and self-limiting. Life-threatening causes of chest pain are very rare. Stress, asthma, GOR and musculoskeletal aetiologies are, by far, the most common causes of chest pain in children.
  - Review, with the family, signs and symptoms of more serious problems and when to seek care.

⇨ FOLLOW-UP

- Follow-up is an essential component in the management of chest pain and should be discussed with the family: this may include further diagnostics, referral or watching/waiting.

⇄ MEDICAL CONSULT/ SPECIALIST REFERRAL

- Any child that is in severe distress and has vital sign changes or positive findings on physical examination and/or diagnostic testing.
- Any child in whom a cardiac, pulmonary or other significant aetiology is suspected.
- Any child requiring intervention for drug or cocaine abuse.

- Any child who is experiencing acute distress.
- Any child with an ill or anxious appearance, history of significant trauma or family history of sudden death.
- Any child experiencing pain with exercise, syncope, palpitations, and/or dizziness.
- Any child with serious emotional upset.
- Any child with a suspected foreign body and/or caustic ingestion.

🜨 PAEDIATRIC PEARLS

- A good history and thorough physical examination is the key to problem identification; avoid expensive and invasive diagnostics with chronic pain, benign history and normal examination.
- Be sure to review normal findings as part of the examination in order to reassure the child and family.
- Chest pain during exercise is a red flag for organic disease.
- Fever with chest pain requires consideration of organic aetiologies such as pericarditis, myocarditis or pneumonia.
- Analgesics (e.g. paracetamol or ibuprofen), rest and relaxation may be all that is needed for musculoskeletal chest pain.

- A trial of antacids may be both therapeutic and diagnostic in cases of reflux and oesophagitis.
- For the anxious child, teaching relaxation techniques or yoga classes may alleviate the chest pain.
- Follow-up is the key if the first visit does not reveal anything specific after a careful history and physical examination. Use of a symptom diary can be a useful adjuvant and may reveal a potential cause.

🗒 BIBLIOGRAPHY

Allen H, Golinko R, Williams R. Heart murmurs in children: when is a workup needed? Contemp Pediatr 1994; 11(11):29–52.

Daford D. Clinical and basic laboratory assessment of children for possible congenital heart disease. Curr Opin Pediatr 2000; 12(5):487–491.

Feit L. The heart of the matter: evaluating heart murmurs in children. Contemp Pediatr 1997; 14(10):97–122.

Kaden G, Shenker I, Gootman N. Chest pain in adolescents. J Adolesc Health Care 1991; 12:251–255.

Moody Y. Pediatric cardiovascular assessment and referral in the primary care setting. Nurse Pract 1997; 22(1):120–134.

Pelech A. The cardiac murmur: when to refer? Pediatr Clin Am 1998; 45(1):107–121.

Selbst S. Chest pain in children. Pediatr Rev 1997; 18(5):169–173.

CHAPTER 12

Gastrointestinal and Endocrine Problems

12.1 ACUTE ABDOMINAL PAIN

Katie Barnes

📖 INTRODUCTION

- The overall incidence of acute abdominal pain (AAP) is unknown, as the vast majority of episodes are managed successfully at home. It has been estimated that 1–2% of children presenting to emergency settings with AAP will have serious disease (acute appendicitis being the most common surgical diagnosis). The patient's age has important implications for the expression of pain (see Sec. 13.3) as well as for the potential aetiology of the pain (Table 12.1).
- The primary objective in the evaluation of AAP is the accurate and timely differentiation of those conditions which are benign, self-limiting and within the nurse practitioner's (NP's) scope of practice from those that represent more significant pathology and therefore, require medical consultation and referral.

🔬 PATHOPHYSIOLOGY

- AAP results from the stimulation of nerve fibres from the parietal peritoneum (e.g. peritoneal lining and mucosa) and/or the abdominal viscera (e.g. deep muscular wall and the associated structures of the visceral cavity). Parietal pain is characteristically sharp, localised and stimulated by inflammation, whereas visceral pain is usually dull, poorly localised and triggered by tension and stretching. However, there is common enervation of many abdominal organs and referred pain can result when there is mixing of signals or when there is an overflow of signals from the visceral to the parietal pathways.
- For the most part, *epigastric pain* usually results from pathology in the foregut (stomach, pancreas, liver and upper small bowel) whereas *periumbilical pain* is generated from the midgut (distal small bowel, caecum, appendix and ascending colon). *Suprapubic pain* is typically related to the hindgut (distal intestine, urinary tract, pelvic organs).
- *It is important to remember that progressive pathology can change the symptomatology:* visceral stretch receptors stimulated in early appendicitis would likely cause diffuse non-specific epigastric pain that later becomes localised to the right lower quadrant and sharper as the inflammation of the appendix increased (i.e. stimulation of the parietal fibres).

⬅ HISTORY

- Onset, frequency, distribution and characteristics of the pain (if child able to describe). Include information on aggravating/relieving factors and whether the pain has awoken the child from sleep.
- Where the pain started, whether it is shifting/changing, whether it is worsened by movement and whether other family members are affected.
- Associated nausea, vomiting, diarrhoea/bloody stool, fever or other symptoms (e.g. rashes, dysuria, constipation, weight loss, anorexia, sore throat and/or joint pain).
- Previous history of AAP, relationship of pain to meals (or specific foods) and what has been done to relieve pain.
- Age-related history (Table 12.1).

Table 12.1	Age-related AAP History
Age group	Query
Infants	• Unusual facial expression, cry, and activity/sleep pattern disruption (thrashing, restless, motionless)
Toddlers/pre-school	• Aggressive behaviour and/or disturbed sleep patterns
School-age	• Child's description and 'one-finger' localisation (e.g. asking the child to point to the pain 'using only 1 finger') • Bullying or trauma at school
Adolescents	• Sexual and menstrual history (consider obtaining history without parent)

PHYSICAL EXAMINATION

- It is vital that the initial contact with the child is *not* painful. Likewise, careful observation of the child during the physical examination is imperative; useful manoeuvres to assess the degree of peritoneal inflammation and visceral pain include asking the child to 'hop on each leg' or 'climb' onto the examination table (or carer's lap). In addition, it is useful to establish the child's baseline level of response by touching an arm or leg and comparing complaints of 'how much that hurts' with the discomfort associated with the abdominal examination.

- **Skin:** examine for rashes, petechiae and/or purpura.

- **Head, ear, nose and throat (ENT) and lymph examination:** careful examination as pharyngitis in school-aged children often presents as AAP.

- **Cardiopulmonary:** note respiratory symptoms as pneumonia in young children can present as AAP.

- **Neurological and musculoskeletal:** limit examination to assessment of pain on movement and overall level of alertness.

- **Abdomen:** should be done last; include rectal examination as it is integral to evaluation of the suspected appendicitis. However, it should only be performed *once*, accompanied by careful explanation and consent from child and carer. Observe abdomen for distension and/or visible peristalsis. Palpate the abdomen carefully, starting with the least painful area and include a careful feel for masses (remove nappy). Rebound tenderness, psoas and obturator signs (as performed in adults) usually not helpful (even with older children/adolescents); much more helpful is an assessment of the child's ease of movement (hopping, walking, climbing).

- Determination of abdominal tenderness can likewise be ascertained during auscultation for bowel sounds by pressing firmly with the stethoscope or through percussion of the lower chest and abdomen (beginning in an area that is unlikely to be tender). Include assessment of costovertebral angle (CVA) and suprapubic tenderness, liver, spleen and inguinal canal.

- If history suggests gynaecological aetiology, pelvic examination should be considered.

- *Repeat examinations (with careful documentation at regular intervals) are a mainstay of early assessment and management.*

DIFFERENTIAL DIAGNOSES

- Numerous and often age-related (Table 12.2). Although the majority of aetiologies are benign, it is *crucial that surgical emergencies are distinguished from medical conditions* (Table 12.3).

MANAGEMENT

- **Additional diagnostics:** usefulness limited to excluding the likelihood of other aetiologies (Table 12.3).

- **Pharmacotherapeutics:** use of medication is aetiology-specific; pain relief often deferred in early evaluation to prevent masking of pain levels and/or fever.

- **Behavioural intervention:** aetiology-specific; often includes dietary changes, fluids and symptom management.

- **Patient education:**
  - strong NP/family communication and follow-up is vital; *families must clearly understand the importance of returning/ringing if symptoms are worse or unresolved*
  - discuss with them the potential aetiologies that are under consideration and be sure that they are clear on their role in home management

- additional patient education is aetiology-specific.

FOLLOW-UP

- Return visit or phone call if pain has not settled (see Patient education).
- No further follow-up required if symptomatology resolves with supportive care.

MEDICAL CONSULT/ SPECIALIST REFERRAL

- Any child in whom there is any suspected surgical, gynaecological or urogenital emergency.
- Any child with a gravely ill appearance or one requiring a more extensive evaluation.
- Any child in whom a diagnosis is unclear.
- Any child who has not responded to initial management.

PAEDIATRIC PEARLS

- Appendicitis can occur concomitantly with another illness: i.e. gastroenteritis, upper respiratory tract infection (URTI).
- With recurrent acute abdominal pain that occurs repeatedly over a prolonged period, always consider the possibility of child protection issues.
- History and physical examination findings are the basis for additional diagnostics, consultation and/or referral; *do not* delay referral if physical findings are suspicious. This is especially important if preliminary laboratory results are not conclusive. The early presentation of appendicitis in children often has unremarkable results—high normal white cell count (WCC),

Table 12.2	Age-related AAP Aetiologies
Age	Consider
All ages	Gastroenteritis, constipation/gas, appendicitis, urinary tract infection (UTI), child abuse/non-accidental injury (NAI) and intestinal obstruction
0–2 years	Intussusception, incarcerated hernia, volvulus
3–12 years	Pneumonia, acute non-specific abdominal pain (ANSAP), pharyngitis, Henoch–Schönlein purpura
>12 years	ANSAP, ectopic pregnancy, pelvic inflammatory disease (PID), testicular or ovarian torsion, ovarian cyst

Table 12.3 Common Differential Diagnoses of Acute Abdominal Pain (AAP)

Cause	Fever	Vomit	↑WCC	↑ESR	FOB	AXR	U/S	U/A	Other
Appendicitis	+/−	+/−	+/−	+/−	+/−	• + in approx. 25% of cases • Majority with non-specific findings	• Especially helpful in diagnosing equivocal cases • Can also detect other causes of pathology (renal or gynaecological) • U/S is imaging test of choice	+/− WBC +/− RBC +/− protein +/− ketone	• Peak incidence at 12 years of age; uncommon <4 years • "Classic" presentation = **LAMENT:** **L**eucocytosis, **A**norexia, **M**igration of pain, **E**levated temperature, **N**ausea and vomiting, **T**enderness (right lower quadrant and rebound) • Vomiting often occurs *after* onset of pain • 50–70% of paediatric cases present atypically and may have concurrent tonsillitis, upper respiratory tract infection (URTI), urinary tract infection (UTI) symptoms with white blood cells (WBCs) in urine, diarrhoea, intermittent pain/diminished pain, and hunger • Accurate and *timely* diagnosis is *crucial*
Volvulus	−	+	+/−	−	+/−	• Often with non-specific findings	• Upper gastrointestinal series is diagnostic of choice • U/S helpful	−	• Usually <1 month old with palpable right upper quadrant (RUQ) mass • Triad of bilious vomiting, abdominal distension and gastrointestinal bleeding • 30–60% may have other gastrointestinal abnormalities
Intussusception	+	+	+	+	+/−	• May show soft tissue mass or distended bowel	• Helpful in diagnosis	−	• Can occur at any age, although 70% of cases occur in first year of life (usually 3–10 months old with a peak incidence at 7 months) • Classic triad of intermittent pain (90% of cases), vomiting (75%) and frank or occult blood on rectal examination (75%) • Currant jelly stool often late finding along with septic appearance • 80–90% of cases with RUQ mass • Pain-free periods alternate with severe, colicky-type pain
Gastroenteritis	+/−	+	+/−	−	+/−	• May show non-specific dilated bowel loops with air fluid level	• Usually not indicated	• Dipstick may be + for ketone • Check specific gravity	• Diarrhoea is prominent feature • Vomiting usually precedes pain • Child may be quite ill secondary to dehydration • Average no. of episodes among children 0–5 years is 1.3–2.3 episodes/year with duration of 3–7 days
Constipation/gas	−	+/−	−	−	−	• May show retained stool with significant constipation	• Usually not indicated	−	• Caecum is most common point of gas collection causing epigastric pain without migration • Rectal exam with hard stool in ampulla

(continued)

Table 12.3 continued

Cause	Fever	Vomit	↑WCC	↑ESR	FOB	AXR	U/S	U/A	Other
									• Stool often palpable on abdominal examination • History of straining and/or constipation in past
Acute non-specific abdominal pain (ANSAP)	+	+/−	+/−	+/−	−	• Often with non-specific findings • May show multiple small bowel fluid levels	• May have non-specific findings	−	**Diagnosis of exclusion** • Often these children are admitted for observation based on history and examination; subsequently discharged after 24 hours when condition improved/settled • Often history of viral URTI during preceding week • May also find inflamed tonsils and enlarged deep cervical glands • Pain may be less precisely defined than 'classical' appendicitis and may be more medial • If treated surgically and appendix found to be normal with mesenteric nodes enlarged, then mesenteric adenitis is the diagnisis • Mesenteric adenitis found in approx. 11% children treated surgically for appendicitis
UTI	+	+/−	+	+/−	−	• Normal	• Helpful with diagnosis of renal pathology	• Dipstick + esterase or nitrites • + culture	• Check costovertebral angle (CVA) tenderness/back pain • May have pelvic pain/bladder pain • Dysuria and pyuria in approx. 10% of appendicitis cases
Ectopic pregnancy	Rare	+/−	+/−	−	−	• Contraindicated	• Very helpful; often times diagnostic	−	• Triad of abdominal pain, vaginal bleeding, amenorrhoea • Increased risk if history of ectopic pregnancy, pelvic inflammatory disease (PID), or intrauterine contraceptive device (IUD) use
PID	+	+/−	+	+	−	• Normal	• Very helpful; may show adnexal mass, salpinx thickening, and/or cystic structure • Useful to assist in differentiation of appendicitis versus PID	• May have pyuria, and UTI	• Risk factors include multiple partners, IUD use, history of PID • Often follows onset of menses • Most important infection to differentiate from appendicitis in sexually active adolescents • Pain may be lower abdominal/pelvic with fever, chills and vaginal discharge • Most common causes *Chlamydia trachomatis* and *Neisseria gonorrhoea* • Also will exhibit cervical motion and adnexal tenderness

Common extra-abdominal causes of AAP: pneumonia, pharyngitis, URTI/otitis media.

Uncommon extra-abdominal causes: Henoch-Schönlein purpura, Hgb SS disease, child abuse/NAI, ectopic pregnancy, testicular torsion, duodenal ulcer and other intestinal obstructions.

Key: + = positive; − = negative; +/− = positive or negative; WCC = white cell count; ESR = erythrocyte sedimentation rate; FOB = faecal occult blood; AXR = abdominal X-ray; U/S = ultrasound; U/A = urinalysis or dipstick.

urinalysis that may/may not be normal); the child who looks ill probably is.

- A single negative finding (e.g. soft, non-tender abdomen when child asleep) is worth many positive/equivocal findings.
- It is useful to establish the child's baseline level of response (palpating an arm or leg) and compare it with the discomfort associated with the abdominal examination.
- Illnesses with marked lymph involvement may inflame mesenteric nodes, resulting in acute non-specific abdominal pain (ANSAP).
- Progressive nature to pain: think appendicitis.
- Apley's law: the further from the umbilicus, the more likely a discernible

cause; therefore, periumbilical pain is less likely to be pathogenic.

- Repeat examinations at regular intervals (with specific and clear documentation of findings) are a mainstay of early assessment and management.
- Acute abdominal pain with purpura on ankles and buttocks, hypertension and abnormal urinalysis or dipstick: think Henoch–Schönlein purpura (HSP).
- Bloody stools are always of concern (HSP, dysentery, intussusception).

BIBLIOGRAPHY

Ashcraft K. Acute abdominal pain. Pediatr Rev 2000; 21(11):363–367.

Davenport M. Acute abdominal pain in children. BMJ 1996; 312:498–501.

Garcia Peña B, Taylor G, Lund D. Appendicitis revisited: new insights into an age-old problem. Contemp Pediatr 1999; 16(9):122–131.

Hatch EI. The acute abdomen in children. Pediatr Clin North Am 1985; 32(5): 1151–1164.

Montgomery D. Practice guidelines: acute abdominal pain: a challenge for the practitioner. J Pediatr Health Care 1998; 12(3):157–159.

Rudolf M, Levene M. Paediatric child health. Oxford: Blackwell Science; 1999.

Woodward MN, Griffiths DM. Use of dipsticks for routine analysis of urine from children with acute abdominal pain. BMJ 1993; 306:1512.

12.2 CHILDHOOD CONSTIPATION AND ENCOPRESIS

Linda Smith and Cheryl Ward

INTRODUCTION

- *Constipation* is defined as difficulty or delay in defecation with the passage of hard stool commonly accompanied by pain. The development of chronic constipation is often the result of a series of events. Typically, there are a few episodes of constipation; these lead to stool retention (related to the child's fear of painful defecation), more constipation, greater retention, resultant chronic constipation, further retention and continued pain. Thus, a cycle of dysfunctional defecation patterns occurs.
- *Encopresis* is defined as faecal soiling and/or the passage of faeces in clothes (day or night) after the age of 4.
- Childhood constipation is very common, accounting for significant primary and secondary care resources. Children with chronic constipation may go on to develop faecal overflow, which often can be prevented with appropriate treatment at symptom onset.
- A genetic predisposition towards constipation is likely, given that there is

often a family history of motility disturbances. Constipation in early infancy can be a feature of lower intestinal obstruction and may increase the risk of enterocolitis and gut perforation. Constipation in pre-school and older children can be associated with extreme fear and avoidance of defecation. It is, however, invariably associated with intra-family stress.

- Encopresis is six times more common in boys; however, there does not seem to be an association between encopresis and family size, ordinal position in family, age of parents or income.
- There is a common misconception that a high-fibre diet will automatically eliminate the problem; professionals who deal with the problem are only too aware that the solution is not quite so simple.
- Physical effects of constipation include abdominal pain and distension, poor appetite, headaches, halitosis, vomiting and general feeling of ill health. Psychosocial effects include aggression or withdrawal and hiding for

defecation; bullying and/or school refusal among children who soil at school; denial of recreational hobbies and/or social isolation for family (parents judged as incompetent); and revolving of family life around bowel habits of one child.

PATHOPHYSIOLOGY

- Faecal retention or decreased motility allows water to move out of stool, increasing size and firmness. Passage of large, hard stool can trigger painful defecation and/or anal pain/fissures that lead to intentional or subconscious withholding. Rectal dilatation with decreased sensation, shortening of the anal canal and decreased tone of the external anal sphincter (often with leakage of stool/overflow continence) occur as a result of the chronic constipation.
- Less commonly, anatomical anomalies of the lower intestinal tract, anus and rectum or neurological conditions can result in chronic constipation. Likewise, endocrine abnormalities (hypothyroidism), medications or

electrolyte imbalances can cause chronic constipation.

- Chronic constipation and encopresis have multiple aetiologies, some of which are common to all ages in addition to those that are age-related (Table 12.4).

← HISTORY

- Usual bowel routine (where, when and how difficult) and use of suppository, enema or rectal stimulation to produce a bowel movement.
- Size, frequency, consistency and appearance of stool (stool diary for 1 week documenting date, time and amount of stool passed is helpful in assessment).
- Complaints of painful defecation, refusal to stool or stool leakage/soiling.
- Associated bed-wetting, frequent urination and/or urinary tract infections.
- Anal fissures, blood on toilet roll after defecation.
- Recent stressful events and family dynamics at home.
- Unsteady or clumsy gait (or any suggestion of neuromuscular problems).
- Difficulty with toilet training.
- Intake of fluids, milk, caffeine and fibre.
- Age-specific information (Table 12.5).

◌ PHYSICAL EXAMINATION

- Assess for evidence of systemic illness; child should have normal growth parameters.
- Careful abdominal examination, looking for evidence of distension, masses and/or abnormal bowel sounds (palpation often reveals hard stool in ascending, transverse and, occasionally, the descending colon).
- Inspection of anal area for fissures/skin tags or erythema, anal tone and signs and symptoms of abuse.
- Neurological functioning in lower extremities (reflexes, gait, strength and tone).
- Inspect spine for sacral dimple and/or tufts.

Table 12.4 Causes of Constipation

Age	Cause
All ages	Insufficient fluid intake; inappropriate diet; disturbed parent–child relationship
Infants (0–18 months)	Overfeeding with milk; mild illness or fever; anal fissure
Toddlers/pre-schoolers (18 months to 4 years)	Anal fissure; inappropriate treatment of earlier episode of constipation; anxiety associated with potty training; environmental change, i.e. new sibling, house move
School-age/adolescents (4–16 years)	Inappropriate/inadequate treatment of earlier episode of constipation; illness; lack of exercise; refusing the call to stool due to lifestyle; lack of adequate/private toilet facilities at school

Table 12.5 Age-specific Historical Information

Age	History
Infants (0–18 months)	Blood in nappy following defecation; grunting while defecating; composition of diet, i.e. breast or formula fed, recent change to cows' milk
Toddlers/pre-schoolers (18 months to 4 years)	Parent–child relationship; potty training; environmental changes
School-age/adolescents (4–16 years)	Lifestyle (?Refusing the call to stool); fear of using school toileting facilities due to lack of privacy; consumption of junk food

℗ DIFFERENTIAL DIAGNOSES

- Differential diagnoses are numerous and can be divided into different categories:
  - *functional:* faecal retention/withholding, irritable bowel syndrome
  - *neurological:* Hirschsprung's disease, spinal cord dysplasia/hypotonia syndromes
  - *obstructive:* anal ring stenosis, meconium ileus/cystic fibrosis, adenocarcinoma, pelvic tumour or mass
  - *drug-related:* lead poisoning, laxative abuse, opioids (e.g. morphine, codeine), vincristine
  - *other:* collagen-vascular/systemic lupus erythematosus (SLE), diabetes, graft versus host disease.

✚ MANAGEMENT

- Management of chronic constipation and/or encopresis is summarised in Table 12.6. Interventions centre around initial bowel clean out followed by dietary and behavioural changes to establish normal pattern of bowel function. In all age groups, it is important to address psychological and family issues and in many cases, behavioural and/or psychotherapeutic interventions are useful (especially in alleviating any fears with regard to defecation). Likewise, parental attitudes (and expectations) regarding toileting habits need to be discussed. Both parents and children need reassurance concerning the benign nature of the condition. However, education regarding the physiology of normal defecation, management strategies and toilet training as a developmental process are prerequisites to a successful outcome.

- **Additional diagnostics:** consider abdominal X-ray (presence/location of stool and to rule out bowel obstruction). If Hirschsprung's disease or cystic fibrosis are suspected, numerous other diagnostics are indicated.

- **Pharmacotherapeutics:** see Table 12.6.

- **Behavioural interventions:** see Table 12.6.

- **Patient education:** see Table 12.6.

⇨ FOLLOW-UP

- See Table 12.6.

Table 12.6   Management of Chronic Constipation and Encopresis

Age	Management			
	Pharmacotherapeutics[a]	Behavioural interventions	Patient/parent education	Comments/follow-up
1 month to 2 years of age	• Lactulose – 2.5 ml twice daily (under 1 year of age); 5 ml twice daily (1–2 years of age). Should be continued until normal bowel function resumed and then dose gradually reduced over a period of time • In severe cases it may be necessary to administer an enema to loosen impacted stool: glycerin (5–10 ml); micro enemas; or a solution of equal parts phosphate and saline (10–25 ml) • Note: all dosages dependent on severity of condition and weight/age of child	• Parents to provide comfort and reassurance to child • Increase fluid intake (water, very dilute juices)	• Adequate fluid intake/supplementary clear fluids • Increase dietary fibre • Explain and discuss physiology of bowel and normal defecation so parents understand how interventions will work to improve bowel functioning	• Medication is only given under strict supervision • Follow-up is ongoing • Frequency of contact dependent on progress (often intensive during initial treatment moving onto wider spaced monitoring visits)
2–12 years of age	• Glycerin enema (10–15 ml); micro enemas; or a solution of equal parts phosphate and saline (25–50 ml) to clear impacted stool • Lactulose to soften stool: 5 ml twice daily (<5 years of age); 10 ml twice daily (5–10 years of age); 15 ml twice daily (10–12 years of age) • Senna (large colon stimulant to increase bowel motility): 2.5–5 ml once daily at bedtime (2–6 years of age); 5–10 ml once daily at bedtime (6–12 years of age) • Docusate: 2.5 mg/kg (all ages) • Bisacodyl: 5 mg orally at night or 5 mg rectally in the morning (under 10 years of age); 10–20 mg orally at night or 10 mg rectally in the morning (>10 years) • Sodium picosulphate: 2.5–5 ml at night for a period of 3–5 days (4–10 years of age); 5–10 ml (over 10 years of age)[b]	• Age-appropriate toilet training/toilet ritual • Behaviour modification techniques (positive reinforcement, praise)	• As above	• Important to alleviate feelings of guilt for child and parent • Follow-up as above • Medication is only given under strict supervision
12–18 years of age	• Glycerin enema (10–15 ml); micro enemas; or a solution of equal parts phosphate and saline (25–100 ml) • Lactulose: 10–15 ml twice daily • Methylcellulose: 1–2 tablets daily • Senna: 10–20 ml or 2–4 tablets once daily (bedtime) • Sodium picosulphate: 5–10 ml daily for a period of 3–5 days[b] • Persist with medication over a period of 1 year	• As above • Lifestyle changes to accommodate the call to stool • Child to accept responsibility regarding management strategy and medications (age-appropriate)	• Parents to take joint responsibility with child in implementing management strategy • Record keeping of stools passed and medications taken • Education of the effects and why medication is required	• As above • Discuss with school about management strategy and toilet facilities • Medication is only given under strict supervision

[a] As with other medications used in childhood there are only a few laxatives licensed or recommended. Dosages must be checked against existing formularies.
[b] Only given in cases of severe constipation as a boost to the child's usual medication regimen.

⇄ MEDICAL CONSULT/ SPECIALIST REFERRAL

• Indicated for all ages if constipation is associated with vomiting, abdominal distension and evidence of failure to thrive.

• For infants 0–18 months of age: if long-standing constipation (rule out organic causes such as Hirschsprung's disease, hypothyroidism, strictures).
• For children 18 months to 16 years of age: persistent and unresolved constipation/encopresis. Likewise, consider behavioural referral (paediatric psychology, psychiatry or family therapy), especially in difficult cases or those in which the family dynamics require additional support.

PAEDIATRIC PEARLS

- Concordance, good follow-up and close family support are key to successful management of chronic constipation.
- Infants who cry, grunt and/or scream with legs pulled up during bowel movement and yet have consistently soft stool are *not* constipated: it is a contraction of the pelvic floor in response to rectal distension.
- Increasing dietary fibre alone will not 'cure' constipation; there needs to be a significant increase in fluid intake and regular defecation routine to accompany other interventions.
- A child's recommended daily allowance of fibre can be estimated (in milligrams) by adding '5' to the child's age. For example, a 6-year-old child should have an approximate daily intake of 11 mg of fibre.
- Chronic constipation is chronic; it interferes more or less in a child's life but interventions (especially adequate fibre and fluid intake and regular patterns of defecation) need to be maintained throughout childhood, adolescence and probably adulthood.
- Families may expect 'instant' results; careful discussion/explanation of

normal bowel functioning and the rationale behind specific interventions often improves concordance with treatment.
- Rule out organic cause for constipation, especially in infants or young children with a history of delayed passage of meconium, abdominal distension, vomiting, failure to thrive, alternating constipation and diarrhoea, explosive stools and/or family history of Hirschsprung's disease.

BIBLIOGRAPHY

Abi-Hanna A, Lake A. Constipation and encopresis in childhood. Pediatr Rev 1998; 19(1):23–30.

Anonymous. Managing constipation in children. Drug Therap Bull 2000; 38(8):57–59.

Blum N, Taubman B, Osbourne M. Behavioural characteristics of children with stool toileting refusal. Pediatrics 1997; 99(1):50–53.

Castiglia P. Constipation in children. J Pediatr Health Care 2001; 15(4):200–202.

Clayden G. Managing the child with constipation. Prof Care Mother Child 1991; 1(2):64.

Clayden G. Management of chronic constipation. Arch Dis Child 1992; 67:340–344.

Clayden G. Childhood constipation. London: British Paediatric Association Standing Committee on Paediatric Practice Guidelines; 1994.

Dern M, Stein M. He keeps getting stomach aches, doctor. What's wrong? Contemp Pediatr 1999; 16(5):43–54.

Felt B. Guideline for the management of pediatric idiopathic constipation and soiling. Arch Pediatr Adolesc Med 1999; 152:380–385.

Issenman R, Filmer R, Gorski P. A review of bowel and bladder control development in children: how gastrointestinal and urological conditions relate to problems in toilet training. Pediatrics 1999; 103:1246–1352.

Lennard-Jones L. Clinical management of constipation. Pharmacology 1993; 47(1):216.

Loening-Baucke V. Chronic constipation in childhood. Gastroenterology 1993; 105:1557–1564.

Muir J, Burnett C. Setting up a nurse led clinic for intractable childhood constipation. Br J Comm Nurs 1999; 4(8):395–399.

Seth R, Heyman M. Management of constipation and encopresis in infants and children. Gastro Clin North Am 1994; 23(4):621–636.

Staiano G. The long term follow-up of children with chronic idiopathic constipation. Arch Dis Child 1993; 67:340.

12.3 ACUTE GASTROENTERITIS (VOMITING AND DIARRHOEA)

Sally Panter-Brick

INTRODUCTION

- Acute gastroenteritis (AGE) is defined as the sudden onset of diarrhoea (with or without vomiting) *that is limited to less than 2 weeks in duration*.
- AGE is often transmitted through poor hygiene, with lack of handwashing and incorrect storage of foodstuffs likewise contributing. In 2000 there were 86,710 reported cases of food poisoning in the UK; thus, the extent of the problem and the

potential implications for hospital admission.
- Viral infections such as rotavirus and adenovirus are the most common causes of AGE in children. Rotavirus accounts for approximately 60% of cases of gastroenteritis during the winter among children less than 2 years old. Bacterial infections are less common and are more likely to occur during the summer months, while giardiasis is the most common protozoal cause of sudden onset

diarrhoea. A summary of some bacterial, viral and protozoan causes of AGE are outlined in Table 12.7.

PATHOPHYSIOLOGY

- Vomiting can be considered a defence mechanism to expel toxins and/or a response to gastrointestinal inflammation, whereas diarrhoea is an impairment of the normal *secretory* and/or *absorptive* functions of the

Table 12.7 Bacterial, Viral and Protozoan Causes of Acute Gastroenteritis (AGE)

Organism	Source	Incubation	Features	Transmission	School/nursery attendance
Bacterial					
• Escherichia coli (enterotoxigenic, enteropathogenic, enteroinvasive strains)	• GI[a] tract	• Variable	• Explosive stools, pyrexia, usually self-limited (7–10 days)	• Person-to-person (faecal–oral route) • Undercooked meat • Contaminated foods	• 24 hours from last episode of diarrhoea
• E. coli 0157 (enterohaemorrhagic strain of E. coli)	• GI tract of cattle and possibly other domestic animals	• 1–6 days	• Haemorrhagic colitis with haemolytic uraemic syndrome (HUS) occurring in 5% of cases with 10% mortality	• Contaminated food (beef, milk and vegetables) • Person-to-person • Contact with infected animals (especially on farms and animal sanctuaries)	• Following two negative stools
• Shigella (bacillary dysentery)	• Human GI tract	• 1–7 days	• Copious bloody diarrhoea, abdominal pain and fever	• Faecal–oral transmission from infected contacts • Occasionally spread by contaminated food and water	• <5 years of age seek advice • >5 years of age requires 24 hours since last episode
• Clostridium difficile	• 3% of healthy humans and 10–20% of hospital patients are carriers	• Variable	• Bloody diarrhoea stool with abdominal pain • History of antibiotic use (damage to normal gut flora by antibiotics allowing organism to produce toxins) • May present during antibiotic course or 2–6 weeks after (especially with clindamycin and ampicillin) • Oral vancomycin or metronidazole used to treat	• Patient-to-patient spread or via health care workers • More common in elderly and immunocompromised patients	• <5 years of age seek advice • >5 years requires 24 hours since last episode
• Salmonella	• Contaminated food and water • Infected humans (chronic carriers) • Animals and animal by products	• 6–72 hours	• Rapid onset of diarrhoea with blood/mucus possible, abdominal pain, fever, nausea and vomiting • Salmonella spp. can be responsible for salmonella bacteraemia (especially in young children) • Most mild cases recover spontaneously (5 days)	• Undercooked food (especially poultry and eggs) • Poor food preparation techniques or person hygiene (faecal–oral route)	• <5 years of age seek advice (prolonged shedding in stool of young children) • >5 years requires 24 hours since last episode
Viral					
• Rotavirus	• Human GI tract	• 48 hours	• Copious watery diarrhoea with vomiting • Fever often >38°C	• Faecal–oral transmission after environmental contamination • Infants and children at increased risk • Seasonal outbreaks common (winter)	• 24 hours from last episode of vomiting and diarrhoea • Careful handwashing and infection control in nurseries/day-care centres
• Adenovirus	• Respiratory tract	• 2–24 hours	• Associated with URTI[b] • Largely diarrhoea	• Person to person • Faecal–oral • Aerosolised droplets	• 24 hours from last episode of diarrhoea
Protozoan					
• Giardia	• GI tract of humans and animals	• 5–25 days	• Watery diarrhoea with foul smell, complaints of cramping and bloating • Stool may be 'frothy'	• Ingestion of giardia cysts from faecally contaminated food and water or direct faecal–oral transmission (poor hygiene) • Spread within families is common	• <5 years of age seek advice • >5 years requires 24 hours since last episode
• Cryptosporidium	• GI tract of animals and humans	• 2–5 days	• Watery or mucoid diarrhoea	• Contact with infected animals • Outbreaks associated with contaminated water supplies, farm visits, handling of lambs • May be transmitted in swimming pools, lakes, water parks	• <5 years of age seek advice • >5 years requires 24 hours since last episode • Note that oocysts can be shed for prolonged period after clinical resolution • Careful handwashing and infection control in nurseries/day-care centres

[a]GI = gastrointestinal.
[b]URTI = upper respiratory tract infection.

intestine (secondary to viral, bacterial or protozoal invasion).

- Diarrhoea resulting from *decreased absorption* is related to any one, or sometimes a combination of (1) a surface area reduction of the brush border membrane; (2) villus atrophy (or immaturity) with resultant enzyme deficiency (especially lactase); and (3) decreased bowel length.
- *Secretory diarrhoea* is related to increased ion excretion; it is triggered most commonly by bacterial enterotoxins (cholera, *Staphylococcus*, etc.), but likewise implicated in the high-volume stools of rotavirus and others. Secretory diarrhoea is characterised by large watery stools with increased sodium and chloride concentrations.

← HISTORY

- Onset of symptoms (with resultant effect on activity/playfulness).
- Frequency, consistency and appearance of stool (colour, smell, presence of blood or mucus). *Note: bloody diarrhoea is an indication for consultation (rule out haemolytic uraemic syndrome or bacterial diarrhoea).*
- Presence of vomiting and, if so, how often, how much, with what force (i.e. projectile) and with what appearance (colour, blood, bile). *Note: bile-stained or projectile vomiting is a warning of intestinal obstruction and should be referred immediately.*
- Other family members/contacts affected (school or nursery outbreaks).
- History of foreign travel, recent antibiotic use and/or day-care/nursery attendance.
- Recent visits to farms or animal sanctuaries.
- Prodrome or preceding symptoms (URTI, headache, malaise or other).
- Associated symptoms (rashes, joint pains or fever).
- Urinary symptoms (dysuria, frequency, oliguria, enuresis), time of last void and frequency of voiding. *Note: no urine output for 6 hours in infant (or 8 hours in an older child) is cause for concern and indicative of some dehydration.*

- Abdominal pain (distribution, type, shift and temporal relationship to vomiting and/or diarrhoea).
- Oral intake (what and how much of both foods and fluids, including any recent changes in diet).
- Home management (including use of antipyretics and antidiarrhoeals).

🫁 PHYSICAL EXAMINATION

- Assessment of child's general appearance (note presence of tears), temperature and hydration status are *key* (Table 12.8). Inspect and palpate mucous membranes (which will have a slippery feel when hydrated) and test for skin turgor (<2 s) on the abdomen or along the midaxillary line.
- Examine stool (colour, consistency, blood, mucus, smell).
- **Skin:** check head to toe for rashes and *obtain unclothed weight* (compare to pre-morbid weight).
- **Head and ENT:** careful examination, including tympanic membranes as acute otitis media or URTI can present concurrently with vomiting and diarrhoea. Assess hydration status in mouth as above.
- **Cardiovascular (CV):** without abnormalities or signs of shock (thready, weak pulses, changes in heart rate). Check capillary refill time (<2 s).
- **Abdomen:** may reveal hyperactive bowel sounds but should not reveal signs of distension or obstruction. There may be slight discomfort on palpation, but no significant

tenderness. Likewise, liver/spleen enlargement, CVA tenderness and abdominal masses are not consistent with uncomplicated AGE and, as such, probably require consultation.

- **Neurological:** level of consciousness/mental status, utilising **AVPU (A**lert? Responds to parental **V**oice? Responds to **P**ain only? or **U**nresponsive?). In young infants, note level of engagement with environment, playfulness and interaction with carer.

℗ DIFFERENTIAL DIAGNOSES

- Conditions that present with diarrhoea and/or vomiting are numerous. It is vital to determine whether the cause is of a *medical* or *surgical* nature (Table 12.9).

⊕ MANAGEMENT

- For uncomplicated cases of mild AGE, determination of the specific aetiology is unimportant, as the illness is typically brief, self-limited, and management is irrespective of the causative agent with few exceptions (some invasive bacterial or protozoal infections). As such, early re-feeding and adequate fluid intake are cornerstones of management and are usually sufficient to manage the vast majority of children presenting with AGE (see Behavioural interventions).
- **Additional diagnostics:** Usually not required; however, stool can be examined for blood, WBC, ova and parasites, rotavirus, *Clostridium difficile*, *Shigella* and *Escherichia coli*

Table 12.8	Assessment of dehydration		
Clinical signs	Mild (<5%)	Moderate (5–10%)	Severe (>10%)
Appearance	Miserable/irritable	Irritable/lethargic	Drowsy/unresponsive
Tissue turgor	Normal to minimally decreased	Noticeably decreased	Obviously decreased (tenting for >2 s)
Mucous membranes	Dry	Dry	Very dry
Capillary refill	Normal	Normal/prolonged	Prolonged (>2 s)
Pulse	Normal	Rapid	Rapid, thready
Blood pressure	Normal	Normal/low	Low/unrecordable
Urine output	Decreased	Decreased	Oliguria
Eyes	Normal	Sunken	Very sunken
Anterior fontanelle	Normal	Depressed	Very depressed

Table 12.9 Conditions That Can Present with Vomiting and/or Diarrhoea

Medical conditions		Surgical conditions
• Toxic ingestion	• Respiratory tract infection	• Pyloric stenosis
• AGE (viral, bacterial, protozoal)	• Otitis media	• Intussusception
• Septicaemia	• Hepatitis A	• Acute appendicitis
• Haemolytic uraemic syndrome	• Urinary tract infection	• Necrotising enterocolitis
• Coeliac disease	• Diabetic ketoacidosis	• Hirschsprung's disease
• Cows' milk protein allergy	• Reye's syndrome	
• Adrenal insufficiency	• Antibiotic use	
• Meningitis		

if history or physical examination indicate. Children referred for further evaluation may receive abdominal X-ray, ultrasound or endo/colonoscopy (see Sec. 12.1). Blood work (FBC, blood culture, urea, electrolytes and glucose) will not be diagnostic but may be helpful in management. Children that present with moderate-to-severe dehydration, an atypical presentation, or an extremely ill appearance should have blood work checked.

- **Pharmacotherapeutics:** *There is no need to give any medication to alleviate the symptoms of diarrhoea and vomiting.* Antidiarrhoeals are generally ineffective and may prolong the excretion of bacteria and/or toxins from the stool. Antibiotics may be used in specific infections such as *Shigella*, cholera and *Giardia, but choice of antibiotic is organism-dependent and, therefore, antibiotics should not be used presumptively or without consultation.*

- **Behavioural interventions:**
  - *Feeding:* institute as soon as vomiting stabilised—*do not starve.* Small frequent feedings of bland soft foods (complex carbohydrates, fruits and lean meats) are recommended for older children; for breast-fed infants, increase feeding frequency. Efficacy of formula or milk dilution remains controversial. There may be some temporary lactose intolerance during the acute phase (especially in more severe cases of diarrhoea) related to depletion of lactase from the villus; however, milk should not *routinely* be discontinued or changed.
  - *No dehydration:* encourage extraoral fluids with oral rehydration salts

(ORS) and supplement intake with additional ORS (5–10 ml/kg) after each watery stool/emesis. Advance to regular diet if vomiting has stopped/decreased (as above).
  - *Mild dehydration:* Give 50 ml/kg of ORS plus a replacement of 10 ml/kg for each loose stool and/or emesis. The aim is to rehydrate over a 4-hour period. If vomiting, give ORS in 3–5 ml volumes (spoon, syringe or dropper) at 2-min intervals and reasses hydration status every 1–2 hours. Once vomiting has stopped/decreased, re-feeding as above.
  - *Moderate dehydration:* Rehydrate with 100 ml/kg of ORS (over 6-hour period) and add 10 ml/kg for each loose stool/emesis. ORS can be given orally or via nasogastric tube and hydration status should be assessed hourly. Once dehydration corrected, initiate re-feeding. If there is no improvement in the child's condition within 2–3 hours, intravenous fluids should be initiated (with appropriate bloodwork – see below).
  - *Severe dehydration:* hospital admission and intravenous fluids are always required. A cannula should be inserted and blood samples obtained for urea, electrolytes and glucose. Intravenous fluids are determined using the child's pre-morbid weight, electrolyte levels and fluid requirements. If the child is showing signs of shock, then resuscitation fluids (colloid or 0.9% saline) should be bolused at 20 ml/kg. Correct the fluid deficit (plus maintenance fluids and any ongoing losses) over the next 24 hours using appropriate

intravenous fluids. Special care needs to be taken if the child is hypernatraemic, as rapid rehydration can cause a shift of fluid into the cerebral cells, which can result in convulsions and cerebral oedema. Consequently, the hypernatraemic child should be rehydrated slowly over 36–48 hours. If the child is oliguric, then the addition of potassium chloride should be omitted. Check electrolyte levels in 24 hours (or more frequently if they are abnormal). Once the child is able to tolerate oral fluids, they should be increased gradually and the amount of intravenous fluids given can then be reduced. Institute re-feeding as soon as the child's condition improves.
  - *Replacement of fluid deficit:* per cent dehydration × weight (kg) = fluid deficit (ml): e.g. if a 10 kg child is 7.5% dehydrated, the fluid deficit is 750 ml (which is usually replaced over 12–24 hours, hypernatraemia excepted).
  - *Calculation of maintenance fluid requirements/24 hours:* 100 ml/kg for first 10 kg body weight; plus 50 ml/kg for next 10 kg body weight; plus 20 ml/kg for each following kg body weight.

- **Patient education:**
  - Parents need information regarding prevention of AGE through careful storage and preparation of food and the importance of careful handwashing after nappy changes, etc.
  - *Be sure parents are clear on signs/symptoms of decreasing hydration status (tears, dry mouth, decreased urine output, etc.); they should be instructed to seek help immediately if their child's condition is deteriorating.*
  - Clarify the home management of vomiting and diarrhoea (fluids and re-feeding) in order to prevent even mild dehydration from developing. Stress the importance of *appropriate* oral intake (e.g. ORS with amounts) to prevent dehydration (and potential hospitalisation); give *explicit* instructions regarding the avoidance of *inappropriate* fluids (fruits juices, squashes, sodas, etc.).

⇨ FOLLOW-UP

- Not usually necessary unless diarrhoea is persistent or condition is not improving after 1 week of appropriate home management. Occasionally, there can be an intolerance to cows' milk, disaccharides and/or gluten post-AGE episode.
- Parents should be warned that they will receive a visit from a public health official if the cause of the AGE is a reportable one.
- A follow-up visit by the health visitor or community paediatric nurse may be helpful in reinforcing information given about home management of AGE and its subsequent prevention.

⇄ MEDICAL CONSULT/ SPECIALIST REFERRAL

- Any child with severe dehydration and/or an ill appearance.
- Any child with a suspected surgical aetiology.
- Any child with persistent oliguria or bloody diarrhoea (rule out haemolytic uraemic syndrome).

- Any child with symptoms or examination findings inconsistent with typical AGE.
- Any child less than 3 months of age or those in whom initial management has been unsuccessful.

⊙ PAEDIATRIC PEARLS

- Do not forget ABC if severely dehydrated.
- Shock does not automatically equal dehydration (i.e. shock can be due to septicaemia, toxaemia or blood loss).
- Early re-feeding of children during oral rehydration therapy is important; children should eat as normally as possible (avoiding high-fat and high-sugar foods). Breast-feeding should always continue.
- Oral rehydration therapy tastes unpalatable: disguise with a *few drops of juice* (blackcurrant works well) or use the ORS to make flavoured ice-lollies. Both of these interventions can make the ORS more acceptable to the child.
- Classifying degree of dehydration as *'none'*, *'some'* or *'severe'* rather than with a percentage value can simplify decision making. The fluid to be replaced is approximately

60–100 ml/kg for 'some dehydration' and 90–150 ml/kg for 'severe dehydration'.

▤ BIBLIOGRAPHY

American Academy of Pediatrics. Practice parameter: the management of acute gastro-enteritis in young children. Pediatrics 1996; 97(3):424–435.

Anonymous. APLS the practical approach. London: BMJ Publishing; 1997.

Armon K, Lakhanpaul M, Stephenson T. An evidence and consensus-based guideline for acute diarrhoea management. Arch Dis Child 2000; 86(2):138.

Duggan C, Nurko S. Feeding the gut: the scientific basis for continued enteral nutrition during acute diarrhoea. J Pediatr 1997; 131(6):801–808.

Hugger J, Harkless G, Retschler D. Oral rehydration therapy for children with acute diarrhea. Nurse Pract 1998; 23(12):52–62.

Lasche J, Duggan C. Managing acute diarrhea: what every pediatrician needs to know. Contemp Pediatr 1999; 12(2):74–83.

Milner A, Hull D. Hospital paediatrics. Edinburgh: Churchill Livingstone; 1998.

Murphy MS. Guidelines for managing acute gastro-enteritis based on a systemic review of published research. Arch Dis Child 1998; 79:279–284.

Public Health Laboratory Service: http://www.phls.co.uk/facts

12.4 JAUNDICE

Gill Brook

▭ INTRODUCTION

- *Jaundice* is a yellow discoloration of the sclera, skin and other elastic tissues. It is caused by an accumulation of bilirubin and reflects an alteration in its normal metabolism and/or excretion. *Bilirubin* is a waste product derived from the breakdown of red blood cells; it is the predominant pigment of bile.
- The causes of jaundice are numerous, but for the most part they are attributable to an increased rate of haemolysis or a decreased rate of bilirubin conjugation and/or abnormalities of the biliary tree.

- Jaundice is a common finding in the newborn period, as 30–50% of term infants have transient jaundice for 3–5 days after birth. This is unconjugated hyperbilirubinaemia and is related to immature conjugation processes. However, neonatal jaundice that continues past 14 days of life in a healthy term infant requires further evaluation.
- The first objective in the evaluation of the infant or child that presents with jaundice is to determine whether the cause originates from a haematological or hepatological problem. This is determined by undertaking a total bilirubin measurement and including

split conjugated and unconjugated levels.
- Approximately 1 in 500 babies has a potentially life-threatening form of liver disease. Liver disease often presents with jaundice. Recognition and prompt diagnosis are important in avoiding complications (i.e. vitamin-K-dependent haemorrhage), allowing prompt treatment and improving long-term outcomes.

⊗ PATHOPHYSIOLOGY

- Bilirubin is a breakdown product of red blood cell destruction and has two forms: *unconjugated bilirubin* (*indirect bilirubin*) and *conjugated bilirubin* (*direct bilirubin*).

- *Unconjugated* bilirubin is fat soluble and bound to proteins; it is a toxic and unstable compound. In very high levels it will bind to brain cells within the basal ganglia causing kernicterus. Kernicterus will result in significant brain damage or even death; it is prevented by phototherapy, which causes isomerism of the excess unconjugated bilirubin for excretion.

- *Conjugated* bilirubin is water soluble and is the predominant pigment in bile (gives bile its green colour). It can be eliminated from the body via stool and can also be reabsorbed from the gut and excreted as urobilinogen via the kidney.

- *It is important to understand the pathophysiology of bilirubin breakdown:*
  - The haem part of bilirubin is broken down to *unconjugated* bilirubin.
  - The liver converts (conjugates) the unconjugated bilirubin to the more stable, water-soluble *conjugated* bilirubin, which is excreted in bile. The conjugation process is undertaken by the enzyme *glucuronyl transferase.*
  - *Glucuronyl transferase* activity is low in newborn babies (hepatic function is activated once the baby is born). Consequently, the severity and duration of physiological jaundice may be increased in premature infants as a result of their immature liver function.

- Conjugated bilirubin is nearly always elevated in liver disease and is particularly vital in the differential diagnosis of neonatal jaundice. Other functions of the liver (and signs of liver dysfunction) are outlined in Table 12.10.

- Jaundice, can therefore be caused by:
  - high red blood cell breakdown (increased haemolysis)
  - immature liver function or conjugation enzyme deficiency (the latter is very rare); these problems are manifested by *unconjugated* hyperbilirubinaemia.
  - inability to excrete bile, which results in *conjugated* hyperbilirubinaemia (defined as conjugated bilirubin level ⩾20 µmol/l).

Table 12.10 Functions of the Liver and Examples of Dysfunction

Function	Examples of dysfunction
Metabolism of all nutrients	• Failure to thrive • Hypoglycaemia • Metabolic disturbances
Synthesis of protein (albumin)	• Poor albumin production • Decreased serum albumin levels • Oedema, ascites
Storage of glycogen	• Hypoglycaemia

Synthesis of vitamins A, D, E, K	• Vitamin deficiencies:
	  • vitamin A: poor healing
	  • vitamin D: rickets
	  • vitamin E: impaired nerve function
	  • vitamin K: abnormal prothrombin time

Synthesis of most clotting factors	• Prolonged prothrombin time +/− prolonged partial thromboplastin time, haemorrhage, bruising
Toxin removal	• Encephalopathy
Bile production and conjugation of bilirubin	• Jaundice with elevated conjugated bilirubin that is ⩾20 µmol/l • Acholic (white or grey) stools, fatty stools, dark urine, bilirubin present in fresh urine (conjugated hyperbilirubinaemia)

⬅ HISTORY

- General state of health: age, appetite, feeding, weight gain/loss, growth patterns. Note that infants and children with liver disease may have poor appetites or may feed/eat excessively, but weight gain may be poor.
- Time of onset (including age of infant/child when jaundice presented) and duration of jaundice.
- Unexplained bruising, bleeding (nose bleeds or umbilical remnant bleeding in infants) and/or poor healing.
- Colour of stool and urine (observe if possible).
- Unexplained itching (cholestatic liver disease and/or conjugated hyperbilirubinaemia may be accompanied by marked pruritus).
- History of previous illnesses and family history of illness: cystic fibrosis, haemolytic conditions, liver disease, infectious contacts, exposure to blood and blood products, surgeries, intravenous drug use.
- History of a sibling with prolonged neonatal jaundice.
- History of unprotected sexual intercourse (adolescents).
- History of international travel (where and when).
- Developmental history: achievement of milestones (infants), behaviour, school performance and/or handwriting changes (older children). Note that some liver diseases in children may present with neurological deficits (e.g. Wilson's disease).
- Birth history (newborns and infants): maternal infections, medications, type of delivery, gestational age at delivery, neonatal history, rhesus state of mother, height, weight, head circumference at birth.

🩺 PHYSICAL EXAMINATION

- Observation of the infant or child, including general well-being (plot height, weight, head circumference and note relationship to birth measurements); presence of pallor, level of alertness; degree of visible jaundice (check for degree of jaundice in natural light if possible and note distribution); and presence of petechiae, scratch marks or bruising.

- **Examine stool:** pale, fatty or offensive stools are indicative of a liver problem. Stools that are totally without colour (acholic) indicate a total lack of biliary flow.

- **Examine urine:** note that infant urine is classified as colourless. If it is yellow it can be an indication of liver disease (requires further testing, see Additional diagnostics).

- **Head and ENT:** palpate head in infants to rule out cephalohaematoma. There may be pallor of palpebral conjunctivae if marked anaemia is present.

- **Cardiopulmonary:** listen carefully for heart murmurs, as peripheral pulmonary stenosis may be heard in Alagille syndrome. Children with marked anaemia may have a physiological flow murmur.

- **Abdomen:** careful examination to identify liver size/consistency, presence of ascites and palpation of spleen. Note that the lower liver edge is normally palpable 1–2 cm below the right costal margin (midclavicular line) in infants/young children and rarely exceeds more than 1 cm below the right costal margin in older children (except on deep inspiration). If the lower liver edge is palpable, it is important to determine the upper border through light percussion and compare this to age-appropriate liver span measurements (see Further reading). Deep palpation is useful to determine the consistency of the liver edge and its surface. Normally this is soft, fairly sharp and not tender. A round edge with a smooth surface is indicative of an enlarged, swollen liver caused by infection, infiltration and/or congestion. Tenderness is often experienced during the acute phase of an illness. Cirrhosis will be palpable as a hard, enlarged liver with irregular surface and edge.

- **Abdomen (spleen):** palpate for the spleen. The tip (1–2 cm) can normally be felt in some children less than 5 years of age just underneath the left costal margin. Palpation of the spleen may be facilitated by rolling the child onto their right side, which may tip the spleen anteriorly. The spleen edge is very distinct, often feeling like a water balloon just underneath the pads of the fingers. An enlarged spleen may reflect an infectious process or portal hypertension (especially when combined with an enlarged, congested liver), a sign of established liver disease or abnormal storage of metabolites.

- Routine neurological examination (age-specific) to identify any altered neurological function.

Table 12.11 Differential Diagnosis of Jaundice by Type of Hyperbilirubinaemia[a]

Type	Potential causes			
	Congenital and/or obstructive	Infectious	Genetic, metabolic or endocrine	Other
Conjugated	• Biliary atresia • Bile duct stenosis • Gallstones • Choledochal cyst	• Sepsis • UTI • CMV infection • HIV infection • Hepatitis A, B, C • Toxoplasmosis • Syphilis	• Alagille syndrome • Alpha-1 antitrypsin deficiency • Tyrosinaemia • Galactosaemia/fructosaemia • Wilson's disease • Metabolic abnormalities • Cystic fibrosis • Hypothyroidism • Hypopituitarism	• Medications • Idiopathic neonatal hepatitis • TPN
Unconjugated	• Placental dysfunction • Upper GI obstruction • Congenital hypothyroidism • Infants of diabetic mothers	• Sepsis	• Red cell enzyme deficiency (G6PD) • Sickle cell anaemia • Spherocytosis • Defect in hepatic bilirubin conjugation (Crigler–Najjar syndrome) • ABO or rhesus incompatibility	• Physiological jaundice • Breast-milk jaundice

CMV = cytomegalovirus; G6PD = glucose 6-phosphate dehydrogenase; GI = gastrointestinal; HIV = human immunodeficiency virus; TPN = total parenteral nutrition; UTI = urinary tract infection.
[a]This is not a definitive list: refer to Kelly (1999) for a comprehensive discussion.

Table 12.12 Causes of Pathological Jaundice by Age[a]

Age	Consider
Newborn and early infancy	• Extrahepatic biliary atresia • Choledochal cyst • Idiopathic neonatal hepatitis • Alpha-1 antitrypsin deficiency • Infection
Older children	• Autoimmune hepatitis • Viral hepatitis • Wilson's disease • Biliary obstruction (e.g. gallstone or choledochal cyst) • Diseases of increased haemolysis (sickle cell anaemia, G6PD[b] deficiency)

[a]This is not a definitive list: see Kelly (1999).
[b]G6PD = glucose 6-phosphate dehydrogenase.

🔎 DIFFERENTIAL DIAGNOSES

- **Numerous:** can be categorised by type of hyperbilirubinaemia (Table 12.11). In addition, there are some aetiologies of jaundice that are more common in certain ages (Table 12.12).

➕ MANAGEMENT

Specific management of jaundice is aetiology-dependent. In addition, with the exception of initial evaluation (to rule out mild cases of physiological, breast-milk and infectious/viral-related jaundice) management is likely to be coordinated in specialist centres. Consequently, management principles outlined below are largely limited to diagnostics useful at presentation, management of physiological/breast-milk jaundice and the importance of early investigation of conjugated hyperbilirubinaemia in the newborn (Table 12.13).

- **Additional diagnostics:**
  - Largely determined by clinical setting, differential diagnoses, patient age, history and clinical presentation.

Table 12.13   Conjugated and Unconjugated Hyperbilirubinaemia in Infancy Basic Management[a]

Type	Comments	Management
Unconjugated (physiological and breast-milk jaundice)	• *Physiological jaundice* related to high red blood cell breakdown and liver immaturity (liver can't keep up with conjugation process) • Presents within the first few days of life and should be returned to normal in approximately 2 weeks • *Breast-milk jaundice* probably overlaps with physiological and is multifactorial in its aetiology. Breast-milk jaundice continuing longer than 1–2 months should be investigated further • Clinical findings in physiological and breast-milk jaundice: unconjugated component of total bilirubin elevated while conjugated level normal (≤20 μmol/l); normal haemoglobin, reticulocyte count and stool colour; no maternal blood group incompatibility or physical examination findings (jaundice excepted); urine negative for bilirubin • Unconjugated hyperbilirubinaemia can indicate a haemolytic problem or physiological deficiency of glucuronyl transferase (e.g. Criglar–Nijjar syndrome)	• Phototherapy may be required in term infants with unconjugated bilirubin >300 μmol/l • Weight, gestational age, and postnatal age are considered (in addition to bilirubin levels) in decision to initiate phototherapy • Exchange transfusion may be required to prevent kernicterus if unconjugated levels are extremely high • It is very important that the infant is well hydrated and feeding adequately; urine output should be >2 ml/kg/h
Conjugated	• Clinical findings include pale stools, dark urine, bilirubin (on dipstick) in fresh urine • Serum levels of conjugated bilirubin ≥15% of total bilirubin should be considered abnormal • Increased levels imply an impairment of bile excretion, which occurs in severe parenchymal disease and damage to portal tracts • *Requires urgent investigation and referral* as early detection allows prompt treatment and management; both of which directly affect outcome • Early diagnosis is vital to the outcome of biliary atresia as surgical repair prior to 8 weeks of age optimises the outcome • In addition to above, biliary atresia may present with failure to thrive (despite feeding well) and hepatomegaly with firm liver. Note that splenomegaly is a later sign that indicates significant liver damage (fibrosis or cirrhosis)	• Infants with conjugated hyperbilirubinaemia will require supplementation with fat-soluble vitamins (A, D, E and K) and increased monitoring • Prevention of failure to thrive through growth plotting (weekly weight, length and head circumference checks) • Specialist dietary consultation is important • Breast-feeding is encouraged but caloric supplementation may be required • Formula feeds should have increased medium-chain triglycerides: e.g. Pregestimil

[a]In jaundiced newborns, differential bilirubin levels at 14 days of age.

COMMON PAEDIATRIC PROBLEMS

• An important first step is establishing whether jaundice is due to *conjugated* or *unconjugated* hyperbilirubinaemia. This is determined by measuring the total serum bilirubin level and, *specifically,* requesting a split bilirubin (i.e. conjugated and unconjugated levels). *Direct bilirubin exceeding 15% of the total indicates conjugated hyper-bilirubinaemia and should be urgently investigated.*

• Urine 'dipstick' for bilirubin should be performed in all patients presenting with jaundice. This is especially important in the evaluation of the newborn with marked jaundice (who should also receive a total serum bilirubin with split to rule out conjugated hyperbilirubinaemia). Note that urobilinogen is a normal finding in urine but bilirubin is *not*.

• In addition, the following tests should be considered: liver function tests (Table 12.14), FBC with reticulocyte count and peripheral smear, blood cultures, urea/ electrolytes, creatinine, urinalysis (with microscopy, reducing substances, amino acids and organic acids), viral infection screens (Epstein–Barr, cytomegalovirus and hepatitis A, B, C, D) and abdominal ultrasound (liver, gall bladder, spleen, kidney and biliary tract).

• Further diagnostics for newborns: blood type and rhesus factor (infant and mother), Coombs' test, sweat test (rule out cystic fibrosis), congenital infection screens (TORCH titres), metabolic screen (hypothyroidism, galactosaemia and hypopituitarism) and clotting screens, abdominal ultrasound. Note that the presence of a normal gall bladder nearly always excludes extrahepatic biliary atresia but it is important to rule out choledochal cyst. Radionuclear scanning and liver biopsy will be performed in specialist centres.

• **Pharmacotherapeutics:** aetiology-specific.

• **Behavioural interventions:** aetiology-specific.

• **Patient education:** largely aetiology-specific. Information on procedures, liver function and disease management are available from the specialist national referral centres (below). In addition, the Children's Liver Disease Foundation has information leaflets written in conjunction with the centres (tel: 0121-212-3839) and a Family Support Officer:
   - Birmingham Children's Hospital NHS Trust
   - Kings College Hospital
   - Leeds Royal Infirmary NHS Trust.

⇨ FOLLOW-UP

• Physiological jaundice must be followed closely for resolution. Jaundice continuing after 14 days needs to be investigated.

Table 12.14   Liver Function Tests

Test	Comments
Total serum bilirubin with conjugated and unconjugated values	• Elevated levels cause jaundice • Ratio of unconjugated to conjugate (split) is crucial in diagnostic decision making
Aspartate transferase (AST) Alanine transaminase (ALT)	• AST and ALT are enzymes found in hepatocytes; elevated levels indicate cellular inflammation and damage • ALT is more specific to liver damage
Alkaline phosphatase (ALP)	• ALP is associated with the cell membranes lining the biliary tree • Increased levels occur in inflammation or necrosis of these cells • Increased levels also occur when bile flow is impeded • Caution with interpretation as levels are age-dependent; check age-specific reference ranges
Serum albumin	• Made by the liver from other proteins • Reflects the ability of the liver to synthesise these proteins • Reduced in chronic liver disease
Prothrombin time Partial thromboplastin time	• Prolonged in vitamin K deficiency and when there is reduced hepatic synthesis • Both tests reflect the ability of liver to synthesise this protein
Blood glucose	• May obtain serum value or obtained with finger prick (BM Stix) • Levels reflect ability of the liver to metabolise nutrients

• Infants, children and adolescents with viral hepatitis must be followed closely. Any sign of decreasing liver function requires admission to hospital (including specialist referral). This includes changes in behaviour such as drowsiness, irritability and 'naughty'/aggressive behaviour which may indicate encephalopathy and cerebral oedema (acute/fulminant) liver failure.

⇄ MEDICAL CONSULT/ SPECIALIST REFERRAL

• Any infant or child in whom the aetiology of jaundice is not readily apparent from history, physical examination and initial diagnostics.
• Any infant or child in whom there is conjugated hyperbilirubinaemia.
• Any child with an alteration in liver function or in whom there are any signs of liver disease.
• Jaundice in the newborn that is not resolved within 14 days.

♀ PAEDIATRIC PEARLS

• Jaundice is common in the neonatal period and is likely to be 'physiological'. However, be careful not to ignore it or give false

reassurance and watch for spontaneous resolution within 14 days (*further investigations required if not resolved*). Surgery-based urine dip sticks for bilirubin (*urine must be fresh*) can be a useful, cheap and quick screening tool.
• Request total and split bilirubin levels as one of the first investigations.
• Jaundice in the newborn which persists after 14 days *must* be investigated.
• Pale stools and dark urine are physical symptoms to be specifically enquired into; note that urine in newborns should be colourless.
• Breast-milk jaundice may develop during the first week of life in exclusively breast-fed infants and usually peaks at the end of the second week of life. However, occasionally it may persist as long as 1–2 months. The diagnosis is clinical, with differential bilirubin levels (checked at 14 days of age) revealing elevated unconjugated bilirubin and normal conjugated bilirubin ($\leqslant 20\,\mu mol/l$). Physical examination is without findings (jaundice excepted) as are haemoglobin, reticulocytes and compatibility of maternal blood group. Breast-feeding can continue but jaundice should be monitored until resolved. If jaundice persists after 1–2 months, further studies should be instituted.
• Early diagnosis of liver disease is vital and has a direct effect on outcome.

While initial investigations should be commenced in primary and secondary care, expedient referral to a specialist centre is important. Early diagnosis of extrahepatic biliary atresia is especially important as the operation to facilitate biliary drainage (Kasai procedure) must be undertaken in a specialist centre by 8 weeks of age. Infants who undergo this procedure significantly later (or those in whom the procedure has failed) often require transplantation within 1–2 years.

• The Children's Liver Disease Foundation publishes the information leaflet *Early Identification of Liver Disease in Infants*, which is available free of charge from the foundation (tel: 0121-212-3839).
• Not all liver disease presents with jaundice in the early stages (especially older infants and children); careful history, physical examination and basic diagnostics (liver function tests, bilirubin levels that include split levels, FBC, urine dipstick and infection screens) are vital.
• High turnover of red blood cells due to haemolysis can cause jaundice. Serum bilirubin levels will be elevated, with an increase in the *unconjugated* component.
• Elevated total serum bilirubin levels with an elevated conjugated component $\geqslant 20\,\mu mol/l$ are signs of liver disease: *refer immediately*.
• Abnormal feeding (voracious appetite or anorexia) can be signs of chronic/ progressive liver disease and may precede obvious jaundice.

☰ BIBLIOGRAPHY

Beath SV, Booth IW, Kelly DA. Nutritional support in liver disease. Arch Dis Child 1993; 69:545–549.

Hull J, Kelly DA. Investigation of prolonged neonatal jaundice. Curr Paediatr 1991; 89:228–230.

Jarvis C. The abdomen: developmental considerations in the infant and child. In: Jarvis C. ed., Physical examination and health assessment, 2nd edn. London: WB Saunders; 1996: 628–631.

Kelly DA. Diseases of the liver and biliary system in children. Oxford: Blackwell Science; 1999.

Mieli-Vergani G, Howard ER, Portman B, et al. Late referral for biliary atresia: missed opportunities for effective surgery. Lancet 1989; 8635:421–423.

Mowat AP. Liver disorders in childhood, 3rd edn. Oxford: Butterworth-Heinemann; 1994.

Mowat AP, Davison LL, Dick MC. Early identification of biliary atresia and hepatobiliary disease: selective screening in the 3rd week. Arch Dis Child 1995; 72:90–92.

12.5 THREADWORMS

Diane Norton

📖 INTRODUCTION

- Infection by *Enterobius vermicularis* (threadworms) is the most common parasitic infection in developed countries and a common cause of rectal itching in families with young children.
- Threadworm infection predominantly affects pre-school and school-aged children between 5 and 10 years of age.
- Characteristically, the child or parent will complain of rectal itching (starting about 1 hour after going to bed). There is continued disruption of sleep through the night and girls may additionally complain of vulvar itching and dysuria.
- If the anus is inspected during the night, ova or white, thread-like worms (approximately 1 cm long) may be seen. In this scenario, parents will (understandably) be upset.

🔬 PATHOPHYSIOLOGY

- Transmission of threadworms is via the faecal–oral route, with fomite spread common (the eggs can survive in bedding, clothing and house dust for many days).
- Once ingested, the eggs hatch in the intestine and mature worms subsequently migrate to the rectum where eggs are laid in perianal skin (and become infectious within 2–4 hours).
- Perianal itching is caused by the gravid worm exiting from the anus to lay eggs. The migrating female causes the child to scratch, which also results in the harbouring of eggs under the fingernails.

- The worms trigger a minimal inflammatory response in the lower bowel mucosa, which correlates with few gastrointestinal symptoms.
- Humans are the only known host and the entire cycle (from ingestion of eggs to perianal egg-laying) takes approximately 4–6 weeks.

⬅ HISTORY

- Temporality of symptoms (typically, perianal itching, occurs at night or early morning), physical complaints and an assessment of infection and transmission risk. More specifically, the history should address:
  - onset, frequency and extent of 'itching'
  - day-care attendance, handwashing routines and any history of foreign travel or other exposures
  - other family members with symptoms and previous home management
  - any additional symptoms or visualisation of ova or worms.

🐛 PHYSICAL EXAMINATION

- Assessment of the abdomen and inspection of the rectum and external genitalia may be negative or, in severe cases, there may be some slight rectal irritation or excoriation from scratching round the anus.
- In pre-pubescent girls it is not uncommon to find some slight inflammation of the vulva (especially if there is secondary infection). It is unlikely that threadworms or ova will be seen.

- Physical examination requires careful explanation and consent from both parent and child.

🔍 DIFFERENTIAL DIAGNOSES

- Additional aetiologies for rectal itching that should be considered include other parasitic infections, mild gastroenteritis, bacterial or fungal vulvovaginitis, chemical dermatitis, nappy rash, vulvitis from soaps or lotions, poor hygiene or sexual abuse.

➕ MANAGEMENT

- **Additional diagnostics:** a definitive diagnosis of *Enterobius vermicularis* infection can be made by microscopic identification of the worms collected via a 'tape test' (a small piece of transparent Sellotape is wrapped around the carer's finger, sticky side out, and patted over the anus in the early morning before the child rises). If other aetiologies are under consideration, stool for culture and ova/parasite and FBC may be of diagnostic help.
- **Pharmacotherapeutics:** threadworm infection is treated with mebendazole, given as a single dose (for all children over 2 years of age) of 100 mg. Repeat dose after 2 weeks if reinfection is suspected. Note that chewable tablets of 100 mg are available and can be purchased from a pharmacy or a suspension is available on prescription. Consider treatment of all family members (with exception of pregnant women and children <2 years) as threadworm communicability is high. Piperazine (Pripsen) can be given to

children over 3 months of age but it is contraindicated for patients with epilepsy, renal failure or hepatic failure. Symptoms should resolve within a few days of treatment. The dosing schedule is as follows: 3 months to 1 year (2.5 ml of powder); 1–6 years (5 ml of powder); and for children over 6 years of age (1 sachet or 7.5 ml of powder). The dose should be repeated after 14 days.

- **Behavioural interventions:**
  - Good hygiene practices with frequent warm baths if rectal itching/vulvar irritation is marked.
  - Careful handwashing routines are vital and nails should be kept short.
  - Laundry should be washed in hot water and care should be taken to avoid shaking the bedding and clothing before laundering; toys taken to bed may also require washing.
  - Discourage nail-biting and ensure those infected sleep alone.
  - Wearing cotton pants and gloves may help to discourage scratching while asleep.
  - Complications of threadworm infection are uncommon, but typically are related to secondary infection and irritation from the pruritus; these should be treated symptomatically.
- **Patient education:**
  - Threadworm infection is very upsetting to families. Stress the

benign course and simple treatment in addition to addressing specific concerns (likely to be related to transmission, communicability, day-care attendance and environmental control).
- If microscopic confirmation is required, parents will need 'tape-test' instructions.
- Remind the family that threadworms are contracted through human contact only and they are not 'worms' from domestic or farm animal contact.
- Reassure family members that threadworm is not a sign of poor hygiene. However, it is an opportune time to review the role of handwashing in preventing not only threadworm infection but also as an important, good health practice.

⇨ FOLLOW-UP

- Follow-up is generally not indicated unless symptoms persist or reappear.

⇄ MEDICAL CONSULT/ SPECIALIST REFERRAL

- Any infection in a child <2 years of age (or households with a pregnant woman).
- Any child with a history or physical findings suggestive of sexual abuse.
- Any child who experiences complications such as urethritis,

vaginitis, salpingitis or pelvic peritonitis.

⚲ PAEDIATRIC PEARLS

- The diagnosis of parasitic infection can only be made if the possibility is considered.
- Reinfection is common if close contacts are not treated.
- Threadworm infection can be spread through nursery or child care centres; be sure to inform the carer(s) if infection occurs.
- The physical examination may not be helpful in determining the diagnosis and, therefore, a thorough history with a high index of suspicion is the key to an accurate diagnosis.

🗐 BIBLIOGRAPHY

Butler M. A guide to nurse prescribing of insecticides and anthelmintics. Nurs Times 1998; 94(22):56–57.

Finn L. Threadworm infections. Community Nurse 1996; 2(7):39.

Gilbert P. Skin problems and parasites in children 2: parasitic worms. Prof Care Mother Child 1998; 8(4):105–106.

Mead M. Common conditions. London: Churchill Livingstone; 1999.

Mead M. The complaint threadworm. Pract Nurse 2000; 20(3):169–170.

Tanowitz HB, Weiss LM, Wittner M. Diagnosis and treatment of common intestinal helminths II: common intestinal nematodes. Gastroenterologist 1994; 2(1):39–49.

12.6 DIABETES MELLITUS

Adele McEvilly

📖 INTRODUCTION

- Diabetes mellitus (DM) is a severe metabolic condition: it is a disorder of absolute (*Type 1*) or relative (*Type 2*) insulin deficiency that results in disruption of normal energy storage and metabolism. Type 1 Diabetes is caused by a cessation of insulin production, whereas Type 2 Diabetes is caused by a relative

insulin deficit (e.g. insulin resistance at the tissue level). In childhood, the prevalence of Type 1 is far greater than Type 2 and, therefore, is more likely to be encountered in paediatric practice.
- The reduction in insulin production in Type 2 disease is very gradual and it may take up to 2 years before symptoms present. Insulin production has usually decreased as much as 70% by the time clinical symptoms of insulin

deficiency are apparent (e.g. polydipsia, polyuria, ketonuria, nocturia, enuresis, glycosuria, hyperglycaemia and weight loss). In addition, the lack of blood glucose control and hyperglycaemia can result in ketosis, acidosis, dehydration, shock and death (e.g. diabetic ketoacidosis or DKA).
- Type 2 Diabetes is the third most common chronic medical problem in childhood (most common endocrine

problem), with the incidence increasing at all ages and across races. Boys and girls are equally affected, with an estimated 16 new cases per 100,000 children per year. Prevalence is estimated at 1:400 children of school age with diabetes.

PATHOPHYSIOLOGY (TYPE I DIABETES)

- Diabetes is caused by an autoimmune response in a child who is born with a genetic risk for Type 1 DM; the trigger is either an infection and/or something within the environment. This autoimmune response results in (1) recruitment of cytotoxic lymphocytes and (2) production of anti-insulin and anti-islet cell antibodies which progressively destroy the beta cells of the Islets of Langerhans in the pancreas (the site of insulin production).
- Subsequently, there is a failure of the insulin-producing capacity of the pancreas, with consequential loss of the body's ability to utilise glucose (e.g. transport it from the bloodstream into cells).

HISTORY

- *Onset and duration of symptoms.*
- *Family history of diabetes.*
- Typical physical symptoms of new onset Type 1 Diabetes:
  - *Polyuria and enuresis:* excessively wet nappies that soak the cot; bed-wetting in a child who was previously dry at night; rising several times a night to go to the toilet; leaving lessons to use the toilet.
  - *Polydipsia:* child will drink *excessively* from any fluid source they can reach; continually ask for drinks; leaving lessons to get drink; getting up at night for a drink.
  - *Lethargy:* a toddler who does not want to leave the pushchair; reduced interest in playing with friends; decreases/stops outside activities.
  - *Ketone breath:* commonly described as smelling like 'pear drops', although not everyone can smell pear drops.
  - *Weight loss:* a symptom often missed by parents, as it is attributed to

Table 12.15	Physical Examination Findings in Diabetic Ketoacidosis (DKA)
Symptom	*Physical examination findings*
Dehydration	• Mild (3–5%): dry mucous membranes, slightly reduced skin turgor • Moderate (10%): as above, with sunken eyes and decreased capillary refill • Severe (>10% with signs of shock): very ill with poor perfusion, thready, rapid pulse, reduced blood pressure, markedly reduced urine output
Decreased level of consciousness (LOC)	• Age-related findings, but infants would be listless with decreased responsiveness to stimuli. Older children display disorientation and/or decreased responsiveness to questions. Use modified Glasgow Coma scale to assess
Acidosis	• Ketone smell to breath (pear drops) • Acidotic respirations (increased rate with sighing) • Electrocardiogram (ECG) may show T-wave changes indicative of altered electrolyte status

growth changes of the adolescents who wish to lose weight.

- Frequently there are vague complaints of abdominal pain, constipation, hunger, thrush or other infections (e.g. candidal vulvovaginitis).
- More serious complaints associated with related acidosis include changes in behaviour, mental status and/or school performance; malaise and/or muscular weakness; Kussmaul breathing (sighing respirations); and coma/death (rare).

PHYSICAL EXAMINATION

- General observation of the child is important, including the degree of thirst and polyuria exhibited during the visit. Note weight (assess for changes if parent has recent weight), vital signs (including presence of Kussmaul respirations and ketone breath), hydration status, activity level and degree of interactiveness.
- A physical examination in early Type 1 DM presentation is typically normal; however, a full assessment should be performed, including evaluation of the musculoskeletal and neurological systems, looking for abnormalities in tone, strength and level of consciousness.
- Assess degree of hydration in mouth (palpating inside cheek for sandpaper-type feel) and skin turgor by checking the skin on the abdomen.
- Rule out signs and symptoms of shock.
- If left untreated, early symptoms of Type 1 DM give way to rapid onset of DKA, a potentially life-threatening

complication. Physical signs and symptoms of DKA are outlined in Table 12.15.

DIFFERENTIAL DIAGNOSES

- Numerous: urinary tract infection (UTI), renal glycosuria, hypercalcaemia, other chronic illness (especially with children presenting with fatigue, malaise and weight loss), stress-related hyperglycaemia, drug-induced hyperglycaemia (steroid use), pneumonia, sepsis and acute abdominal event. Note that glycosuria (that is not diabetes-related) may occur following an acute infection.

MANAGEMENT

The management of diabetes mellitus is complex and involves medical, educational and psychosocial support. These should be provided on a 24-hour basis by the paediatric diabetes team, who maintain links with primary care. The diagnosis will have an impact on all family members, who will each cope in their own individual way. Some parents will grieve for their normal healthy child and struggle with feelings of guilt at the diagnosis. Support provided must recognise and empathise with any difficulties the family may feel, as they have to come to terms with insulin injections, blood glucose monitoring, dietary adjustment, achievement of good blood glucose control and management of a chronic illness. The targets for care must be individual, taking into account

Table 12.16	Management of Diabetic Ketoacidosis
Management	Details
Initial management	• General resuscitation, including 100% oxygen, and intravenous fluid (to correct hypokalaemia and dehydration) • Treat shock with 20 ml/kg boluses of 0.9% saline • Once rehydration has commenced, insulin therapy is initiated
Ongoing management	• Hourly blood glucose monitoring • Confirm correction of dehydration • Strict fluid balance monitoring/recording • Regular monitoring of serum potassium • Urine testing for glucose and ketones • Frequent neurological observations (Glasgow scale) • Cardiac monitoring • Observations for signs of cerebral oedema, including irritability, slowing of pulse, increasing blood pressure and papilloedema

Table 12.17	Insulin Therapy
Treatment	Details
Administration	• Twice daily administration for a majority of children and adolescents • Administered via subcutaneous injection with 5–8 mm needle and syringe or pen injector • Insulin is absorbed at different rates from different sites; routine is required for consistent absorption (i.e. injections into arms or stomach in the morning and legs or buttocks in the evening) • Usual regimen is a combination of rapid-acting lispro insulin or short-acting soluble insulin, with an isophane intermediate-acting insulin • These may be free mixed in the syringe or given as a fixed mixture, which is more popular now with the increased use of pen injectors • A basal bolus regimen of three injections of rapid-acting insulin prior to main meals and an injection of isophane prior to bed is increasingly used in older children
Dosage	• At diagnosis there is (presumed) residual insulin production and dose is calculated at 0.5 units/kg/24 hours, usually distributed as two-thirds in the morning and one-third in the evening • Dosage increases to 1 unit/kg as residual insulin production decreases • In adolescence, due to insulin resistance, insulin requirements increase to 1.5 units/kg/24 hours and in some cases 2 units/kg/24 hours • The higher insulin doses are reduced at the end of growth and puberty
Side-effects	• Hyperglycaemia • Hypoglycaemia • Hypertrophy local site irritation (soreness, bruising)

age, intelligence, family stability and personal targets. Diabetic ketoacidosis is the most life-threatening complication of Type 1 DM and, therefore, requires high dependency care. Basic management of DKA is outlined in Table 12.16.

• **Additional diagnostics:** an index of suspicion is raised with positive urine glucose and ketones findings followed by capillary (fingerprick) measurement of blood glucose (normal range is 3–7 mmol/l). Diagnosis is confirmed with results from venous glucose, urea and electrolytes, arterial blood gases and full blood count (FBC). In addition, glycosylated haemoglobin can be considered as it gives an idea of blood glucose levels over the previous 2–3 months. Note, however, that it is used for monitoring and is not diagnostic on its own. Glycosylated haemoglobin is also useful in routine follow-up as it provides an objective index of diabetic control. Consider an electrocardiogram (ECG) if there is suspicion of acidosis.

• **Pharmacotherapeutics:**
  • Insulin therapy is the basis of medical treatment. Characteristics of therapy and dosage guidelines are outlined in Table 12.17. Note that in cases of DKA, hospital admission for continuous insulin infusion is often required.

• **Behavioural interventions:** these are outlined in Table 12.18.

• **Patient education**
  • Home management at the time of diagnosis provides the ideal opportunity for education of the child, siblings and *both* parents; education should be adapted to suit the individual family and provided at a rate that suits them as they come to terms with the shock of diagnosis.
  • Knowledge and understanding of the family (including their individual dynamics) must be continually updated; therefore, the family's management of DM must be reviewed and discussed at each visit.
  • Review with parents the chronic nature of the disease. A frequently encountered diabetes 'myth' is that children grow out of diabetes or are able to go onto tablets when they are older. It is important that parents come to terms with the lifelong implications of DM.
  • Stress the importance of continuing education that is adapted to the child and family's individual needs and abilities; negotiation, partnership and the development of self-care are vital.
  • Discuss with parents the positive support the child will need throughout childhood and into adolescence; this must include a period of interdependence that allows the young person to take on more responsibility as he becomes more confident and capable.
  • Reinforce with parents that education of all carers is essential: the child must always be in a safe environment; this includes educating staff in the school and nursery. The health professionals caring for the child and family should have some sort of provision to ensure this collaboration.

⇨ FOLLOW-UP

• Children with diabetes will be followed up for the rest of their lives and, while young, this will involve 3–4 monthly paediatric diabetes hospital clinic appointments where their height, weight and urine is checked.
• Five years after diagnosis or from puberty onwards, an annual clinic

Table 12.18   Behavioural Interventions in Diabetes Mellitus

Action	Comment
Hyperglycaemia intervention	• In children, defined as pre-prandial blood glucose >10 mmol/l • Signs include those experienced prior to diagnosis and most parents notice a change in temperament • Treatment depends on the causes, which include growth, inappropriate insulin or dietary management, stress, illness or exercise-related • Full history required before advice is given and referral to diabetes team is essential if hyperglycaemia is persistent or ketones are present in urine
Hypoglycaemia intervention	• Defined as blood glucose ≤4 mmol/l • Signs include pallor, shaky feeling, headache, blurred vision, tingling, tiredness and/or twitching • Initial treatment consists of increasing blood glucose level by increasing oral intake of refined glucose (10–20 g). Glucose (10 g) is available from one of the following: 2 teaspoons sugar, 3 sugar lumps, 3 glucose tablets, 200 ml milk, 50–55 ml of non-diet versions of Lucozade Sparkling Glucose Drink, or 90 ml of Coca-Cola • Repeat treatment if no improvement after 5–10 min and continue until better • Once feeling better: unrefined carbohydrate required (biscuit or sandwich) • If unable to give glucose by mouth, Hypostop Gel (glucose 10 g) can be rubbed into gums provided the child is conscious • If unconscious or fitting, glucagon (1 mg) can be given by intramuscular injection
Dietary intervention	• Healthy eating is mainstay of dietary management • Unrefined (starchy) carbohydrates should be eaten as part of 3 main meals and 3 snacks each day with avoidance of refined carbohydrate (except at appropriate times) • Other nutritional requirements (protein, fats, fruit and vegetable intake, etc.) as for non-diabetic children
Blood glucose monitoring	• Most effective way of monitoring metabolic control on a day-to-day basis • Link between blood glucose control and long-term complications • Blood glucose targets must be individual and realistic (i.e. ideal blood glucose levels may lead to frequent and severe hypoglycaemic episodes that can result in developmental delays in young children) • Parental stress can arise from the control/complication link, especially during adolescence when the two management styles may be at odds (e.g. the adolescent wanting to forget about the diabetes and parent more concerned with long-term implications of erratic control) • Glycosylated haemoglobin measurement is a longer-term index of blood glucose control as the amount of glucose attached to the red cell for its half-life is measured. As such, an overview of metabolic control over the preceding 6–8 weeks is obtained • Note that there are different measures for this test and target ranges will vary across centres, as will values for individual patients
Exercise	• Beneficial to metabolic control but must be managed effectively (i.e. prevention of hypoglycaemia) • Extra refined carbohydrate should be eaten before and sometimes during exercise • For particularly strenuous or prolonged exercise, insulin may be reduced and extra unrefined carbohydrate taken • Management should be discussed with the diabetes team
Illness	• Illness may affect blood glucose levels and early contact should be made to the diabetes team to discuss appropriate management • Stomach upset may require a reduction in insulin, while a feverish illness could lead to the development of high glucose levels and ketones, which would require an increase in insulin and referral to the diabetes team • Carbohydrate intake needs to be maintained and this is often taken initially as small, frequent sweet drinks; increase volume as soon as well tolerated to avoid dehydration. If carbohydrates are not tolerated, urgent hospital referral is required • Links with primary care should be maintained during illness

check should include eyes (through dilated pupils), microalbuminuria, blood pressure and examination of the feet. Periodically, blood tests should be carried out for thyroid and coeliac antibodies.

- A paediatric diabetes team should also offer home support, with visits either once or twice a year.

MEDICAL CONSULT/ SPECIALIST REFERRAL (including the paediatric diabetic nurse specialist)

- Any child in whom there is an exceptionally high blood glucose level

associated with ketones, vomiting and/or dehydration as there is a suspicion of DKA and *urgent* referral is necessary.
- Any child in whom an episode of illness is affecting blood glucose levels and parents are unsure about how to, or reluctant to, adjust insulin under guidance from the diabetes nurse.
- Any child who has persistently high blood glucose levels over 2 or 3 days should be reviewed by the diabetes nurse and then referred to the consultant if the problem continues.
- Any child who experiences frequent episodes of hypoglycaemia (more than 1 per week or more than 1 severe episode within a short space of time).

- Any child who is planning to travel abroad or attend organised activity weeks.

PAEDIATRIC PEARLS

- Assess the family's sophistication with the Internet at the time of diagnosis; there is a tremendous amount of information available and families may need help interpreting it all. In addition, they can be overwhelmed by the complications of diabetes so soon after diagnosis.

- Anticipatory guidance with regard to parenting skills is important; encourage parents to avoid making diabetes a point of conflict.

- There is a link between diabetes control and the later development of complications. Intensive management and tight maintenance of blood glucose can significantly reduce the risk of diabetic retinopathy, nephropathy and neuropathy. However, a balance must be found to ensure that the young person is not traumatised by the pressure.

- Without an index of suspicion, the diagnosis of Type 1 DM is occasionally missed and a child may instead be treated for chest infection, UTI or candidiasis. The likelihood of a child in general practice presenting with DM, while uncommon, is not rare; be alert for this possibility to assure a diagnosis is not overlooked. Likewise, an increasing number of young people are developing Type 2 Diabetes; consider this possibility and make use of surgery-based screening tools (urine dipsticks, fingerprick glucose).

- There is usually a period of remission following initial stabilisation of blood glucose after diagnosis. This is referred to as the 'honeymoon period' and is a reflection of residual β-cell insulin production. While this period usually lasts weeks to months, it can persist for longer. Insulin doses need to be reduced accordingly and families need to be warned of this possibility as they

may think the diagnosis was incorrect and 'is going away'.

- The goals of glucose control are (1) to feel well; (2) to maintain pre-prandial blood glucose levels <10 mmol/l; (3) to avoid hypoglycaemic episodes; (4) to promote normal growth and development; and (5) to attain a reasonable non-restrictive lifestyle while maintaining positive psychosocial and emotional development.

- The National Service Framework (NSF) for diabetes has been published. The framework includes recommendations on diagnosis, management and follow-up of diabetes. The NSF is likely to have a big impact on diabetes in general, although the extent that it will affect paediatrics remains to be seen.·

- Internet diabetes resources:
  - **Diabetes UK:** www.diabetes.org.uk (email: balance@diabetes.org.uk)
  - **Juvenile Diabetes Foundation:** www.jdf.irg.uk
  - **Audit Commission:** www.audit-commission.gov.uk
  - **Diabetes National Service Framework:** www.doh.gov.uk./nsf/diabetes

📖 BIBLIOGRAPHY

Audit Commission. Testing times: a review of diabetes services in England and Wales. Abingdon: Audit Commission; 2000.

Brosnan C, Upchurch S, Schreiner B. Type 2 diabetes in children and adolescents: an emerging disease. J Pediatr Health Care 2001; 15(4):187–193.

Craddock S, Avery L. Nurse prescribing in diabetes. Prof Nurse 1998; 13(5):12–13.

Diabetes Control and Complications Trial Research Group. The effect of intensive treatment of diabetes and the development and progression of long-term complications in insulin-dependent diabetes mellitus. N Engl J Med 1993; 329:977–986.

Diabetes UK Report. Dietary recommendations for children and adolescents with diabetes. Diabetes Med 1993; 10:874–885.

Harrop M. Improving paediatric diabetes care. Nurs Stand 1999; 13(51):12–13.

Hatton D. Parents' perception of caring for an infant or toddler with diabetes. J Adv Nurs 1995; 22:569–577.

International Society for Paediatric and Adolescent Diabetes. Consensus guidelines 2000. Netherlands: Public Medical Forum International; 2000.

Kaufman F. Diabetes in children and adolescents, areas of controversy. Med Clin N Am 1998; 82(4):721–738.

McEvilly A. Paediatric care in the community. Pract Diabetes Int 1998; 15(6):167–169.

Newton R. Dilemmas and directions in the care of the diabetic teenager: the Arnold Bloom Lecture. Pract Diabetes Int 2000; 17(1):230–234.

Partanen TM, Rissanen A. Insulin injection practices. Pract Diabetes Int 2000; 17(8):321–323.

Swift P. A decade of diabetes: keeping children out of hospital. BMJ 1993; 307:96–98.

12.7 DELAYED SEXUAL DEVELOPMENT (DELAYED PUBERTY)

Angela Casey

📖 INTRODUCTION

- 'Normal' puberty is difficult to define as there is great variation with regard to the timing and rate of pubertal changes. Influencing factors include social, genetic, environmental, nutritional and gender-related factors.

- Among girls, puberty usually begins between the ages of 8 and 13 years, whereas pubertal changes for boys occur slightly later (9–14 years of age).

Delayed puberty in females is defined as the absence of initial pubertal changes (i.e. Tanner stage 2) after 14 years of age or an interval of greater than 5 years between the initiation of breast growth and menarche. Amongst males, delayed puberty is the absence of initial pubertal changes after 14.5 years of age or a gap of greater than 5 years between the start of genital growth and its completion (i.e. Tanner stage 5).

- Note that the appearance of axillary or pubic hair without concomitant breast or genital growth is not necessarily indicative of the start of pubertal changes. It is termed premature adrenarche and often reflects maturation of the adrenal gland.

- Delayed puberty is one of the most common reasons for growth clinic referral, which is seen more often in boys than in girls (due to differences in the sensitivity of the hypothalamo–pituitary–gonadal axis).

PATHOPHYSIOLOGY

- Puberty describes the process by which a child's body matures into adulthood. Following a period of steady growth in childhood, puberty is distinguished by rapid and dramatic body changes. These include (1) the development of secondary sexual characteristics; (2) the achievement of fertility; and (3) an adolescent growth spurt that is completed by the fusion of the long bone epiphyses and attainment of final adult height. It is important to note that while there can be wide variation in the timing and rate of pubertal changes, they occur in a predictable sequence and well-documented pattern (see Tanner staging, Figs 12.1–12.3).
- The onset of puberty is activated by an increase in gonadotrophin-releasing hormone (GnRH) from the hypothalamus to the pituitary gland, which subsequently secretes the pituitary gonatrophins, luteinising hormone (LH) and follicle-stimulating hormone (FSH). These hormones initiate egg production in the ovaries and sperm production in the testes and are responsible for the secretion of the additional sex hormones (testosterone, oestrogen and progesterone).
- Note that a delay in the onset or progression of sexual development can be caused by numerous factors, each with their own specific pathophysiology.
- Figure 12.4 outlines the endocrine glands and their specific hormones.

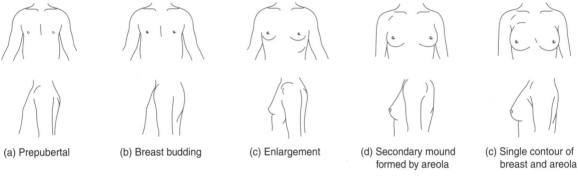

| (a) Prepubertal | (b) Breast budding | (c) Enlargement | (d) Secondary mound formed by areola | (c) Single contour of breast and areola |

Figure 12.1   Tanner's stages of breast development in puberty. Reproduced with permission from Butterworth-Heinemann.

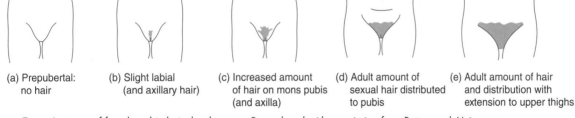

| (a) Prepubertal: no hair | (b) Slight labial (and axillary hair) | (c) Increased amount of hair on mons pubis (and axilla) | (d) Adult amount of sexual hair distributed to pubis | (e) Adult amount of hair and distribution with extension to upper thighs |

Figure 12.2   Tanner's stages of female pubic hair development. Reproduced with permission from Butterworth-Heinemann.

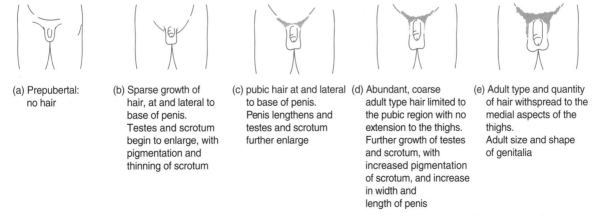

| (a) Prepubertal: no hair | (b) Sparse growth of hair, at and lateral to base of penis. Testes and scrotum begin to enlarge, with pigmentation and thinning of scrotum | (c) pubic hair at and lateral to base of penis. Penis lengthens and testes and scrotum further enlarge | (d) Abundant, coarse adult type hair limited to the pubic region with no extension to the thighs. Further growth of testes and scrotum, with increased pigmentation of scrotum, and increase in width and length of penis | (e) Adult type and quantity of hair withspread to the medial aspects of the thighs. Adult size and shape of genitalia |

Figure 12.3   Tanner's stages of male genital development and pubic hair growth. Reproduced with permission from Butterworth-Heinemann.

159

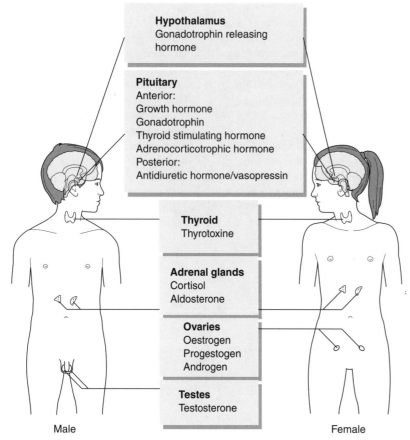

Figure 12.4 Endocrine glands and their respective hormones.

HISTORY

- Growth record (see also Sec. 12.9).
- Review of systems, including enquiries regarding chronic illness or medication use.
- History of genital irradiation, surgery, infection or trauma.
- Nutrition and eating habits (both malnutrition and anorexia nervosa can delay puberty).
- Exercise/activity.
- Family or school stressors, including marked deprivation. Note that extreme psychological stress can delay puberty and growth.
- Age of puberty for parents and/or family history of delayed puberty or growth (especially among older siblings and parents).

PHYSICAL EXAMINATION

- General appearance of the child (see also Sec. 12.9), including overall assessment of health, nutritional status and body proportions.
- Accurate height and weight measurement (with plotting of height and weight).
- Assessment of thyroid.
- Tanner staging of sexual maturity: depending on the child's age there should be early breast bud appearance in females (Tanner stage 2) and testicular volume of at least 4 ml in boys (Tanner stage 2). The Prader orchidometer is a useful tool for assessing testicular development. Each testicle should be manually palpated and its size compared to the Prader bead closest in size.
- General physical examination to rule out a potential disorder outside the genital/reproductive system that could contribute to the lack of development (evidence of cardiac, pulmonary, liver, renal or neurological problems).

DIFFERENTIAL DIAGNOSES

- See Table 12.19.

MANAGEMENT

- **Additional diagnostics:** consider basic diagnostics to rule out other illness (urinalysis, full blood count, erythrocyte

Table 12.19	Differential Diagnoses of Delayed Puberty
Aetiology	*Comments*
Constitutional delay of puberty and growth (CDPG)	• About 90–95% of delayed puberty is constitutional delay of puberty and growth (CDPG) • Diagnosis of exclusion • Criteria include otherwise well and healthy child (i.e. negative review of systems); evidence of appropriate nutrition; linear growth of at least 3.7 cm/year; normal physical examination (including genital anatomy, sense of smell and upper and lower body proportions); normal diagnostics (urinalysis, full blood count, C-reactive protein or erythrocyte sedimentation rate); normal thyroxine (T4), follicle-stimulating hormone (FSH) and luteinising hormone (LH) values; and bone age delayed 1.5–4 years compared with chronological age • Findings supportive of CDPG include family history of CDPG and height between the 3rd and 25th percentiles for age
Chronic illness	• Important to identify abnormal findings on physical examination and basic diagnostics (urinalysis, full blood count, electrolytes and urea, etc.); rule out diseases such as Crohn's, asthma, renal failure, etc. • Height and weight curves often fall off at onset of disease
Gonadotrophin deficiency	• May have history of neurological symptoms • Adolescents with Kallmann's syndrome may have an absent sense of smell • May have low FSH and LH, particulary if bone age is >13 years
Gonadal disorders, including congenital syndromes	• Often history of genital irradiation, surgery, infection or trauma • Very high levels of FSH and LH (especially at pubertal ages) • Males often with gynaecomastia, hypogonadism (testes rarely exceed 4 ml volume in congenital syndromes) • Abnormal chromosomal profile • Turner's syndrome one of the most common causes of maturational delay (CDPG and chronic illness excepted)

sedimentation rate or C-reactive protein, urea and electrolytes). A bone age X-ray of the left wrist is helpful as it can compare chronological age with physiological age. Chromosomal and hormonal analyses are considered in cases of suspected gonadal failure and often performed in specialty care. Pelvic ultrasound may also be considered if there is suspicion of absent gonads or underdevelopment.

- **Pharmacotherapeutics:** the use of medications in delayed puberty is related to the degree of stress experienced by the child/family and the aetiology of the delay. Low-dose oxandrolone (anabolic steroid) can be used to stimulate the pubertal growth spurt in boys with CDPG, whereas testosterone is used when there is concern over delayed secondary sexual characteristics. Girls with CDPG can be prescribed a low-dose oestrogen (ethinyloestradiol) to stimulate breast development for 6–12 months. It should be noted that hormonal or steroid therapy is a decision that requires careful consideration and is likely to only be taken within the context of specialty consultation.

- **Behavioural interventions:**
  - Ongoing support is required for the adolescent and the family.
  - Children with an underlying pathology will require additional interventions specific to their illness (gluten-free diet in coeliac disease, treatment of anorexia nervosa, etc.).
  - Reassure the adolescent and family regarding the self-limiting nature of CDPG; they will require support and practical advice with issues such as identity cards for proof of age.

- **Patient education:**
  - Discuss honestly with the adolescent the expected course the puberty delay will (likely) take and the aetiology behind the delay. Adolescence is a time of great upheaval (even when its course runs as expected), so that for those with an unanticipated delay there is potential for extreme stress.
  - In cases of CDPG, remind patients and their families that puberty and growth will occur, especially as other

causes for the delay have been investigated/ruled out. Reassure them that follow-up will check that no abnormality was missed and that they *will* experience growth and sexual maturation.
- Provide patients and their families with anticipatory guidance regarding unwanted effects of hormonal treatment in CDPG (secondary sexual characteristics, acne, mood swings).
- The Child Growth Foundation, 2 Mayfield Avenue, London W4 1PW is a potential resource for practical advice on topics such as identity cards, bullying, clothing shops, etc.

→ FOLLOW-UP

- Follow-up is largely determined by the treatment course. If watchful waiting is planned, follow-up in 3–6 months is advisable.
- If pubertal changes have not started in girls over 14 years of age and boys over 15 years of age, specialist referral is indicated.

⇄ MEDICAL CONSULT/ SPECIALIST REFERRAL

- Any child with a delay in pubertal development (clear-cut constitutional delay excepted).
- Any child in whom the aetiology of the delay is unclear.
- Any child or family experiencing significant stress related to the delayed puberty.
- Any child in whom hormone or steroid treatment is being considered.

⊘ PAEDIATRIC PEARLS

- Faulty measuring techniques or poorly calibrated measuring equipment often result in mistakes on the child's growth chart; careful attention must be paid to measurement technique and equipment.
- Treat the child according to his/her age not size; it is important not to 'baby'.
- Children with delayed pubertal development are at risk of bullying; address this issue in the assessment and anticipatory guidance with the child and family.

- Excluding chronic illness and constitutional delay, Turner's syndrome is one of the more common causes of maturational delay (see also Sec. 12.9).
- In eliciting information with regard to pubertal development of family members, it is useful to enquire about mother's age at menarche, older sisters' age at menarche, age at which father started to shave and whether father (or mother) were much shorter than their classmates as a teenager.
- It is helpful to consider the following in the evaluation of pubertal delay: (1) evidence of any disorder that may be responsible for the growth failure (e.g. undiagnosed chronic illness); (2) the extent to which skeletal maturation has progressed; and (3) evidence of disruption of gonadal or hypothalamic–pituitary function.

▤ BIBLIOGRAPHY

Albanese A, Stanhope R. Investigation of delayed puberty. Clin Endocrinol (Oxf) 1995; 43(1):105–110.

Algranati PS. The pediatric patient: an approach to history and physical examination. Baltimore: Williams & Wilkins; 1992.

Buckler JMH. Growth disorders in children. London: BMJ Publishing; 1994.

Buckler JMH. A reference manual of growth and development, 2nd edn. Oxford: Blackwell Scientific Publications; 1997.

Mazur T, Clopper RR. Pubertal disorders: psychology and clinical management. Endocrinol Metab Clin N Am 1991; 20(1):211–230.

Rieder J, Coupey SM. Update on pubertal development. Curr Opin Obstet Gynecol 1999; 11(5):457–462.

Stanhope R. Constitutional delay of growth and puberty: a guide for parents and patients. Middlesex: Serono Pharmaceuticals; 1995.

Tanner JM. Growth at adolescence, 2nd edn. Oxford: Blackwell Scientific; 1962.

Zachmann M, Prader A, Kind HP, et al. Testicular volume during adolescence. Helv Paediatr Acta 1974; 29:61.

ACKNOWLEDGEMENT

The author would like to acknowledge the expertise of Dr Jeremy Kirk, Consultant Paediatric Endocrinologist, Birmingham Children's Hospital, in the preparation of this section.

COMMON PAEDIATRIC PROBLEMS

2

12.8 PREMATURE SEXUAL DEVELOPMENT (PRECOCIOUS PUBERTY)

Pam Hayes

📖 INTRODUCTION

- The physical signs of puberty are often the first change noticed by parents, although hormonal activation will have been occurring for several years. When the physical changes of puberty occur prematurely, the cause of the precocious sexual development should be investigated (i.e. specialist referral).
- True *precocious puberty* (also called gonadotrophin-dependent, central or idiopathic precocious puberty) is defined as pubertal changes (i.e. pubic hair growth, breast development, or penile and testicular growth) occurring in the expected sequence, but at an unexpected age (i.e. earlier than 8 years of age in girls and 9 years in boys).
- *Premature thelarche* is early breast development that occurs in the absence of other pubertal changes; it may be unilateral or bilateral. It most commonly affects girls between 2 and 4 years of age, is self-limiting and does not require treatment.
- *Premature adrenarche* is the early growth of pubic hair that can affect both boys and girls. It is caused by the premature production of androgens and may be accompanied by an acceleration of growth and slightly advanced bone age. Although most often it is benign and self-limiting, specialist evaluation should be completed to rule out endocrine pathology.
- Children with precocious puberty will often initially be taller than their peers (due to an earlier pubertal growth spurt and an advanced bone age). However, if left untreated, this tall stature in early childhood may result in short stature in adulthood, related to premature fusing of the long bone epiphyses. If the physical changes of puberty continue, girls will experience the onset of menses, which can be very distressing to parents and children alike.
- Despite physical advancement, children with precocious puberty rarely exhibit accelerated psychosocial development; social interaction is usually age-appropriate. If they try to develop associations with older children (i.e. those whose appearance is similar to their own) they are at a disadvantage because of their lack of social skills. Behavioural problems (of differing degrees) and inappropriate sexual behaviour in children with precocious puberty have often been reported. Because the reasoning capabilities of children with premature sexual development do not usually match their more advanced physical appearance, they may be at risk for inappropriate relationships and/or abuse.

🔬 PATHOPHYSIOLOGY

- The cause of premature sexual development is often idiopathic, especially in girls. There is however, an association between precocious puberty and central nervous system (CNS) problems such as trauma, surgery, chemotherapy and radiotherapy. It is also important to rule out CNS disease and malignancies (see Differential diagnoses).
- Peripheral precocious puberty, also known as gonadotrophin-independent precocious puberty (GIPP), is more common in boys than girls. In this condition, hormones are produced directly by the gonads and not by the usual hypothalamic–pituitary route. This results in elevated levels of sex hormones but low gonadotrophin levels (requires specialist evaluation).
- Note that there may be a familial trend towards early sexual development.

⬅ HISTORY

- Complete past medical history, including any problems at birth, past illnesses, trauma (especially head trauma) and any intercurrent disease.
- History of drug ingestion (especially the possibility of sex steroids), including products that may contain hormones (creams, make-up or oils).
- Family history of pubertal changes (including early development in family members).
- Chronology of growth and development, including growth rate increases, development of secondary sexual characteristics (breast or genital development, axillary hair, pubic hair, and/or menses).
- Other changes (acne, body odour, emotional changes/mood swings, etc.).
- Social history, including interactions at home and school (with assessment of risk for inappropriate relationships and abuse).

🔬 PHYSICAL EXAMINATION

- Children with premature sexual development are likely to be very shy with regard to their atypical appearance. Consequently, extreme sensitivity should be exercised during the physical examination, including preservation of privacy and consent from both parent and child.
- Accurate measurement of height and weight with charting on appropriate centile charts.
- Evaluation of sexual maturity using the Tanner classification (see Figs 12.1–12.3 in Sec. 12.7).
- Careful neurological examination to identify CNS abnormalities.
- Careful testicular examination in boys to rule out gonadal masses.
- Examine for signs of hypothyroidism, café au lait patches and cutaneous neurofibromata.

DIFFERENTIAL DIAGNOSES

- In addition to an idiopathic cause (diagnosis of exclusion), sexual precocity can be the result of organic brain disease (including brain tumours, hypothalamic hamartomas, hydrocephalus, and cranial irradiation), gonadotrophin-secreting tumours, gonadal or adrenal tumours, hypothyroidism (rare) and McCune–Albright syndrome in girls (uncommon).

MANAGEMENT

- **Additional diagnostics:** include the possibility of hormone levels (serum levels of sex hormones and dynamic endocrine testing), thyroid function, bone age X-ray and ultrasound scanning to assess ovarian and uterine development. In view of the high incidence of intracranial abnormalities, all patients should have a magnetic resonance imaging (MRI) scan of the brain and hypothalamo–pituitary region.
- **Pharmacotherapeutics:** the mainstay of drug therapy in precocious puberty are gonadotrophin-releasing hormone (GnRH) analogues such as goserelin, administered by monthly or 3-monthly subcutaneous implants. Note that with the start of treatment, physical changes may temporarily advance. Cyproterone acetate may also be given as an oral preparation. This medication does slow the advance of puberty but can have unwanted effects (headaches and weight gain). It is usually administered for a short period of time. Medications are typically discontinued when the child's peers would be entering puberty, although factors such as bone age and hormone levels would be simultaneously considered.
- **Behavioural interventions:**
  - As children with precocious puberty are often tall, problems can present in relationships, particularly with peers. Adults may have raised expectations of behaviour and achievement; it is important that children are treated appropriately for their age.

- There does not seem to be long-term psychological sequelae related to increased height and physical development. However, because children who appear physically mature probably do not possess the same degree of emotional maturity, care must be taken to protect them from inappropriate relationships.
- **Patient education:**
  - Discuss openly and honestly with both parents and children the diagnosis of precocious puberty, including its consequences and treatment. It is important to discuss potential problems that may arise from the diagnosis (i.e. the possibility of inappropriate relationships or bullying at school).
  - Reassure parents (and children) that the condition is treatable and has a very good prognosis (if appropriate).
  - Review behavioural interventions (above).
  - Information from sources such as the Child Growth Foundation (2 Mayfield Avenue, London W4 1PW) are often very helpful for families. Support can also be provided from meeting other families with similar conditions.

FOLLOW-UP

- Initial follow-up may be as often as 3-monthly in order to monitor the effects of treatment and/or to observe for continued development.
- For children and families that have additional concerns or need additional support, follow-up contact may be more frequent.

MEDICAL CONSULT/ SPECIALIST REFERRAL

- Any child in whom there is a suspicion of premature sexual development.
- Any child in whom there is a suspicion of endocrine pathology or CNS involvement.
- Any child (or family) who is significantly distressed by the diagnosis, treatment or management of premature sexual development.
- Any child in whom final height is likely to be restricted.

- Any child who is experiencing behavioural difficulties related to the diagnosis.

PAEDIATRIC PEARLS

- Always check the age of a child; do not rely on physical appearance.
- Although premature adrenarche and thelarche can be self-limiting and benign, it can also be the first sign of true precocious puberty; it requires careful assessment and observation.
- Bone age and stimulated gonadotrophin levels are important parameters upon which management decisions are made.
- Both play specialist and/or psychology referral can be very helpful with children and families who are experiencing significant issues related to their diagnosis.
- Rule out hypothyroidism among children with a retarded bone age and short stature, although a bone age consistent with chronological age is often seen among children with incomplete precocious puberty (i.e. premature thelarche and adrenarche).
- Given their potential fertility, it is important to consider early sex education among children with true precocious puberty. This should be discussed carefully with parents and children.

BIBLIOGRAPHY

Buckler JMH. Growth disorders in children. London: BMJ Publishing; 1994.
Buckler JMH. A reference manual of growth and development, 2nd edn. Blackwell Scientific; 1997.
Fry V, Stanhope R. Premature sexual maturation – series No. 4. London: Child Growth Foundation; 1996.
Lee PA. Central precocious puberty: an overview of diagnosis, treatment and outcome. Pediatr Endocrinol 28(4): 901–918.
Mazur T, Clopper RR. Pubertal disorders. Psychology and clinical management. Endocrinol Metab Clin North Am 1991; 20(1):211–230.
Merke DP, Cutler GB Jr. Evaluation and management of precocious puberty. Arch Dis Child 1996; 75(4):269–271.
Partsch CJ, Heger S, Sippell WG. Management and outcome of central

precocious puberty. Clin Endocrinol (Oxf) 2002; 56(2):129–148.

Rieder J, Coupey SM. Update on pubertal development. Curr Opin Obstet Gynecol 1999; 11(5):457–462.

Tanner JM, Whitehouse RH. Atlas of children's growth: normal variations and growth disorders. London: Academic Press; 1982.

Tato L, Savage MO, Antoniazzi F et al. Optimal therapy of pubertal disorders in precocious/early puberty. J Pediatr Endocrinol Metab 2001; 14(suppl 2): 985–995.

Wales J, Rogal DD, Wit JM. Color atlas of pediatric endocrinology and growth. London: Mosby-Wolfe; 1996.

ACKNOWLEDGEMENT

The author would like to acknowledge the expertise of Dr Jeremy Kirk, Consultant Paediatric Endocrinologist, Birmingham Children's Hospital, in the preparation of this section.

12.9 SHORT STATURE

Emma Murphy

📖 INTRODUCTION

- A child's height measurement can be an excellent indicator of his state of health; however, it is often neglected in preference to measurement of weight.
- An abnormal growth pattern (which requires a series of measurements to identify) in children should never be ignored, as it can be indicative of compromised physical, psychological or emotional health.
- Short stature has been defined as 'height below the third centile'. This definition is problematic for several reasons: (1) a healthy child with a normal growth rate and height below the third centile may have a 'normal height' given his genetic potential (i.e. when parental heights are taken into consideration); (2) centile charts may be derived from longitudinal data (Buckler–Tanner) or cross-sectional data (Child Growth Foundation) and therefore differ slightly; and (3) racial differences should be taken into account.
- In the UK, by definition, approximately 1 in 33 children will have measurements below the third centile. Whereas most short stature is not associated with pathology, the further away from the normal range the measurement is, the greater the likelihood that the cause is pathological. However, it is important to distinguish short stature from *growth failure* (downward crossing of growth percentiles that can lead to short stature) and *failure to thrive* (failure to meet appropriate standards for weight, and in extreme cases, height). Note that diagnostic evaluation of growth failure should be initiated when the child begins to cross percentiles (regardless of whether short stature is present) and that failure-to-thrive children may or may not be short.
- Each child's growth should therefore be assessed on an individual basis. This assessment includes (1) accurate measurement of the child's height; (2) careful plotting on an appropriate centile chart; (3) calculation of the child's genetic height potential and height velocity; and (4) the child's pubertal staging (see Sec. 12.7). Only with this information can the diagnosis of 'short stature' begin to be considered and therefore, a distinction made between short children who are within their expected height potential and short children who have an underlying pathology.

🔬 PATHOPHYSIOLOGY

- Before an abnormal growth pattern is recognised, it is important to appreciate the characteristics of normal growth in childhood. Growth charts provide the simplest and most effective representation of a child's growth pattern; by plotting a child's measurements over a period of time it is easy to distinguish a normal pattern of growth from an abnormal one.
- Growth hormone (GH) is responsible for the stimulation of growth in children whose long bone epiphyses are not yet fused. GH is released, among other stimuli, in response to sleep, exercise and hypoglycaemia.
- Prior to the onset of puberty, a healthy, well-nourished child's rate of growth is constant and relatively slow. Surprisingly, there is little variation between the height and weight of the average prepubescent boy and girl.
- Due to differences in the timing and initiation of puberty (e.g. girls typically begin puberty earlier and therefore experience an earlier growth spurt) girls of average height are slightly taller than their male classmates between the ages of 11 and 13 years.
- However, by the end of puberty when no further growth is possible (i.e. the long bone epiphyses are fused) the average adult male is 12.5 cm taller. This height differential is due to the extra growth boys achieve before (their slightly later) puberty and their greater peak height velocity of 10–12 cm/year (vs 8–10 cm/year in girls).

⬅ HISTORY

- Prenatal history (exposure to alcohol, cigarettes or drugs; maternal nutrition and/or illness).
- Birth weight, height and head circumference.

- Problems in the neonatal period, including problems of hypoglycaemia (can be indicative of pituitary deficiency) or lymphoedema (Turner's syndrome).
- Feeding and/or diet history (includes information related to body image and consider anorexia) and possibility of malnutrition.
- Previous growth and development (if serial height measurements are not available, enquire about changes in clothing sizes).
- Review of systems, including presence of any chronic illness or medication use (e.g. recurrent otitis media associated with Turner's syndrome; long-term steroid use for asthma management; congenital cardiac abnormalities; malabsorption syndromes, gastrointestinal problems, etc.).
- Absence or presence of pubertal changes (if menarche achieved, enquire about age at presentation, regularity of cycles, symptoms of dysmenorrhoea or menorrhagia).
- Family circumstances and psychosocial history (emotional stresses can affect growth either directly through abnormal GH production or indirectly through inadequate nutrition).
- Family history of short stature, endocrine disorders, chronic illness or chromosomal abnormalities (e.g. skeletal dysplasia, diabetes, thyroid disorders, inborn errors of metabolism, inflammatory bowel disease, trisomy 21 or Turner's syndrome).
- Parental ages of puberty.

🫁 PHYSICAL EXAMINATION

- Note the child's general appearance, including an impression of body proportions and dysmorphic features that may be indicative of a chromosomal abnormality: e.g. Turner's syndrome, the features of which are outlined in Box 12.1. Note that limb length and sitting height should be measured if skeletal dysplasia is suspected (reference values available).
- *Accurate* height, weight and head circumference measurements are imperative.
- Note presence (or absence) of secondary sexual characteristics and

---

Box 12.1   Physical features of Turner's syndrome[a] (Note: not listed in order of frequency)

- Broad chest with widely spaced nipples
- Chronic middle ear infections
- Constriction or narrowing of the aorta (coarctation)
- Cubitus valgus (increased carrying angle of the elbows)
- Feeding difficulties in early life (usually associated with the high arched palate)
- Folds of skin on the ridge of the eye
- Hearing problems
- High blood pressure
- Hypothyroidism (reduced thyroid function)
- Infertility
- Kidney and urinary tract problems
- Learning difficulties
- Low hairline
- Low set ears
- Lymphoedema (build up of fluid in the limbs)
- Micrognathia (small jaw)
- Narrow high-arched palate
- Non-functioning ovaries
- Pigmented naevi (moles)
- Short fingers and toes
- Soft spoon-shaped nails which turn up at the tips
- Squint
- Webbed neck

[a]It is important to remember that it is unlikely for any girl to have all the associated features. Parents of a baby that is newly diagnosed with the syndrome may be concerned that their daughter will attain additional physical characteristics as she gets older. This is not so, as the physical characteristics do not change markedly through life.

Tanner staging (e.g. pubertal status). Tanner staging is outlined in Section 12.7 (Figs 12.1–12.3).
- A general physical examination of all systems to identify any potential abnormalities. Careful observation in any girl with short stature to identify symptoms of Turner's syndrome (Box 12.1).

🔎 DIFFERENTIAL DIAGNOSES

- See Table 12.20.

➕ MANAGEMENT

- **Additional diagnostics:** consider basic diagnostics to rule out infection, anaemia, inflammation and leukaemia (e.g. urinalysis, full blood count, C-reactive protein, erythrocyte sedimentation rate, urea and electrolytes). Additional diagnostics (e.g. GH measurement, metabolic panel, thyroid function, karyotyping and analysis of other hormones) are usually performed at the discretion of specialist care. Bone age is extremely useful. If bone age is delayed, additional growth potential remains (consider constitutional delay or chronic disease). If bone age is advanced, there is decreased growth potential remaining and these children can end up as short adults (consider premature puberty and other causes of short stature).

- **Pharmacotherapeutics:** aetiology-dependent and almost always under the supervision of specialty care (e.g. paediatric endocrinology). In children with GH insufficiency, exogenous GH can be given by subcutaneous injection. A lesser but variable response is found with other aetiologies of short stature (e.g. chronic renal failure, Turner's syndrome or skeletal dysplasias, small for gestational age). Children with deficiencies of other hormones are replaced as necessary (e.g. thyroxine in patients with hypothyroidism).

- **Behavioural interventions:**
  - accurate measurement and plotting of height, weight and head circumference is imperative
  - use of age-appropriate scales (balanced correctly), stadiometers and correct head circumference measuring technique is very important
  - use of an age- and gender-appropriate growth chart and height velocity chart
  - racial differences need to be considered
  - calculation of mid-parental height and target centile range (Table 12.21).

Table 12.20	Differential Diagnoses of Short Stature	
Classification	Aetiology	Comments
Variations of normal growth	• Familial short stature	• Short parents • Normal height velocity (around 25th percentile) • Normal age of pubertal onset • Normal bone age • Short stature throughout childhood and adolescence • Final adult height close to the mid-parental height and usually around the 3rd or 5th percentile
	• Constitutional short stature/delay of growth and puberty	• Height percentile below the target range defined by parental heights • Delayed bone age • Reduced height velocity (especially in late childhood, usually <25th percentile) • Associated with delayed pubertal maturation • Positive family history of delayed puberty (more common in boys) • Final adult height in normal range and within genetic target height
	• Idiopathic short stature	• *Diagnosis of exclusion;* these children are otherwise normal but cannot be diagnosed with any variant of normal growth or any other cause of short stature • Used with children whose height is below the 5th percentile and whose calculated *predicted* height is 2 standard deviations below mid-parental height (>10 cm). These children also have a delay of skeletal maturation but no family history of constitutional delay of growth or adolescence
Primary short stature[a]	• Skeletal dysplasia	• Genetic transmission or mutation • Defects in growth of tubular bones and/or axial skeleton • Typical findings on radiographic skeletal survey • More common forms: achondroplasia (disproportionately short with large heads and short limbs) and hypochondroplasia (similar condition but more subtle presentation)
	• Error of metabolism	• Diffuse skeletal involvement • Mostly autosomal recessive inheritance • Dysmorphic features • Typical biochemical abnormalities • Mucopolysaccharidosis, while rare, is the most common error of metabolism
	• Chromosomal abnormality	• Variations in height related to autosomes or sex chromosomes • Usually associated with other somatic abnormalities and/or learning disabilities • Clinical findings may be subtle • More common forms: trisomy 21, Turner's syndrome
	• Intrauterine growth retardation (IUGR)	• Often associated with poor postnatal growth • Cause for IUGR may be related to mother, placenta or fetus • Seen in fetal infection, fetal exposures, placental abnormalities, maternal disease and fetal hormone abnormalities • Primordial dwarfism due to intrinsic fetal defect leading to prenatal and postnatal growth failure (may be associated with a genetic anomaly) • Majority will not reach full genetic potential but will be in normal range of adult height • Consider Russell–Silver syndrome if child is small for dates, continues small and has little subcutaneous fat and elf-like face. May also have a limb length discrepancy
Secondary short stature	• Malnutrition	• Malabsorption syndromes (inhibited absorption of food depresses child's growth) • More common under 2 years of age and especially in first 6 months of life • Can be related to caloric and/or protein malnutrition • Can be a result of vitamin and/or mineral deficiency (vitamin D, iron or zinc deficiency)
	• Chronic illness	• Many chronic illnesses present first with poor growth (congenital cardiac disease, asthma, Crohn's disease, cystic fibrosis, inflammatory bowel disease, coeliac disease, chronic gastroenteritis, renal disease, diabetes mellitus, HIV, anaemia, leukaemia, sickle cell disease, etc.)
	• Drugs	• Long-term and/or high-dose corticosteroid use • Use of sex hormones
	• Psychosocial growth delay	• Children who experience extreme stress: homelessness, maltreatment, neglect • Is likely related to stress-induced decrease in growth hormone (GH)
	• Endocrine short stature	• Relatively uncommon cause of short stature • Includes GH insufficiency (present with normal skeletal proportions, facial appearance and intelligence; often overweight with delayed bone age) and Cushing's disease (present short and overweight due to excess corticosteroid secretion) • Children who have undergone pituitary surgery or radiotherapy (for treatment of malignancies) can be rendered GH-deficient

[a]Note: usually an abnormality of the skeletal system (bone age often normal or slightly delayed). Skeletal defect can be a primary defect or secondary to a metabolic disorder. Note that the skeletal defect may result in short stature and/or dysmorphism.

Table 12.21 Calculation of Genetic Height Potential	
Females	Males
1. Calculate an average of father's and mother's height (cm)	1. Calculate an average of father's and mother's height (cm)
2. Calculate mid-parental height (MPH) by subtracting 7 cm from the averaged parental heights	2. Calculate MPH by adding 7 cm to the averaged parental heights
3. Obtain mid-parental centile (MPC) by plotting the MPH on the girl's height chart (5–20 years) at the 18-year axis	3. Obtain MPC by plotting the MPH on the boy's height chart (5–20 years) at the 18-year axis
4. Calculate the target centile range (TCR)^a by adding and subtracting 8.5 cm from the MPH and obtaining corresponding percentiles on the girl's height chart (5–20 years) at 18-year axis	4. Calculate the TCR by adding and subtracting 8.5 cm from the MPH and obtaining corresponding percentiles on the boy's height chart (5–20 years) at 18-year axis

^{a}The TCR subsequently serves as a benchmark for determining the percentile parameters for a child's expected growth given their genetic make-up. Note that these calculations are not appropriate if either parent is not of normal stature.

- **Patient education:**
  - Discuss with the child and the family the aetiology of the short stature, the long-term prognosis and available treatment options.
  - Reassure parents of a short child that has a height below the 3rd percentile but normal growth velocity, pattern and target centile range. It is often helpful to calculate the child's height potential with the parents so that the genetic influence can be better appreciated.
  - Talk openly with the child and family about the implications of short stature as the child matures. Short stature in childhood can be associated with psychological and/or social problems. Children who are short can be targeted by bullies and experience problems with self-esteem and social interaction. It is important that families understand that support and/or counselling can be helpful if problems arise.
  - Review any medications to be used (if appropriate) including administration, adverse effects and rationale behind their use. Careful education with regard to medications can also improve concordance with treatment.
  - Girls with Turner's syndrome (and their families) may require additional support and counselling as they come to terms with the short stature, delayed/absent physical maturation, infertility and the implications of a genetic disorder.

⇨ FOLLOW-UP

- If concerns are unresolved, review growth again in 3–6 months time.

⇄ MEDICAL CONSULT/ SPECIALIST REFERRAL

- Any child with a growth delay that is potentially pathological in its aetiology.
- Any child in whom the diagnosis is uncertain.
- Any child who is inappropriately short given parental height.
- Any child in whom the short stature has become a focal disruption for the family structure or the child's life (counselling referral).
- Any child whose height falls below the 0.4th centile line.
- Any child <5 years of age whose growth veers downwards over the width of one centile band during a 12–18-month period.
- Any child >5 years of age whose growth veers downwards over the width of two-thirds of one centile band during a 12–18-month period.

⚲ PAEDIATRIC PEARLS

- Although most short stature is not associated with pathology, it is important to think broadly with regard to the list of differential diagnoses and eliminate different aetiologies systematically.
- To evaluate the child with questionable growth, it is imperative that special attention is paid to accuracy of height, weight and head circumference measurements.
- Any girl with short stature of unknown cause should have a chromosomal analysis to rule out Turner's syndrome.
- Growth patterns are important. After 2–3 years of age and until puberty, shifts from an established growth curve suggest a pathological aetiology and require careful investigation.
- Specialist growth charts are available for children with Turner's syndrome, Down's syndrome and achondroplasia.
- Charts are available to monitor growth velocity, body mass index and head circumference throughout childhood.
- Child Growth Foundation, 2 Mayfield Avenue, London W4 1PW.

🕮 BIBLIOGRAPHY

Chinn S. Growth charts for ethnic populations in the UK. Lancet 1996; 347:839–840.

Cole TJ. Do growth charts need a facelift? BMJ 1994; 308:641–642.

Freeman JV. Cross-sectional stature and weight reference curves for the UK, 1990. Arch Dis Child 1995; 73:17–24.

ACKNOWLEDGEMENT

The author would like to acknowledge the expertise of Dr Jeremy Kirk, Consultant Paediatric Endocrinologist, Birmingham Children's Hospital, in the preparation of this section.

COMMON PAEDIATRIC PROBLEMS

2

12.10 INGESTIONS AND POISONINGS

Peter Wilson

📖 INTRODUCTION

- The two groups most at risk of toxic ingestions are adolescents and children under 5.
- Sixty per cent of all ingestions occur in children under 5, and 90% of all cases occur in the home.
- Household substances, cosmetics and medications (especially analgesics, cough and cold preparations, and vitamins or iron preparations) account for 60% of all poisonings.
- The majority of these accidental ingestions are harmless, with only 10% being admitted to hospital, although deaths do occur. Deaths are mainly due to analgesics, iron, hydrocarbons and corrosive cleaning products.
- About 5% of poisonings are deliberate. These occur more regularly within the adolescent population. Although adolescents make up a much smaller number of those taking overdoses, they are much more likely to take a potentially toxic dose and therefore, require treatment and hospitalisation.
- The commonest drug used in deliberate self-harm is paracetamol. It is implicated in 40% of all cases. There are an estimated 70,000 cases per year, with a mortality rate of 11% and a transplant rate of 15%.
- There is however, an increase in the number of hospitalisations/fatalities due to recreational drugs, such as ecstasy and ketamine, in the adolescent population.

🔬 PATHOPHYSIOLOGY

The specific pathophysiology of overdoses is dependent on the drug ingested. There are far too many drugs to examine each individually, so a brief overview of important points to be considered is outlined below:

- **Route of absorption** (e.g. ingestion, skin contact, inhalation): this is important as some drugs may have a delayed effect.
- **Mechanism of injury:** inflammatory response (e.g. chemical pneumonitis); and/or cellular damage (e.g. paracetamol overdose).
- **Dose-related response:** is the degree of injury proportional to amount ingested? This is important to decide if drug levels will be of assistance in management.
- **Excretion of toxin:** through what mechanism is the drug metabolised and excreted (e.g. urine, gastrointestinal tract, degraded by liver enzymes). An understanding of the drug's excretion process will facilitate faster decontamination (if known) and enable correct treatment.

⬅ HISTORY

- It is very important to get a clear history of what the child has taken or inhaled. Lack of information will hinder the accurate and timely treatment of patients. If possible, examine the drug's packaging or container (helpful in estimating amount taken and ingredients).
- The name of the drug, including the brand name.
- The number and strength of tablets supposedly ingested. Important to ask how many tablets were originally in the container, as well as how many are now left.
- If alcohol or solvent abuse, an estimation of the exposure.
- When did the incident occur?
- What is the child's age and weight? This will allow an assessment of whether the dose ingested is toxic.
- What has occurred since the ingestion and/or whether the child has vomited? It is important to tell parents *not* to induce vomiting. This is especially important if the child has ingested paraffin or any other substance that could cause a chemical pneumonitis if inhaled.
- Is the child taking any medication(s) or have any past medical history that would be relevant to the ingestion/inhalation?
- Does the child have any other symptoms? Specifically enquire about drowsiness, dry mouth, blurred vision, seizures, palpitations, respiratory difficulties and diarrhoea. It is important to remember that many of these symptoms are caused by more than one drug.

🩺 PHYSICAL EXAMINATION

- **General examination of the child**: this includes any evidence of drug ingestion. For example, stained hands or tongue, or smell of solvent on breath. Many drugs are associated with distinctive clinical signs. Tables 12.22 and 12.23 outline the more common ones.

- **Cardiovascular:**
  - pulse rate (can have tachycardia or bradycardia)
  - blood pressure
  - capillary refill time (important in determining presence of shock).

- **Respiratory:**
  - dry mouth or increased secretions
  - respiratory rate and pattern (important to assess respiratory effort in patients with a depressed level of consciousness)
  - ability to maintain a patent airway.

- **Neurological:**
  - Glasgow Coma Scale (useful in determining the level of consciousness). See Section 13.5 for an outline of the Glasgow scale (including an adaptation for infants and young children).
  - Signs of agitation or hallucinations.
  - Abnormal movements (dystonic reactions, twitches).
  - Evidence of seizures.
  - Size of pupils (can be dilated or pinpoint).
  - Muscle tone (can be increased or decreased).
  - Reflexes (can be brisk or absent).
  - Control over bowels and bladder.

Table 12.22   Clinical Patterns and Associated Poisons

Clinical pattern	Consider
Coma, reduced level of consciousness, flaccidity, decreased reflexes	• Benzodiazepines • Barbiturates • Ethanol • Tricyclics • Phenothiazines • Opiates • Chloral • Antihistamines
Coma, agitation, hallucinations, twitches, hyper-reflexia, dilated pupils, tachycardia	• Anticholinergics • Tricyclics • Phenothiazines • Antihistamines
Coma, ventricular tachycardia/fibrillation, hypotension	• Tricyclics • Chloral • Quinidine • Phenothiazines • Anticholinergics • Antihistamines
Seizures, hypertonia, hyper-reflexia, pyrexia, hypokalaemia, hyperglycaemia, metabolic acidosis	• Theophylline • Monamine oxidase inhibitors • Amphetamines

Table 12.23   Drug Class and Clinical Symptoms

Drug	Level of consciousness	Pupils	Vital signs[a]	Other
Sympathomimetics	Agitated, psychosis	Dilated	↑HR, ↑BP, ↑T	Tremors, sweating, seizures, arrhythmias
Anticholinergics	Delirium, hallucinations	Dilated	↑HR, ↑T	Flushed, dry mucous membranes, urinary retention
Opiates	Coma	Pinpoint	↓RR, ↑HR, ↑BP	Shallow respirations
Organophosphates	Sedated or coma	Miosis	↓or ↑HR, ↓or ↑BP	Salivation, lacrimation, bronchorrhoea, diarrhoea, muscle twitching, seizures, diaphoresis
Sedative–hypnotics	Sedated or coma	Miosis	↓RR, ↓T, ↓BP	Ataxia, nystagmus, slurred speech
Phenothiazines	Sedated or coma	Miosis	↓BP, ↓T	Dystonic reactions, ataxia
Tricyclics	Agitation, coma	Dilated	↑HR, ↑T, ↓or ↑BP	Prolonged QRS interval, ventricular arrhythmias, seizures
Salicylates	Disorientated, hyperexcitable	Not affected	↑T, ↑RR	Vomiting, tinnitus, metabolic acidosis, hypokalaemia

[a]BP = blood pressure; HR = heart rate; RR = respiratory rate; T = temperature.

🅟 DIFFERENTIAL DIAGNOSES

- It is important to always consider drug ingestion in any child presenting with a decreased level of consciousness or abnormal neurological signs. It is not uncommon for parents and children to deny administering/taking a drug for fear of punishment.
- Always consider drug ingestion in any adolescent presenting with a decreased level of consciousness.
- Consider encephalitis, meningitis, sepsis, encephalopathy (due to a hepatic, renal, metabolic or infectious cause) and seizures in any child with a decreased level of consciousness.

- Tables 12.22 and 12.23 assist with differentiating between the different drugs ingested.
- In inhalation and/or solvent ingestion consider additional causes of a wheezing such as asthma, viral pneumonitis and foreign body (e.g. peanut inhalation or other).

✚ MANAGEMENT

- Most of the management of ingestions is supportive. It is important to establish what was taken and whether it was a possible toxic dose. General principles of management are outlined below. More specific interventions and development of the management strategy are dependent on the drug(s) ingested and should be discussed with the local Poison Information Centre.

- Initial resuscitation is centred around the ABCs (i.e. airway, breathing and circulation).
  - Ensure patent airway and is ventilating adequately.
  - Intravenous access should be gained.
  - Cardiac monitoring is important if the ingested substance can cause arrhythmias.
  - Obtain a blood glucose urgently. This may be all that is needed in the treatment of an overdose.

- **Additional diagnostics:** in addition to the initial blood glucose, consider blood gas, electrolytes and urine for toxicology screen. Depending upon the likely drugs involved, blood can subsequently be sent for specific assays (e.g. paracetamol, salicylates, iron, theophylline, etc.). Note that only a few drug levels will be of assistance in the treatment of overdoses.

- **Pharmacotherapeutics:**
  - *Prevention of further drug adsorption is important.*
  - Activated charcoal is the method of drug adsorption. It should be administered in a dose of 1 g/kg (max. dose = 50 g). Many children will not tolerate drinking activated charcoal and a nasogastric tube may need to be considered (depending on the seriousness of the ingestion). Potential adverse effects of activated charcoal administration include

emesis and aspiration pneumonia. Consequently, it should be used judiciously and never when the child's airway is unprotected.

- Activated charcoal is most effective within 30 min of ingestion (mean decrease in drug adsorption of 89%), although it can be effective up to 1 hour post-ingestion (mean decrease in drug adsorption of 37%). Drugs that impede gastric emptying (Box 12.2) may require multiple doses of charcoal (they remain in the stomach for longer). In addition, some substances are not readily adsorbed by activated charcoal (Box 12.3). In these cases, other means of gastrointestinal decontamination need to be considered.

- Note that *forced emesis with syrup of ipecacuanha (Ipecac) is no longer part of accepted management*. It has not been shown to decrease morbidity or mortality, and may increase morbidity by causing aspiration and Mallory–Weiss tears (as a result of the forced emesis).

- Drug antidotes can be used in certain circumstances, depending on the drug ingested or inhaled (Table 12.24). Patients requiring an antidote should be admitted to a hospital for observation.

- *Gastric lavage is also largely contraindicated*. It has not been shown to improve the removal of tablets or to improve morbidity or mortality, and in one study was shown to have a complication rate of 3%. *It should only be used within 1 hour of ingestion, and where the airway is already protected*. Its main clinical use is for drugs that are not adsorbed by activated charcoal. It should never be used after the ingestion of corrosive substances, and is considered dangerous after the ingestion of hydrocarbons (such as paraffin) as it could cause a chemical pneumonitis.

- *Whole bowel irrigation is only an option in serious ingestions where activated charcoal is ineffective (e.g. iron, lead or enteric-coated preparations)*. It is potentially dangerous in children, as it can cause large shifts in fluid balance that result in rapid changes in sodium concentrations and/or shock.

- **Behavioural interventions:** Poison centres were set up to give advice to health professionals as well as to monitor poisoning trends. The centres contribute to improved access to specialist expertise, rapid treatment, accurate epidemiological data and the creation of useful prevention strategies. There are numerous poison centres around the country and the nurse practitioner (NP) should be familiar with the number of her local facility. For the UK National Poisons Information Service (which can direct callers to the relevant local centre), tel: 0870-600-6266.

- **Patient education and prevention** (prevention is a key component of drug ingestion management):
  - Children should be taught from a young age about the dangers of medication.

Box 12.2	Indications for multiple doses of activated charcoal

- Slow-release preparations, e.g. theophylline
- Carbamazepine
- Dapsone
- Digoxin
- Paraquat
- Phenobarbital
- Quinine

Box 12.3	Substances not readily adsorbed to charcoal

- Ferrous salts
- Lithium preparations
- Potassium salts
- Ethanol
- Methanol
- Ethylene glycol
- Acids
- Alkalis
- Fluorides
- Organic solvents
- Mercury
- Lead

Table 12.24	Poison Antidotes	
Poison	*Antidote*	*Dose*
Paracetamol	Acetylcysteine	150 mg/kg over 15 min, then 50 mg/kg over 4 h, then 100 mg/kg over 16 h
Organophosphates	Atropine	0.05 mg/kg intravenous (IV) max 2 mg
Dystonic effects of phenothiazines and metoclopramide	Benzatropine (benztropine)	0.02 mg/kg every 15 min
Calcium channel blockers, hyperkalaemia and hypermagnesaemia	Calcium chloride	0.15 mg/kg over 10 min
Lead	Dimercaprol	4 mg/kg/dose 4-hourly for 3–7 days
Iron	Desferrioxamine	Gastric lavage with 2 g in 1 litre of water; then 15 mg/kg/h IV. Note that the *BNF*[a] maximum is 80 mg/kg/24 h
Methanol	Ethanol	0.8 g/kg IV followed by 130 mg/kg hour
Beta-blockers	Glucagon	25 µg/kg IV followed by infusion at 5–20 µg/kg/h
Opiates	Naloxone	0.1 mg/kg IV — shorter half-life than opiates, so will need monitoring
Anticholinergic agents	Neostigmine (IV preparation) Pyridostigmine (oral preparation)	
Arrhythmias due to tricyclics	Sodium bicarbonate	1 mmol/kg IV

[a] *BNF = British National Formulary*, published by British Medical Association and Royal Pharmaceutical Society of Great Britain.

- Parents should be encouraged to keep all drugs in locked cupboards, and to keep all household cleaners out of reach of children.
- Active drug education programmes need to be set up within schools. Teenagers need to be told about the risks of common drugs such as paracetamol, as well as the more serious drugs such as heroin, cocaine and ecstasy. Many adolescents did not intend to kill themselves when taking paracetamol.
- Teenagers need to be encouraged to talk about their problems, and not to resort to overdoses as a cry for help.
- Legislation has already led to bottles having childproof lids, paracetamol being sold in much smaller quantities and manufacturers being forced to put all known side-effects on the drug packets.
- The quest for safer drugs has also decreased fatalities: for example, haloperidol has been replaced with antipsychotics with much fewer side-effects.

➡ FOLLOW-UP

- Most cases of accidental drug ingestion do not need follow-up. However, a single follow-up visit may be useful to reinforce the safety and prevention aspects discussed above.
- Children who have tried to self-harm will need ongoing counselling.

⮁ MEDICAL CONSULT/ SPECIALIST REFERRAL

- If the facilities are available, contact the Poison Information Centre (0870-600-6266) for further information regarding side-effects and treatment. The poison centre will comment on the likelihood of the child requiring ongoing treatment or monitoring.
- Any child with a potentially dangerous ingestion/inhalation.
- Any child requiring cardiac or respiratory monitoring.
- Any child in whom there is a suspicion or admission of self-harm.

⊙ PAEDIATRIC PEARLS

- Always consider drug ingestion in any differential diagnosis. This is especially true when neurological symptoms and signs are present.
- The phone number for the UK National Poisons Information Service (which can direct callers to the relevant local centre) is 0870-600-6266. Local centres include Belfast, Birmingham, Cardiff, Dublin, Edinburgh, London and Newcastle.
- A history of drug ingestion may be related to child protection issues in younger children and/or attempted self-harm (especially in adolescents). Take a careful history so as not to miss these children.
- Always use the highest estimated dose (of the drug ingested) to guide management.
- Forced emesis can have serious consequences, especially if the child has ingested a volatile agent such as paraffin. Therefore, syrup of ipecacuanha (Ipecac) is no longer used.
- Gastric lavage should only be performed on children with protected airways. It is now outmoded and should not be used except in severe/life-threatening poisonings.

- It is important to remember that a good history is always better at detecting drugs than a random drug screen.
- The management of drug ingestions revolves around good, early instigation of the ABCs.

📑 BIBLIOGRAPHY

American Academy of Clinical Toxicology and European Association of Poison Centres. Position statement: ipecac syrup. J Clin Toxicol – Clin Toxicol 1997; 35:699–709.

Anonymous. Canadian hospitals injury reporting and prevention program. CHIRPP News 1995; Issue 5.

Fagan E, Wannan G. Reducing paracetamol overdoses. BMJ 1996; 313:1417–1418.

Jones AL, Volans A. Management of self poisoning. BMJ 1999; 319:1414–1417.

Kilham H, Isaacs D. Acute poisonings and envenomation. In: Kilham H, Isaacs D, eds, The New Children's Hospital Handbook. 1999:302–305.

Morrison A, Stone DH, Doraiswamy N, et al. Injury surveillance in an accident and emergency department: a year in the life of CHIRPP. Arch Dis Child 1999; 80:533–536.

Pond SM, Lewis-Driver DJ, Williams GM, et al. Gastric emptying in acute overdose: a prospective randomised controlled trial. Med J Aust 1995; 163:345–349.

Shannon M. Ingestion of toxic substances by children. New Engl J Med 2000; 342(3):186–191.

Tenenbein M. Recent advancements in pediatric toxicology. Pediatr Clin North Am 1999; 46:1179–1188.

Veltri JC, Schmitz BF. Annual report of the American Association of Poison Control Centers National Data Collection System. Am J Emerg Med 1987; 6:479.

Worthley LIG. Poisoning and drug overdosage. In: Worthley LIG, ed., Synopsis of intensive care medicine. Edinburgh: Churchill Livingstone; 1994:845–870.

CHAPTER 13

Musculoskeletal Problems, Neurological Problems and Trauma

13.1 LIMP AND HIP PAIN
Ruth Johnson

📦 INTRODUCTION

- A limp is an asymmetric deviation from a normal gait pattern resulting from pain, weakness or deformity; it is *not* a normal finding in children. As such, an acute onset of a limp is a cause for concern and requires a systematic approach to the history, musculoskeletal examination and (if appropriate) laboratory or radiological studies.
- Although not an uncommon complaint in paediatric practice, a wide variety of conditions can cause a limp, many of them with a developmental or age-related component (Table 13.1).
- Because a limp, hip pain or refusal to bear weight is not a normal finding in children, the child who presents with any of these symptoms is likely to have an underlying organic cause, including infection, inflammation, trauma, systemic illness or tumours (Table 13.2).

🔬 PATHOPHYSIOLOGY

- Largely aetiology-dependent; however, a basic understanding of the hip structure and vascular supply is important in understanding illness-specific pathological processes.
- The hip bone consists of the ilium, ischium and the pubis, with the three parts meeting at the acetabulum. During puberty, the hip cartilage ossifies and the vascular supply to the hip and head of the femur increases. In prepubertal children, the hip is fused with cartilage (i.e. ossification has not occurred) and the vascular supply is interrupted by the presence of the growth plate, with the resultant implications of diminished vascular supply (i.e. decreased perfusion, decreased penetration of nutrient arterioles compared with an older child).
- Hip disease should always be considered in any child with limp, hip or knee pain, leg length discrepancy, in-toeing or refusal to bear weight or move the leg.

⬅ HISTORY

- Onset, location and duration of pain, limp and/or altered gait (include information on who noticed and where pain presented, etc.).
- Type of pain (painless, acute, mild), relationship to activity and associated limitation of movement.
- Progression (i.e. 'Has it got any worse?').
- Triggers, relievers and home management (include use of medications, complementary therapies, etc.).
- Presence and extent of fever (fever may suggest an infection or inflammatory process; higher temperatures may suggest possible infection, whereas lower fevers can be associated with rheumatological or post-infectious inflammatory disorders).
- Other symptoms (malaise, nausea, swollen joints, pharyngitis) and/or recent history of viral upper respiratory tract infection (URTI) or acute gastroenteritis.
- Recent history of trauma and activity levels/sports participation.
- Brief past medical history (i.e. underlying disease, medication use or developmental delay).
- Family history of hip/joint disease.

Table 13.1	Age-related Cause of Hip Pain and Limp
Age	*Consider*
All ages	Fracture, osteomyelitis (often under 10 years of age), juvenile rheumatoid arthritis (JRA), child abuse/non-accidental injury (NAI), viral illness related arthralgia
0–5 years	Developmental dysplasia of the hip (DDH), sickle cell disease, cerebral palsy, septic arthritis of the hip (generally 3–7 years of age), Perthes' disease, transient synovitis (generally 3–7 years of age), limb length discrepancy, acute lymphocytic leukaemia (ALL)
6–12 years	Septic arthritis of the hip, transient synovitis, Perthes' disease (peaks 6–9 years of age), slipped capital femoral epiphysis (SCFE)
>12 years	SCFE, Osgood–Schlatter disease, osteosarcoma, Ewing's sarcoma, ileac apophysitis

Table 13.2 Differential Diagnosis of Hip Pain/Limp

Condition	Characteristics
Acute lymphocytic leukaemia (ALL)	• Usually presents in children <5 years of age with complaints of bone/joint pain • Physical complaints include lethargy, pallor, bruising, bleeding, purpura, headache, hepatosplenomegaly and infection • Laboratory evidence of impaired haematological functioning (anaemia, neutropenia, thrombocytopenia)
Cerebral palsy	• Should be diagnosed by the time the child is 5 years old • No history of pain but likely history of developmental delay, poor milestone achievement, poor balance, spasticity, prematurity/traumatic birth and hand preference before 18 months of age
Developmental dysplasia of the hip (DDH)	• Usually pain-free and presents birth to 24 months • More common in females, prematurity, breech birth + family history (DDH or foot deformities) • Limited abduction with hip in flexion; shortened leg length on affected side; + Trendelenburg's sign (if ambulatory) or + Ortololani/Barlow manoeuvres (<4 months of age) • Very positive ultrasound findings in infants <3–4 months; dislocation on anteroposterior views in older children
Ewing's sarcoma	• Peak incidence at 12 years of age (range 5–20 years) • Complaints of thigh or knee pain (although can include heel) with increased pain at night or at rest • Radiological examination will disclose bone mass
Fractures	• Moderate-to-severe pain with history of trauma and/or sudden onset • Often signs of inflammation and refusal to bear weight • Positive radiological findings indicative of fracture
Ileac apophysitis	• Overuse syndrome more commonly seen in young distance runners; history usually describes long-distance running • Examination reveals tightened hip musculature and tenderness of iliac crest • Radiological findings normal; laboratory studies not helpful
Juvenile rheumatoid arthritis (JRA)	• Affects adolescents and children <16 years of age; amount of pain is variable • Recurrent pain/inflammation in one or more joints and may be accompanied by malaise, lymphadenopathy and maculopapular rash • Limited range of motion (ROM) with stiffness after inactivity/sleeping • Laboratory evidence of inflammation with history of rash, spiking fevers and hepatosplenomegaly
Limb length discrepancy	• Usually identified by 5 years of age • Unequal measurements from anterior iliac crest to medial malleolus and uneven bony landmarks
Osgood–Schlatter disease	• Primarily affects adolescents; mild-to-moderate pain that is aggravated by activity and is usually activity-related • More common in males and during periods of rapid growth • Painful swelling of anterior aspect of tibial tuberosity that is tender to palpation
Osteomyelitis	• Can affect any age although peak incidence in children <10 years of age • Pain is severe with examination findings of inflammation, +/− fevers; limited ROM; point tenderness and refusal to bear weight/walk
Osteosarcoma	• Presents during adolescence with peak incidence at 14 years of age • Persistent deep pain (most often of distal femur or knee) for a number of weeks that is not activity-related (although worse at night) • Examination may display slight swelling with laboratory evidence of inflammation
Perthes' disease (Legg–Calvé-Perthes, Perthes' disease or idiopathic avascular necrosis of the femoral head)	• Four times more common in Caucasian males and affects children between ages of 2 and 12 (peak incidence between 6 and 9 years of age) • History of persistent hip pain (although limp can be painless) with referred knee pain common; examination with loss of internal rotation, loss of abduction and overall decreased ROM • Laboratory results may be normal; however, anterior posterior hip radiographs reveal widened joint space and flattening of femoral head; lateral hip film with cleft in femoral head. Bone scan shows decrease uptake, whereas magnetic resonance imaging (MRI) will show avascular necrosis (even if radiographs are normal)
Septic arthritis	• Usually affects children <10 years of age • Sudden onset of significant hip pain accompanied by fever and ill/toxic appearance; leg is often held in flexed abduction with decreased ROM (child often refuses to straighten) • Laboratory values with signs of marked inflammation and acute infection; blood cultures considered to isolate organism (positive in 20% of cases) but joint fluid aspiration with better yield (positive in 80% of cases) • Radiological findings reveal increased joint space (secondary to infection) although may be normal in early presentation; bone scan usually positive
Slipped capital femoral epiphysis (SCFE)	• Most common in overweight adolescent males (9–16 years of age) with acute or chronic limp • Pain may vary from mild and persistent 'chronic SCFE' to sudden onset of severe pain (acute SCFE); pain may radiate to hip, groin or thigh • Loss of internal hip rotation (most pronounced with hip in extension); if insidious onset examination may reveal shortening of affected leg and thigh atrophy • Laboratory evidence not helpful • Radiographic studies (anteroposterior and lateral or frog-legged positions) show slipped capital femoral epiphysis over neck of femur
Transient tenosynovitis (irritable hip or toxic synovitis)	• Most common cause of limp and hip pain in children; usually benign and self-limiting (some children go on to develop Perthes' disease); diagnosis of exclusion • Affects children <10 years of age (usually 3–7 years old) and more common in males • Moderate-to-marked pain of sudden onset with history of preceding viral illness; usually unilateral (right hip more commonly affected) but can be bilateral • Child usually appears well but may have low-grade temperature elevation • Decreased ROM (internal rotation and abduction) and child often prefers to hold in flexed, externally rotated position • Laboratory findings provide evidence of mild inflammation • Radiological studies often normal but may show mild joint effusion

- Age-specific history:
  - **Infants:** lack of spontaneous movement (i.e. lying still), rigidity, cry, dislike of handling.
  - **Toddler/Pre-schooler:** increased crying, upset, tantrums and requests to be 'carried'.
  - **School-age/adolescents:** able to articulate much of history (including location of pain).

PHYSICAL EXAMINATION

- **General appearance of the child** (well-appearing, toxic-looking, etc.): height, weight and vital signs.

- **Routine head-to-abdomen assessment:** look for signs of systemic illness (rashes, lymphadenopathy, splenomegaly, etc.).

- **Musculoskeletal:** careful assessment that begins with observation of the child while non-weight bearing (observe the child's gait last if hip is painful). It is important to assess pain and degree of movement of the joint although it is vital that early contacts with the child are not painful. It is often helpful to assess the child's baseline level of pain tolerance by touching a non-painful area and asking the child if that hurts. Palpate all joints for redness, tenderness, swelling, pain and limitation of movement.

- **Spine:** examine carefully for any curvature, tufts or dimples.

- **Hips:** assess the range of motion (ROM) of both hips, including hip flexion, extension, abduction (with hips extended and flexed), adduction (while hips are extended) and internal and external rotation of hips (with hips extended and flexed). Position the infant/child on his back for the examination (see Theophilopoulos & Barrett, 1998 for details). Leg lengths can be determined by measuring from the anterior iliac crest to the medial malleolus (while supine and standing), in addition to comparing bony and surface landmarks. Infants and small children pose a greater assessment challenge and observational skills are even more paramount. Watch for spontaneous movement, response to palpation and passive ROM of

joints/muscles (as above). Assessment of infants <4 months of age should include evaluation for developmental dysplasia of the hip (Ortolani and Barlow manoeuvres), which may reveal limited abduction with flexed hips examination (see Theophilopoulos & Barrett, 1998 for details).

- **Gait:** observe for symmetry, speed, stability of pelvis (including balancing on each leg separately, i.e. Trendelenburg's sign) and balance (while barefoot, undressed and from the front, back and side of the child). There are three types of gait disturbances. (1) *Antalgic gait* is painful gait that increases with stress of walking as the child tries to get weight off the affected side quickly. It is seen not only with painful hips but also with painful knees, toes and ankles. (2) *Trendelenburg gait* is caused by hip problems such as dislocation, dysplasia and inflammation etc. The child tilts over the affected hip with each stride in order to maintain his centre of gravity. (3) *Ataxic gait* is caused by lack of neurological coordination, which creates a wide-based, unsteady gait (i.e. a child with cerebral palsy or neuromuscular disease).

- **Neurological:** examine muscle strength and tone for equality (comparing sides); assess deep tendon reflexes and sensation. Note any suspicion of spasticity.

DIFFERENTIAL DIAGNOSES

- See Table 13.2.

MANAGEMENT

Management of hip pain and limp is aetiology-specific but is likely to include specialist consultation and potential hospital admission (with all but the most self-limiting aetiologies). Consequently, additional diagnostics and pharmaco-therapeutics are largely setting-dependent (i.e. primary or acute care) and may be completed as part of the initial work-up or during hospital admission.

- **Additional diagnostics:** Blood work—full blood count (FBC), erythrocyte sedimentation rate (ESR) and C-reactive protein (CRP)—should

all be considered to separate the infectious from the non-infectious hip. In addition, blood cultures, blood cell morphology and/or rheumatological studies may be helpful in pinpointing the diagnosis. Radiographic studies include anteroposterior (AP) views of the hip and lateral views of the pelvis. The frog-leg position is especially helpful in AP views and in the diagnosis of slipped capital femoral epiphysis (SCFE), Perthes' disease, hip subluxations, dislocations and some fractures. Ultrasound evaluation is especially helpful with infants under 4 months old (as the femur head is not ossified and is poorly seen on radiographs). Ultrasound is also helpful in identification of joint effusions (toxic synovitis or septic hip joint). Consider bone scan to localise an area of infection (osteomyelitis) or areas of poor uptake (Perthes' disease). Computed tomography (CT), magnetic resonance imaging (MRI) and hip joint aspiration are all reserved for specialist intervention.

- **Pharmacotherapeutics:** aetiology-specific and may include non-steroidal anti-inflammatory drugs (NSAIDs) and antibiotics.

- **Behavioural interventions:** aetiology-specific but often include rest and physiotherapy at some point.

- **Patient education:**
  - It is important that parents (and children) understand the cause of the problem and their role in its resolution.
  - Review with the family all diagnostics, medications, behavioural interventions, follow-up care and other professionals likely to be involved in care.
  - After discharge (from general practice or the ward), it is vital that families are advised about the signs and symptoms that necessitate immediate evaluation and are provided with contact information in order to do this (names, phone numbers, etc.).

FOLLOW-UP

- Aetiology-specific: all admissions are likely to be followed up in an orthopaedic clinic 2 weeks after discharge.

MEDICAL CONSULT/ SPECIALIST REFERRAL

- Any child with a painful, swollen joint, refusal to bear weight or complaints of hip pain/limp.
- Any child with a toxic appearance.

PAEDIATRIC PEARLS

- The history and physical examination findings are the basis for consultation and referral; do not postpone consultation in a child with a limp or hip pain while awaiting blood results.
- Carefully inspect *all* joints; repeat of assessments of the child are important to monitor progress (pain, limitation of movement, onset of fever, etc.) and include re-accessing specialist consultation if the situation changes.

- Painful joints can get better with no cause found; however, more serious aetiologies need to be ruled out, especially the possibility of septic arthritis, which can lead to death or permanent disability if the diagnosis is missed.
- A history that is inconsistent with injury, examination and/or diagnostic findings should prompt the suspicion of non-accidental injury (NAI).
- If there is pain in the knee, always look at the hip.
- Complaints of hip pain and limp are *not* expected findings in children; evaluate them carefully.

BIBLIOGRAPHY

Cadou S. Case of a school-aged child with a limp and hip pain. J Pediatr Health Care 2000; 14(5):250, 259–260.

Davids JRD. Paediatric knee: clinical assessment and common disorders. Pediatr Clin North Am 1996; 43(5):1067–1089.

Gunner KB. Practice guidelines: evaluation of a child with a limp. J Pediatr Health Care 2001; 15(1):38–40.

Killam PE. Orthopaedic assessment of young children: developmental variations. Nurse Pract 1989; 14(7):27–36.

Lett AI, Skaggs DL. Evaluation of the acutely limping child. Am Fam Phys 2000; 61(4):1011–1018: www.aafp.org

Milner AD, Hull D. Hospital paediatrics. London: Churchill Livingstone; 1999.

Rudolf MCJ, Levene MI. Paediatrics and child health. Oxford: Blackwell Science; 2000.

Schafer RC. Monograph 8 joint trauma: some perspectives from a chiropractic family physician. Joint trauma 1997: www.chiro.org

Shaw B, Gerardi J, Hennikus W. Avoiding the pitfalls of orthopedic disorders. Contemp Pediatr 1998; 15(6):122–135.

Smart J. Paediatric handbook: the Royal Children's Hospital Melbourne. Australia: Blackwell Science; 2000.

Theophilopoulos EP, Barrett DJ. Get a grip on the pediatric hip. Contemp Pediatr 1998; 15(11):43–65.

13.2 LACERATIONS

Melanie Hutton

INTRODUCTION

- A laceration is a tear in the tissue caused by trauma. It can be classified as a simple laceration (no tissue loss, deeper injury or imbedded debris) or a complicated laceration (rupture of skin caused by blunt force with irregular borders and tearing of tissues). Examples of each include knife/glass cuts (simple) or a laceration after a fall or motor vehicle accident (complicated). *It is useful to consider lacerations with regard to (1) the degree of tissue loss; (2) the extent of contamination; and (3) the depth of the wound.*

- Other types of skin wounds include:
  - abrasion: skin is scraped off due to direct contact with a rough surface
  - contusion: an area of bruising due to blunt force, without a break in the skin
  - penetrating injury: a wound with a fine pathway, caused by a sharp object; it is of variable depth and is often not visible to the naked eye.

PATHOPHYSIOLOGY

- Lacerations are a break in the dermal and epidermal integrity that possibly involve the deeper structures of fascia, muscle, tendons and/or nerves. As such it is important to consider the location of the laceration within the context of its involvement with other structures.
- The location of the laceration and the circumstances that resulted in its occurrence have implications for the likelihood of subsequent bacterial infection. For example, the concentration of normal skin flora in the axilla, perineum, anorectal areas and nail beds are far higher than on the trunk or extremities. Other factors that play a part in the likelihood of wound infection include the vascularity

and anatomy of the area, time elapsed before care is received and the implantation of particulate matter in the wound.
- The goals of wound management are achievement of optimal closure in the area; restoration of function; prevention of infection and adequate cosmetic result.

HISTORY

- Time of injury and time elapsed since injury (important in determining closure and tetanus prophylaxis).
- Witnessed accident.
- Mechanism of injury and what caused the laceration (what happened to cause trauma and what caused the laceration? knife, glass, fall, etc.).
- Likelihood of foreign body in wound.
- Associated injuries: e.g. head, bony involvement.
- Loss of consciousness (see Sec. 13.5).

- Tetanus status (ensure that the child has a full immunisation history and is therefore tetanus immune).
- Allergies to antibiotics and/or anaesthetics.

PHYSICAL EXAMINATION

- Location and size of wound should be accurately documented (type, length and depth of wound); these are best demonstrated by the use of a drawing or diagram.
- Indication of bony injury is important to establish as compound fractures can be overlooked if focus is on the wound alone. If a fracture is suspected, then the limb should be X-rayed.
- Indication of vascular, tendon and/or nerve injury is easily missed. Therefore, it is imperative that *adequate perfusion, along with tendon and nerve and function are tested in the wound area and distal to every limb wound.*
- Determination of foreign body presence/absence is vital. If a foreign body is visible, it should only be removed (in the absence of consultation) if there is no risk of further tissue damage.
- Determination of infection risk and consideration of the need for antibiotics. Assess wound for the likelihood of contamination.

DIFFERENTIAL DIAGNOSES

- Although the child may present with a laceration, it is vital to ensure that there are no other underlying problems. It is therefore essential to rule out bony injury and other structural damage in addition to consideration of child protection issues.

MANAGEMENT

- **Additional diagnostics:** depends on location, size and type of wound. The laceration may require an X-ray if there is bony tenderness and/or to rule out foreign body; note that not all wound debris is radio-opaque. If a foreign

Table 13.3	Wound Closure Options		
Type of closure	*Advantages*		*Disadvantages*
Adhesive strips	• Commonly used for simple, incised wounds • Easy to apply (for the most part) • Less traumatic than other types of closure • Easy for parents to remove at home		• Not suitable over joints • Are difficult to apply to scalp • Require a dry field in order to adhere
Tissue adhesives	• Widely used for closure of minor wounds (often in lieu of sutures) • Reduces trauma associated with sutures • Eliminates need for local anaesthetic • Less time consuming and, if used on scalp wound, no need for hair to be shaved • With skilled application, produces excellent cosmetic results • As glue forms protective seal, no need for dressing • Considered to be ideal medium for closure of cutaneous wounds • Novelty factor is useful: 'You have been glued back together'		• Not useful for wounds where there is risk of foreign body or if wound caused by bite • Debate exists on the use of tissue adhesives for facial wounds. Often they are used only on wounds that are above the eyebrow. However, there are variations in practice
Sutures	• Closure of choice over joints • Wounds with involvement of deeper structures • Deep scalp wounds • Wounds through lip margin • Wounds through eyebrow		• Involves some sort of anaesthesia (local and/or general) possible sedation • Can be traumatic for child • Requires follow-up for suture removal • Likely to involve greater time and expense
Staples	• Not commonly used in paediatrics		• As for sutures

body is suspected in the hand and/or foot, the area may need to be explored (see indications for referral). If antibiotics are to be given, the wound should be swabbed prior to discharge.

- **Pharmacotherapeutics:** Adequate pain relief should be given (see Sec. 13.3). For most types of lacerations, paracetamol is usually adequate for pain relief; however, each individual's level of pain should be measured and analgesia given accordingly. Debridement and/or probing will require local anaesthetic. Consideration should be given regarding the need for antibiotics; however, it should be noted that they are not always necessary. Adequate cleansing and good surgical technique (see Behavioural interventions) are mainstays in preventing wound infection. Wounds that may benefit from prophylactic cover include those associated with fractures, dirty wounds, deep penetrating wounds and those that result from a human or animal bite. If it is determined that an antibiotic is required, choice

of preparation is dictated by the organism most likely to infect the wound.

- **Behavioural interventions:** centre around wound cleansing, debridement and closure.
  - *Cleansing:* normal saline (irrigation or on a swab) is typically used until the wound is clean.
  - *Debridement:* remove dried blood, wound debris and devitalised tissue; trim ragged edges if suturing after local anaesthetic given.
  - *Closure:* depends on the location, size and type of wound. The age of the child should also be taken into consideration. There are many types of wound closure agents available (see Table 13.3).

- **Patient education:** for all children this includes age-appropriate safety counselling. Details of wound care at home, signs and symptoms of wound infection, activity restrictions, bathing and follow-up should be discussed, but these are largely dependent on wound and type of closure used (Table 13.4). Written

Table 13.4 Patient Education

Type of closure	Important information for child and carer
Adhesive strips	• A dry dressing may be applied over the adhesive strips to prevent the child from removing the strips • Both dressing and strips need to stay dry for 3–5 days • If either become wet, they need to be re-applied (send family home with a few extra) • Length of time strips should be in place dependent on location of wound; normally 3–5 days (useful to tell carer to allow strips to fall off on their own after this time) • Follow-up not usually required; however, consider re-attendance for removal/inspection of wound site
Tissue adhesives	• Follow-up not usually required; however, consider re-attendance for inspection of wound site if increased risk of infection • Important to stress with carer and child that wound needs to stay dry for 5 days • Remind child not to 'pick' at wound; scab will fall off on its own (usually in about 10 days)
Sutures	• If dissolvable, then no follow-up necessary • Scalp sutures removed in 5–7 days • Facial sutures removed in 3–5 days • Hand sutures removed in 8–10 days • Arm sutures removed in 7–10 days • Leg sutures removed in 10–14 days • Foot sutures removed in 10–14 days
Staples	• Removal times as for sutures • Removal requires use of dedicated forceps

instructions to accompany discharge should be used and should include a contact phone number for potential questions/concerns.

⇨ FOLLOW-UP

• Dependent on type of wound closure (see Table 13.3).

⇄ MEDICAL CONSULT/ SPECIALIST REFERRAL

• Any child with a wound(s) that is accompanied by a suspicion of a fracture and/or foreign body following X-ray.
• Any child with large, complicated wounds and/or those that would require general anaesthetic/ sedation.
• Any child in whom the circumstances surrounding the injury are suspicious (i.e. child protection issues).

⊘ PAEDIATRIC PEARLS

• Mechanism of injury is vital to establish extent of injury.
• If there is any doubt of foreign body, always X-ray.
• If crushing injury suspected, X-ray to exclude compound fracture.
• Antibiotics are no substitute for meticulous wound cleaning.

▤ BIBLIOGRAPHY

Beattie TF, Hendry GM, Duguid KP. Pediatric emergencies. London: Mosby-Wolfe; 1997.

Ellis DAF, Shikh A. The ideal tissue adhesive in facial plastic and reconstructive surgery. J Otolaryngol 1990; 19(1):68–72.

Guly HR. History taking, examination, and record keeping. In: Guly HR, ed., Emergency medicine. New York: Oxford University Press; 1996.

Quinn JV. A randomised controlled trial comparing a tissue adhesive with suturing in the repair of paediatric facial lacerations. Am Emerg Med 1993; 22:1130–1135.

Simon H. How good are tissue adhesives at repairing lacerations? Contemp Pediatr 1997; 14(11):90–96.

13.3 PAIN ASSESSMENT AND MANAGEMENT

Anita Flynn and Sara Higginson

▭ INTRODUCTION

• Pain is a common complaint in childhood. The most common sources are from everyday incidents that occur during play. Few of these incidents result in significant injury and the pain associated with them is typically of short duration, with the majority of episodes managed successfully at home.
• Some diseases or disorders (e.g. cancer, arthritis, sickle cell disease, etc.) have pain as a predominant symptom of their illness. Similarly, recurrent pain (such as that experienced with migraines and recurrent abdominal pain) is common in children and frequently seen in primary care.
• Acute paediatric trauma (e.g. burns, fractures, etc.) will require analgesic intervention and it is likely that the nurse practitioner (NP) working in the acute setting will likewise encounter these children.
• Therefore, a priority for the NP (in all settings) is to accurately assess and manage pain in children, while also differentiating conditions that are benign and self-limiting from those that represent more significant pathology (and thus require medical consultation and referral). This is especially true for children whose pain is a presenting symptom (e.g. appendicitis, testicular torsion, etc.) and it is the NP that makes the initial assessment.

⊗ PATHOPHYSIOLOGY

• There are many kinds of pain, with each type possessing its own physiology.

Table 13.5	Classification of Pain	
Classification type	Type of pain	Characteristics
Temporal	Acute pain	• Refers to immediate, sudden pain which is caused by actual illness or injury • Resolves when healing has taken place
	Chronic pain (three types)	• Recurrent acute (e.g. migraine) • Chronic acute (e.g. cancer or burn pain) • Chronic non-malignant (e.g. back pain)
Clinical	Mild Moderate Severe	• Minor, slight, subtle pain • Medium, average, modest pain • Intense, great, relentless
Neurophysiologic	Somatic	• Sharp, achy, well-localised and consistent with lesion (e.g. postoperative pain, appendicitis, arthritis)
	Visceral	• Diffuse, dull, deep, poorly localised, crampy often accompanied by nausea and vomiting, diaphoresis and referral to other areas (e.g. intestinal obstruction, perforation)
	Neuropathic	• Burning, radiating or stabbing sensation, abnormal central sensitisation (e.g. nerve injury or irritation, phantom limb pain)
Psychogenic		• May present as any of the above • Important to recognise

- For the most part, however, pain results from the stimulation of pain receptors located throughout the body. These impulses are subsequently conveyed, via the nervous system, to the brain for interpretation.
- Nerves that carry pain impulses can be categorised according to (1) what kind of message they carry; (2) their size; and (3) the conduction rate of the fibres.
- Sharp pain (i.e. somatic pain) is conveyed by thick, myelinated fibres with relatively fast conduction.
- Dull pain (i.e. visceral pain) is conveyed by unmyelinated, slow conduction fibres.
- Other sensations (e.g. warmth, touch, etc.) are conveyed by A beta fibres.
- It is important to classify pain, as it has implications for management (i.e. types of interventions used). Table 13.5 outlines the different ways pain can be classified.

⬅ HISTORY

- The pain history is largely influenced by the child's age and developmental level as well as his capacity to communicate. Involvement of parents/carers is important as they can provide information on their child's usual pain-coping strategies, effective pain relief measures and interpretation of symptoms.

- If pain is not the presenting complaint, it is important to obtain an episodic history (see Ch. 4) in order to place the child's pain within the context of his presenting symptomatology.
- Location of the pain: it is important for the child to identify the painful area (if possible) and this information should be specifically documented: e.g. 'left temporal headache' rather than 'headache'.
- Onset, frequency and duration of pain.
- Intensity and distribution.
- Child and family's perception of the pain's aetiology (e.g. '*Where do you think the pain is coming from?*').
- Does the pain interfere with eating, drinking, sleeping and/or breathing?
- Does the pain hinder the child when walking, sitting, running?
- Does the pain stop the child from going to school, school activities or play?
- Does the child complain of pain on Saturdays and Sundays (i.e. days he does not have to attend school)?
- Does the pain make the child cry and/or awaken from a sound sleep?
- Exacerbating and relieving factors (including pain management strategies tried thus far and the child's response).
- Associated symptoms (nausea, vomiting, rashes, fever, diarrhoea, etc.).
- Previous experiences with pain.

- Family and sociocultural factors, including parental attitudes and sibling experiences with pain.

🩺 PHYSICAL EXAMINATION

- If the aetiology of the pain is not readily apparent (or if the pain is a symptom of the illness) it is important to examine the child from head to toe. This is especially significant when the source of the pain is unknown and the pain is of acute onset.
- Pain assessment is an essential component of the physical examination. It is important that a validated pain tool is used and that the assessment is (1) age and/or developmentally appropriate and (2) the child/family's social circumstances and cultural background are considered. The tool should be used in tandem with the child's self-report of pain, the parent's perspective and the NP's assessment of the pain. Table 13.6 outlines age-appropriate pain assessment.

✚ MANAGEMENT

Successful management of pain depends on identification of the source and aetiology of the pain; aggravating and relieving factors; the severity of the pain (which impacts treatment choice); and the individual needs of the child. Consequently, it is likely that a number of interventions (e.g. pharmacological, psychological, emotional and behavioural) will be utilised (and individualised) in order to provide adequate relief. The sum effect of a combination of interventions is likely to be greater than any one intervention alone.

- **Additional diagnostics:** specific to the aetiology of the pain.
- **Pharmacotherapeutics:** see Tables 13.7 and 13.8 and Fig. 13.1.
- **Behavioural interventions:** see Table 13.9.
- **Patient education:**
  - be sure that the patient understands the pain assessment tool
  - explain to the child that he should not be afraid to tell someone about the pain and that it is very important to do so.

Table 13.6	Age-Appropriate Pain Assessment	
Age	*Rationale*	*Comments and tools*
Neonates and infants	• Behaviour and physiological values are interpreted together	• Observation of facial expression, body position and movement, crying, blood pressure, heart rate, skin colour, oxygen saturation and respiratory rate • Neonates may cry intermittently or continuously and/or be inconsolable when they have pain • CRIES scale (Krechel & Bildner, 1995) • Postoperative Pain Score (Attia, 1987) • Pain Assessment Tool (Hodgkinson, 1995) • Pain Rating Scale (Joyce, 1994)
Pre-verbal children	• A behavioural scale (e.g. one in which pain is identified according to the child's actions) should be used	• Observation of irritability, crying, aggressiveness (biting, kicking, hitting) grimacing and loss of interest in play or eating • Note that the absence of behavioural cues (above) does not exclude pain • Unlike adults who likely decrease their activity when in pain, toddlers typically become restless and overly active (behaviours that may not be recognised as a response to pain) • Memory, physical restraint, parent separation and lack of preparation influence the intensity of the behavioural response • Pain Rating Scale (Joyce, 1994)
Young children (3–7 years of age)	• Behavioural and self-report scales can be used. Specific tool used will depend on child's age and cognitive level	• Child may be restless, fretful, irritable and reluctant to move painful area • Most 3 year olds will be able to differentiate the presence or absence of pain and will point to where their pain is located (roughly) • A 3 year old can usually indicate pain intensity in broad categories ('none, some, a lot') • The FACES scale is widely used. However, younger children may think that they have to choose the 'happy' face rather than the face that relates to their own pain experience. Likewise, children may indicate a particular 'face' as a rating of how they are feeling (e.g. sad, happy, tearful, etc.) rather than their degree of pain • FACES Pain Rating Scale (Wong et al., 1999) • Poker Chip Tool (Hester, 1998)
Older children and adolescents	• Able to use visual and colour analogue scales and self-report measures	• In older children, behaviour may bear no relation to the intensity of pain • Adolescent Pediatric Pain Tool (Savedra, 1993)

Table 13.7	Pharmacotherapeutic Management of Pain	
Class	*Name(s)*	*Use and comments*
Non-opioid analgesic	• Paracetamol	• Effective for relief of mild pain (sore throat, ear ache, sprains, abdominal pain) • Available as an oral suspension or tablets • May be given rectally if nausea or vomiting present, but absorption is less reliable
Non-steroidal anti-inflammatory drugs (NSAIDs)	• Ibuprofen • Diclofenac	• Ibuprofen is available as an oral suspension or tablets • Diclofenac is available as a tablet or suppository • NSAIDs effective for control of pain from inflammation in soft tissues, joints and musculoskeletal trauma. Also useful for postoperative pain • Use NSAIDs with caution in asthmatics • Avoid use in children with history of gastrointestinal bleeding and among children with renal impairment (only with careful monitoring) • May interfere with platelet function and, therefore, may be unsuitable for children with thrombocytopenia and those at risk of haemorrhage from other causes
	• Entonox (nitrous oxide + oxygen mixture)	• Potent analgesic which depends on self-administration and cooperation of child for its successful use • Quick-acting, with an equally rapid offset when administration ceases • Ideal for short-term use and pain of short duration (dressing changes, suturing wounds, applying traction, etc.) • Should not be used with any condition where air is trapped within body and where its expansion might be dangerous (e.g. head injuries with impaired consciousness, air embolism, maxillofacial injuries and gross abdominal distension)
Opioid analgesic	• Codeine • Morphine	• Codeine used to relieve moderate or severe pain (e.g. skeletal trauma, burns, postoperative pain). Available in tablet, liquid and rectal forms • Morphine is the standard opioid for the relief of severe pain in children. Available for oral, rectal and parenteral administration
Topical anaesthetic	• Lidocaine (Emla cream) • Ametop (tetracaine gel)	• Useful in alleviating pain and distress associated with needle insertion and other minor procedures • Emla must be applied under an occlusive dressing for a minimum of 50 min before the procedure

Table 13.8 Analgesic Guidelines in Infants and Children

Analgesic	Dose	Preparations	Comments
PARACETAMOL	**>3 months:** Oral: Loading dose of 20 mg/kg then: Day 1: 15 mg/kg, 4 hourly Day 2: 15 mg/kg, 6 hourly, then 15 mg/kg, 4–6 hourly p.m. Rectal: 3–12 months 60–125 mg, 6 hourly 1–5 years 125–250 mg, 6 hourly 6–12 years 250–500 mg, 6 hourly Over 12 years 500 mg to 1 g, 6 hourly **Maximum dose (oral or rectal) is 90 mg/kg/24 hours or 1 g QDS. Maximum 4 doses in 24 hours** **For Home management:** (oral) 3–12 months, 60–120 mg, 4–6 hourly 1–5 years, 120–240 mg, 4–6 hourly 6–12 years, 250–500 mg, 4–6 hourly Over 12 years, 500 mg to 1 g, 4–6 hourly **<3 months:** Oral: 15 mg/kg, 6 hourly Rectal: 30–60 mg, 6 hourly **Maximum dose (oral or rectal) is 60 mg/kg/24 hours**	Suspension: 120 mg/5 ml (age 5 and under) 250 mg/5 ml (age 6 and older) Tablets: 500 mg and 500 mg soluble tablets Suppositories: 60 mg, 125 mg, 250 mg and 500 mg	Antipyretic and analgesic effect (no anti-inflammatory effect) Avoid in liver impairment Can combine with NSAIDs and opioids
IBUPROFEN	Oral: 4–10 mg/kg/dose, 6–8 hourly. **Maximum 30 mg/kg/day** 6–12 months 50 mg, 6–8 hourly 1–3 years 100 mg, 8 hourly 4–6 years 150 mg, 8 hourly 7–9 years 200 mg, 8 hourly 10–12 years 300 mg, 8 hourly Over 12 years 400 mg, 8 hourly **For Home management:** **Maximum 30 mg/kg/day**	Suspension: 100 mg/5 ml Tablets: 200 mg and 400 mg	Antipyretic, analgesic and anti-inflammatory Give with or after food if possible Do not use if patient has a bleeding disorder or active peptic ulceration. Caution in asthma or renal impairment. Can cause gastrointestinal irritation. Unlicensed in children less than 6 months or less than 7 kg
DICLOFENAC	Oral: 1 mg/kg, 8 hourly Over 12 years, 25–50 mg, 8 hourly or 75 mg SR 75 mg, 12 hourly Rectal: 1 mg/kg, 8 hourly (round down to nearest suppository) Over 12 years, 25–50 mg, 8 hourly **Maximum (po/pr) 3 mg/kg/24 hours or 150 mg/24 hours**	Tablets: 25 mg and 50 mg enteric coated, 75 mg SR (12 hourly dose), 50 mg dispersible (useful for small doses – dissolve in known quantity of water and take appropriate portion) Suppositories: 12.5, 25 and 50 mg	As Ibuprofen Can be used in children aged 6 months or more (6 kg or more) Enteric-coated tablets take 1 hour to work – unsuitable for acute pain
CODEINE	Oral or rectal: 6 months to 1 year, 0.5 mg/kg, 6–8 hourly Over 1 year, 0.5–1 mg/kg/dose **(max. 30 mg)**, 4–6 hourly **Maximum 6 mg/kg/day or 180 mg/day** Over 12 years; 30–60 mg, 4 hourly. **Max. 240 mg/day** (For rectal administration, round down to nearest suppository)	Linctus: 15 mg/5 ml Tablets: 15 mg and 30 mg Suppositories: 2 mg, 3 mg and 15 mg	Opioid analgesic. Do not give with morphine Can cause constipation, sedation, nausea and vomiting **Monitor respiration** Give prophylactic lactulose 0.5 ml/kg twice a day if treatment is longer than 2–3 days
MORPHINE *Note:* The following patients may be more sensitive to morphine: • Infants less than 6 months old • Children recovering from anaesthesia or other depressant drugs • Children with syndromes	IM/SC: (cannulae) 6–12 months, 0.1 mg/kg 3 hourly 12 months to 12 years, 0.1–0.2 mg/kg 3 hourly >12 years, 0.2 mg/kg 3 hourly **Max. 10 mg dose** (Can use IM algorithm for >12 years if >40 kg) Oral or rectal: <1 year, 80 µg/kg >1 year, 0.2–0.4 mg/kg 4 hourly or, 1–5 years, 2.5–5 mg 6–12 years, 5–10 mg Over 12 years, 10–15 mg per dose PCA/ epidural Slow IV (over 5–10 min) 0–3 months, 25 µg/kg 6 hourly 3–6 months, 50 µg/kg 6 hourly 6–12 months, 0.1 mg/kg 4 hourly >12 months, 0.1–0.2 mg/kg 4 hourly **Max. 6 mg dose**	Oral solution: 10 mg/5 ml unit dose vials Tablets: 10 mg, 20 mg and 50 mg Suppositories: 15 mg and 30 mg Injection: 10 mg/1 ml (10,000 µg/1 ml) CONTROLLED DRUG Caution with small doses Can dilute 1 ml (10 mg) to 10 ml with sodium chloride 0.9% to give 1 mg/ml solution for accurate administration 1 mg = 1000 µg	Opioid analgesic. Side-effects and prophylactic lactulose as for codeine, plus antiemetic **Monitor respiration and conscious level** Naloxone is used to reverse opioid-induced respiratory depression if respiratory rate <20/min in patients less than 5 years, or <10/min in patients 5–15 years Dilute 1 ml (400 µg) of naloxone to 10 ml with sodium chloride 0.9% and give 4 µg/kg (0.1 ml/kg) every 1–2 min until respiration recovers. Maximum total dose 2 mg. Analgesic effect will also be reversed

IM = intramuscular; IV = intravenous; NSAIDs = non-steroidal anti-inflammatory drugs; PCA = patient-controlled analgesia. QDS = four times a day; SC = subcutaneous; SR = sustained release.

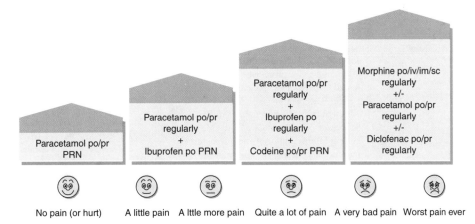

No pain (or hurt)   A little pain   A lttle more pain   Quite a lot of pain   A very bad pain   Worst pain ever

The cause of pain must be considered when analgesics are prescribed

Do not use more than one NSAID at a time (i.e. diclofenac or ibuprofen).
Do not use more than one opioid at a time (i.e. codeine or morphine).
Do not use NSAIDs in:

• Patients with poor renal function or renal failure.
• Patients with gastric duodenal ulceration.
• Patients with coagulation disorders or who are actively bleeding during or after surgery.
• Patients on anticoagulants.
• Moderate or severe asthmatics who require regular prophylactic bronchodilator therapy.
 They may be given with caution to mild asthmatics.
• Patients on methotrexate.

Regular codeine is an alternative analgesic where NSAIDs are contra-indicated.
When morphine is started, continued use of regular paracetamol and a NSAID can have
an 'opioid-sparing' effect.

Please see analgesic pain guidelines for dosage information.
To be used in conjunction with the Clinical Pracice Guidelines "The Recognition & Assessment of Acute Pain in Children"
recommendations (RCN) 1999.

Figure 13.1 Acute Pain Ladder: infants and children. NSAID = non-steroidal anti-inflammatory drug; im = intramuscularly; iv = intravenously; po = orally; pr = rectally; PRN = when required; sc = subcutaneously.

Table 13.9	Behavioural Interventions for Pain Management
Intervention	*Rationale and comments*
Information and preparation	• The experience of pain can be made worse by fear of what the pain will be like • Information giving and preparation are very effective ways to help children cope with painful procedures • The type and amount of information will depend on the child's developmental level • The procedure should be discussed with the parent in order to determine what information has been given to the child • The length of the procedure and the sensation that will be felt should be explained truthfully to the child • Suggestions on how the child can help during the procedure should also be included
Relaxation	• A variety of techniques can be taught to both the parent and the child (e.g. distraction, imagery, play, deep breathing, and positive self-talk) • Play therapy is used to reduce a child's anxiety and help prepare them for threatening events. Note, however, that some children may not be able to play with needles or other equipment before a procedure or examination • The actual type of play should be considered carefully and based on an assessment of the child's developmental and stress levels
Distraction	• Distraction is useful during times of acute distress. However, it needs to be tailored to the child's developmental level. The more interactive the activity, the more it will hold the child's interest and enthusiasm • Infants can be distracted with stroking, nursery rhymes or use of a dummy • Toddlers can blow bubbles while the adult encourages them to blow away painful feelings (with the bubbles) • Children who are able to count can look through a book to count the number of times a certain object appears • Older children can be distracted using games, puzzles or computer games. They can also be taught imagery techniques
Positive self-talk	• Involves the use of statements such as 'I can do this' throughout the procedure
Use of choice and/or control	• Effective coping strategy for pain

⇨ FOLLOW-UP

- Not usually required if pain resolves with supportive care.
- Return visit or phone call if parental anxiety high or pain has not settled.

⇄ MEDICAL CONSULT/ SPECIALIST REFERRAL

- Any child with prolonged crying and/or inadequate control of pain.
- Any child in whom the pain history is inappropriate.
- Any child whose pain becomes worse despite appropriate initial management.
- Any child in whom the cause of the pain is beyond the NP's scope of practice.
- Any child who experiences intense pain, particularly if it is of sudden onset, and/or accompanied with altered vital signs (e.g. hypotension, tachycardia, tachypnoea or fever).

🔍 PAEDIATRIC PEARLS

- Always take note of a mother who reports that 'her baby's cry has changed or is different'.
- Just because a child is not crying does not mean he is pain-free.
- Some children may deny they have pain in order to avoid having treatment or being admitted to the hospital.
- Tell children the truth about pain.
- Focusing on the child's pain without accounting for his cultural background and environment may lead to incorrect conclusion and management.
- Marked pain that awakens a child from a sound sleep is worrying and will likely require some sort of evaluation.
- Principles of pain management are summarised in the acronym *QUESTT*: *Q*uestion the child; *U*se pain rating scales; *E*valuate behaviour and physiological changes; *S*ecure parental involvement; *T*ake cause of pain into account; *T*ake action and evaluate results.

📖 BIBLIOGRAPHY

Attia J. Measurement of postoperative pain and narcotic administration in infants using a new clinical scoring system. Anesthesiology 1987; 67(3A): AS32.

Bernstein BA, Pachter LM. Cultural considerations in children's pain. In: Schechter NL, Berde CB, Yester M, eds, Pain in infants, children and adolescents. Baltimore: Williams & Wilkins; 1993: 122–133.

British National Formulary 43. London: British Medical Association and Royal Pharmaceutical Society of Great Britain; 2002.

Broome ME, Lillis PP, McGahee T, et al. The use of distraction and imagery with children during painful procedures. Eur J Cancer Care 1994; 3: 26–30.

Bruce E, Frank L. Self-administered nitrous oxide (Entonox) for the management of procedural pain. Paediatr Nurs 2000; 12(7): 15–19.

Buchholz M, Karl HW, Pomietto M, et al. Pain scores in infants: a modified infant pain scale versus visual analogue. J Pain Sympt Manag 1998; 15(2):117–124.

Choonara I, Nunn AJ. Paediatric and perinatal drug therapy. Edinburgh: Churchill Livingstone; 1997.

Colwell C, Clark L, Perkins R. Post operative use of pain scales: children's self-report versus nurse assessment of pain intensity and effect. J Paediatr Nurs 1996; 11(6): 375–382.

Cunliffe M. Guidelines on the management of pain in children. Liverpool: Alder Hay Royal Liverpool Children's NHS Trust; 1998.

Duff L, Louw L, McClarey M. Clinical guideline for the recognition and assessment of acute pain in children. Paediatr Nurs 1999; 11(6):18–21.

Fanurik D, Koh J, Schmitz M, et al. Pharmacological and behavioural techniques for paediatric medical procedures. Child Health Care 1997; 26(1): 31–46.

Hester NO. Putting pain measurement into clinical practice. In: Finlay GA, McGrath PJ, eds, Measurement of pain in infants and children, Vol. 10. Seattle: International Association for the Study of Pain Press; 1998.

Hodgkinson K. Measuring pain in neonates: evaluating an instrument and developing a common language. Austr J Adv Nurs 1994; 12(1):17–22.

Joyce BA. Reliability and validity of preverbal pain assessment tools. Iss Comp Pediatr Nurs 1994; 17:121–135.

Krechel SW, Bildner J. CRIES: a new neonatal post-operative pain measurement score: initial testing of reliability and validity. Pediatr Anesth 1995; 5: 53–61.

Lynn AM, Ulma GA, Spieker M. Pain control for very young infants: an update. Contemp Pediatr 1999; 16(11):39–65.

McArthur E, Cunliffe M. Pain assessment and documentation: making a difference. J Child Health Care 1998; 2(4): 164–169.

McClarey M, Duff L, Louw L. Philosophy of care: recognition and assessment of pain in children. Paediatr Nurs 1999; 11(6):15–17.

Morton NS. Acute paediatric pain management: a practical guide. London: Harcourt Brace; 1998.

Royal College of Anaesthetists. Guidelines for the use of non-steroidal anti-inflammatory drugs in the perioperative period. London: Royal College of Anaesthetists; 1998.

Royal College of Nursing. Clinical practice guidelines: the recognition and assessment of acute pain in children. London: Royal College of Nursing; 1999.

Royal College of Paediatrics and Child Health. Medicines for children. London: Royal College of Paediatrics and Child Health; 1999.

Savedra MC. Assessment of postoperative pain in children and adolescents using the Adolescent Pediatric Pain Tool. Nurs Res 1993; 42(1): 5–9.

Southall D. Prevention and control of pain in children. A manual for health care professionals. London: Royal College of Paediatrics and Child Health; 1997.

Tywcross A. Children's cognitive level and perception of pain. Prof Nurse 1998; 14(1): 35–37.

Tywcross A. The management of acute pain in children. Prof Nurse 1998; 14(2): 95–98.

Wong D, Hockenberry-Eaton M, Wilson D, Winkelstein ML, Ahmann E, DiVito-Thomas PA. Family-centered care of the child during illness and hospitalization. In: Wong D, ed., Whaley and Wong's nursing care of infants and children, 6th edn. New York: Mosby; 1999: 1131–1282.

13.4 FEBRILE SEIZURES

Elinor White

📖 INTRODUCTION

- A simple febrile seizure is defined as a brief, generalised, clonic or tonic–clonic seizure that occurs within the context of a febrile illness and lasts less than 15 min, in an otherwise healthy, developmentally normal and neurologically intact child between the ages of 6 months and 6 years. The peak incidence is 23 months of age, and boys and girls are equally affected.
- The two goals of clinical assessment and management are to exclude the possibility of central nervous system (CNS) disease and to identify the source of the fever. Consequently, a careful history, physical examination and thoughtful diagnostics are required.
- Febrile seizures are commonly familial; simple autosomal dominant inheritance with incomplete penetration is postulated as the form of transmission.
- A febrile convulsion is experienced by 3–4% of children. The prognosis for the vast majority of these children is benign. However, approximately 30% of those who experience a simple, first febrile seizure will have a second, with a subsequent febrile illness; one-half of these children will experience a third seizure and less than 9% of children with febrile seizures will have more than three seizures. The majority of recurrences (90%) occur within 2 years, with 50% of recurrences within 6 months of the initial seizure and 75% occurring within 1 year. The risk of recurrence is greater if there is a positive family history of febrile seizures; if the first episode occurred before 1 year of age; and/or the child's body temperature was less than 40°C when the seizure occurred.
- Very few children (2%) whose first seizure was associated with fever are diagnosed with non-febrile seizures by age 7. Children with prolonged or focal seizures and those with a prior neurological deficit and family history

of epilepsy have an increased risk of subsequent epilepsy.
- *There is no evidence that occasional febrile seizure(s) result in neurological damage.*

🧠 PATHOPHYSIOLOGY

- The aetiology of febrile seizures is not well understood. In most children it appears to be the height rather than the rapidity of the temperature elevation that is problematic. The seizure usually occurs during the temperature rise rather than after a prolonged elevation.
- It has been postulated that children who experience febrile seizures have a lower seizure threshold (that is a function of their neurological immaturity) as febrile seizures do not occur after 6 years of age.
- Alternatively, there is support for the theory that the seizures are related to the effects of neurochemicals (usually involved in the production of fever) acting on other parts of the brain (see Sec. 15.4).

← HISTORY

- Establish the presence/absence of precipitating factors and what the child was doing immediately prior to seizure. More specifically, determine whether the child had a fever (including height of the temperature elevation), duration and symptoms of any preceding illness, possibility of a recent head injury and/or the possibility of an ingestion/ intoxication.
- Detailed description of the seizure is required, including eye movement, limb movement, pallor, level of consciousness, excessive salivation, incontinence and duration.
- Presence or absence of postictal sleep.
- Recent onset of other symptomatology (to rule out coexisting neurological problem). This includes headaches, neck stiffness, vomiting, lethargy,

weakness, sensory deficits or changes in vision, behaviour, balance or gait.
- Current medications.
- Past medical history, including previous history of seizures (febrile or afebrile), birth and developmental history.
- Immunisation history, including history of adverse reactions, especially to DTP (diphtheria and tetanus toxoids and pertussis) vaccine.
- Family history of seizures (febrile and afebrile) and/or neurological abnormality.

👀 PHYSICAL EXAMINATION

- Observation of child and assessment of vital signs (including evaluation for temperature elevation, tachycardia, hypotension, tachypnoea and head circumference to rule out signs of sepsis, CNS disease or respiratory infection).
- Careful physical examination to identify focus for infection (see also Sec. 15.1).
- Thorough neurological assessment to rule out meningeal signs (see Sec. 15.8), signs of increased intracranial pressure and focal neurological abnormalities. It is important to include evaluation of mental status, strength, tone, balance and sensation.

❓ DIFFERENTIAL DIAGNOSES

- Consider other causes of seizures (or seizure-like activity), including CNS infection (meningitis, encephalitis), anoxia, hypoglycaemia, breath-holding spells, trauma, stroke/haemorrhage, intoxication/ingestion, metabolic encephalopathy, neurodegenerative disorder, brain tumour, previous brain injury and potential child protection issues.

✚ MANAGEMENT

Emergency management of the seizure focuses on the ABCs (i.e. airway, breathing, circulation). This includes recovery positioning, maintenance of the airway (positioning) and, if seizure is prolonged, activation of the emergency system and/or rectal diazepam (uncommon).

- **Additional diagnostics:** laboratory testing is used to help identify a focus of infection and therefore, a full septic screen may be required to rule out serious infection and/or meningitis (see Secs 15.1 and 15.8). Among children under 18 months of age (in whom signs of serious bacterial infection are often very non-specific) there may be a lower threshold for diagnostics testing. Older children would require lumbar puncture and sepsis screen if they presented with a toxic appearance or signs of CNS infection. Neuroimaging or other more complicated diagnostics are reserved for children that are neurologically abnormal (e.g. focal or complex seizures and/or neurological deficits post-seizure).

- **Pharmacotherapeutics:** No anticonvulsant therapy is required unless there are numerous episodes of seizures and/or the seizure is of prolonged duration (>20 min). For subsequent episodes, rectal diazepam is given and parents instructed in its use at home if subsequent convulsions last longer than 5 min. Management of pyrexia includes antipyretics such as paracetamol and/or ibuprofen. If a focus for infection is discovered, antibiotics should be administered as necessary.

- **Behavioural interventions:**
  - Minimal cotton clothing while febrile. Tepid sponging and a fan to cool the environment are also helpful in decreasing fever.
  - Encourage fluids while febrile.

- **Patient education:**
  - Review with parents the relationship between the fever and the seizure.
  - Discuss with them the likelihood of recurrence (see Introduction) and the lack of evidence linking occasional febrile seizures to long-term neurological sequelae. Stress with parents the strong evidence

that isolated febrile seizures do not result in later problems.
  - Reassure parents (if appropriate) that the risk of non-febrile seizures in the future is minimal.
  - Instruct parents on the first-aid management of febrile seizures in case of recurrence (one-third of children).
  - Review temperature control interventions (both pharmacological and non-pharmacological).
  - Provide written information to supplement all instructions/teaching.

⇨ FOLLOW-UP

- Consider health visitor follow-up to reinforce febrile seizure instructions and provide reassurance and support for the family.
- No further follow-up is required for an isolated, simple febrile seizure.

⇄ MEDICAL CONSULT/ SPECIALIST REFERRAL

- Any child with a first febrile seizure (often admitted to hospital to confirm diagnosis, verify focus of infection and support/reassure parents).
- Any child in whom there is suspicion as to the aetiology of the seizure (i.e. there is doubt as to whether the incident was a simple febrile seizure).
- Any child with a gravely ill or toxic appearance or those in whom an infectious aetiology is suspected.

⊘ PAEDIATRIC PEARLS

- Parental anxiety following the first febrile seizure is understandably very high; reassurance and adequate explanation are very important to allay their fears and gain their cooperation. Review carefully (and clearly) the prognosis and risk of future seizures with families.
- Infants with febrile seizures may have a serious bacterial infection (e.g. meningitis, septicaemia, bacteraemia, etc.) triggering their fever. Consequently, examination of the cerebrospinal fluid and

appropriate cultures should be considered among children <18–24 months of age.

- There is no evidence of permanent neurological damage as a result of a simple febrile seizure.
- A febrile convulsion is considered complex if it is longer than 20 min in duration, recurs within 24 hours and is focal in its presentation (a simple febrile convulsion is usually tonic or tonic–clonic in nature).
- Seizures that continue beyond 6 years of age are no longer compatible with a diagnosis of simple febrile seizures; additional aetiologies need to be considered and explored.
- Children who have experienced a febrile seizure should not be restricted from full participation in activities.
- The child who appears clinically well after a simple febrile seizure does not routinely require any additional diagnostic testing.
- As only one-third of children with an initial febrile seizure have a second seizure, empirical treatment of an isolated episode (in a clinically well child) is not indicated.

▤ BIBLIOGRAPHY

Berg AT, Shinner S, Darefsky AS, et al. Predictors of recurrent febrile seizures: a prospective cohort study. Arch Pediatr Adolesc Med 1997; 151(4):371–378.

Daley HM, Appleton RT. Fits, faints and funny turns. Curr Paediatr 9. London: Harcourt; 2000.

Hirtz DG. Febrile seizures. Pediatr Rev 1997; 18(1):508.

Milner AD, Hull D. Hospital paediatrics. Edinburgh: Churchill Livingstone; 1992: 102–105.

Offringa M, Moyer VA. Evidence based paediatrics: evidence based management of seizures associated with fever. BMJ 2001; 323(7321):1111–1114.

Schmitt BD. Pediatric telephone advice, 2nd edn. Philadelphia: Lippincott Raven; 1999.

Schwatz MW. The 5 minute consult, 2nd edn. Philadelphia: Lippincott, Williams & Wilkins; 1999.

Verity CM. Do seizures damage the brain: the epidemiological evidence. Arch Dis Child 1998; 78(1):78–84.

Vining EP. Gaining a perspective on childhood seizures. New Engl J Med 1996; 338(26):1916–1918.

13.5 HEAD INJURY

Lee M. Ranstrom and Deborah Chadwick

📖 INTRODUCTION

- Trauma is the greatest threat to life in the paediatric population aged 1–14 years. Male children are at twice the risk of female children for sustaining a significant head injury.
- The majority of accidents occur between the hours of noon and midnight as children are often out of their structured environment and these are the hours in which there is likely to be more playtime and less supervision. In addition, children (and carers) may be more tired and less watchful as the day wears on and, therefore, there is an increased risk of injury or accident.
- Roads are the most common location of trauma (43%), whereas trauma in the home accounts for 34% of injuries. Falls are a leading cause of injury (26%), with road traffic accidents (both collisions with other vehicles and pedestrian injuries) accounting for another 35% of injuries.
- The use of bicycle helmets can significantly reduce the risk of a head injury should an accident occur.
- Approximately 25% of fatal head injuries occur without a skull fracture. Intracranial bleeding can occur with or without a skull fracture and is an important risk factor for morbidity and mortality.

🗺 PATHOPHYSIOLOGY

- Infants and children are at greater risk of head injury as a function of their development.
- A child's head is more susceptible to injury due to the proportion of head-to-body size (the head accounts for 15% of total body mass in the neonate vs 3% in the adult).
- The neck musculature in infants and children is not fully developed and, therefore, infants and young children have less head control. In addition, the paediatric scalp is thinner and more elastic and therefore at greater risk for subgaleal haematomas and scalp avulsion injuries. Children also experience increased scalp bleeding post-injury, resulting from the large number of blood vessels in the cutaneous layer of the paediatric scalp.
- The meninges have three layers: the dura mater, the arachnoid and the pia. In children, the dura mater is not adhered tightly to the skull except at the suture lines. Therefore, if bleeding occurs as a result of a head injury, there is increased bleeding into the subdural space (which may result in greater swelling). The subarachnoid space in children is smaller and, therefore, there is less space to act as a buffer for the brain and its bath of cerebrospinal fluid (CSF).
- The paediatric brain has a greater water content than an adult brain (88% vs 77%, respectively). As a result, a child's brain is at greater risk for acceleration/deceleration injuries.
- Head trauma causes damage to the brain and its surrounding structures. Closed head injuries often result in more diffuse or multifocal damage, whereas open head injuries have a greater likelihood of focal injury.
- Primary brain damage is related to mechanical forces that contuse the brain (when it hits the bony skull surfaces during the injury) or tear connections within the brain (both of which can result in bleeding, swelling and obstruction of CSF).
- Secondary brain injury is damage that occurs through the associated hypoxia, bleeding, swelling, ischaemia and/or hypotension of the original injury.

🔁 HISTORY

- A major objective of the history is to determine the possible extent/severity of the head injury, as there are important implications for management and referral. Note that the history should sound plausible and match the clinical examination findings. It is important to always bear in mind the possibility of child protection issues when the presenting complaint is a head injury. This is particularly relevant for children under 2 years of age.
- Full description of the incident, including the mechanism of injury (e.g. moving, stationary, fast, slow, site, walking, road traffic accident, etc.); time and place of injury; and whether the injury was witnessed or not. If a fall occurred, obtain information related to the height of the fall, the surface upon which the child landed and on what part of the head (or other body part) did the child land. It is important to obtain information from the person present at the scene when the child was injured. If the cause of the injury is a road traffic accident, ejection from the car is a very poor prognostic indicator.
- The child's behaviour immediately before the injury (in order to rule out pre-existing seizure activity as a catalyst to the accident).
- The child's recollection of what happened (the child may be unaware of losing consciousness at the time of the injury but is later amnesic with regard to the event).
- Loss of consciousness, presence of seizures and/or any changes in consciousness/alertness since the injury.
- Length of crying after the incident (lack of crying or crying for >10 min are concerning).
- Activity since the accident (including presence of confusion, vomiting, lethargy, sleepiness and slurred speech) and whether the child knows name, mother's name, where he is.
- Weakness, numbness, visual changes, difficulty walking or using arms and/or a headache that seems to be increasing.
- Complaints of neck pain or other pain.
- Use of protective equipment (seat belts, car seat, helmet).
- Body parts other than the head that potentially were injured in the accident.

- Past medical history, including any history of neurological disorders.
- Medication use.
- Immunisation history (i.e. tetanus, especially if scalp or open head injury).

🧠 PHYSICAL EXAMINATION

- **Initial assessment:** the physical examination of the head-injured child begins with an initial assessment of the ABCs (airway, breathing and circulation); if there is compromise, appropriate treatment follows. Note that the cervical spine must be protected (until involvement is ruled out) in all cases of head injury. However, once satisfied the ABCs are acceptable, an overall assessment of the child's level of consciousness (LOC) and body systems should occur. The extent of systemic involvement and/or compromise of the child's LOC have important implications for his long-term outcome and prognosis.

- **Check all vital signs, the child's mental status and level of consciousness:** note that the assessment must be developmentally appropriate. Level of consciousness can be assessed with the Paediatric Advanced Life Support (PALS) standard *AVPU* (*A*lert, *V*ocalising, responds to *P*ain, *U*nresponsive); the *Glasgow Coma Scale* (for use with older children); or the *Modified Glasgow Coma Scale* (for children under 5 and those with special needs). Figure 13.2 includes an example of the modified paediatric coma scale and a format for charting neurological assessment in the acute care setting. Note that a 'grimace score' has been incorporated to improve the assessment of intubated or non-vocalising patients; this provides an invaluable alternative to verbal scoring in neonates, infants and pre-verbal children. Mental status checks in an older child include the ability to answer questions correctly and respond to instructions appropriately. In infants and younger children, check for alertness, activity, social interaction, consistency of response and cry. Signs and symptoms of increased intracranial pressure should be systematically evaluated.

- **Head and ear, nose and throat (ENT):** check pupillary response, ocular movements, red reflex and presence/absence of papilloedema (which may or may not be at an early stage). Assess for periorbital ecchymosis and Battle's sign (mastoid ecchymosis). Any fluid from the middle ear should be checked for glucose to rule out the possibility of CSF leakage. Likewise, the middle ear and nares should be checked for blood.

- **Cardiopulmonary:** assess for signs of injury that may be associated with the original injury.

- **Abdomen:** as above.

- **Neurological:** careful and complete assessment of the neurological system that is developmentally appropriate. Note that it is important to log roll the patient in order to perform a spinal survey.

❓ DIFFERENTIAL DIAGNOSES

- The child with a head injury does not usually present a diagnostic dilemma as there is often a history of trauma/injury and the event is often witnessed. However, the following must be considered: skull fracture, scalp laceration, concussion, contusion or intracranial bleed. If a child is found unconscious and comatose, then in addition to head injury the following should be considered: poisoning/ingestion, metabolic disorders, CNS infection, postictal state and rupture of a vascular malformation.
- *The issue of child protection needs to be ruled out in all cases of head injury.*

✚ MANAGEMENT

The head-injured child with a normal examination, no loss of consciousness and no subsequent vomiting can be safely managed at home, following appropriate advice given to parents/carers. It is important that included in the management of benign head injury is attention to the issue of prevention (car seats, use of safety equipment, cycle helmets, prevention of falls).

- **Additional diagnostics:** none usually required; however, consider a full blood count (FBC) with haematocrit if marked bleeding present. A CT scan of the head should be considered if there is a history of significant head trauma or marked examination findings, including significant scalp swelling, localised neurological signs, significant loss of consciousness and/or the possibility of skull or cervical spinal fracture.

- **Pharmacotherapeutics:** none usually required for benign head injury with the exception of paracetamol. If pain is severe enough for stronger analgesics, then the child should probably receive referral for further evaluation.

- **Behavioural interventions:**
  - Application of ice (or bag of frozen peas) to the site for 20 min to reduce swelling.
  - Observation post-injury for the development of complications includes night-time awakening twice per night for 48 hours (i.e. at parent's bedtime and once 4 hours later). Parents should arouse child sufficiently for him to walk or talk normally. In addition, it is important that parents are alert for any changes in behaviour, activity, appetite, gait, balance, alertness and/or speech. The development of severe headache and/or vomiting should likewise trigger concern.
  - Scalp lacerations, if present, will require irrigation, debridement and closure.
  - All children with the possibility of a spinal injury and/or significant head injury should be treated as though they have a spinal injury (i.e. use of a cervical collar to immobilise the neck until the results of spinal radiographs are known).

- **Patient education:**
  - Discuss with parents the behavioural interventions (above). Stress the importance of their observation of the child over the following 48 hours.
  - Remind parents that they know their child best and it is their opinion that is important with

COMMON PAEDIATRIC PROBLEMS

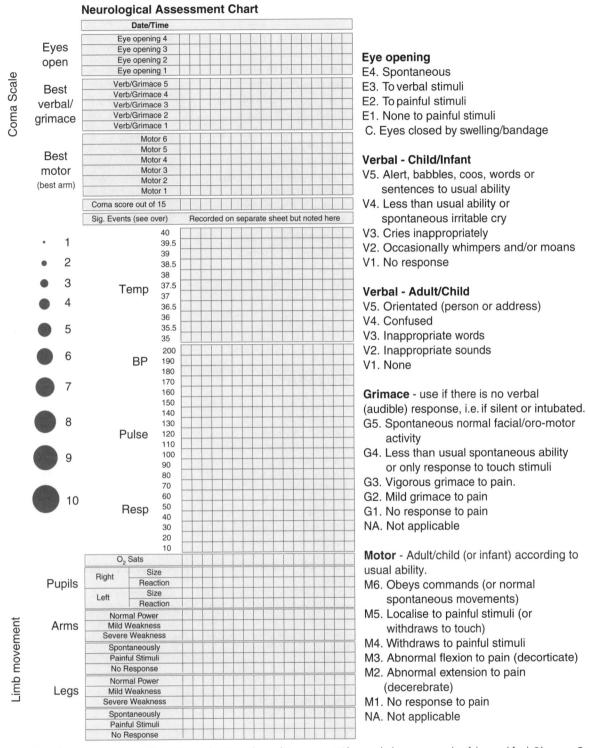

Neurological Assessment Chart

Eye opening
E4. Spontaneous
E3. To verbal stimuli
E2. To painful stimuli
E1. None to painful stimuli
C. Eyes closed by swelling/bandage

Verbal - Child/Infant
V5. Alert, babbles, coos, words or
    sentences to usual ability
V4. Less than usual ability or
    spontaneous irritable cry
V3. Cries inappropriately
V2. Occasionally whimpers and/or moans
V1. No response

Verbal - Adult/Child
V5. Orientated (person or address)
V4. Confused
V3. Inappropriate words
V2. Inappropriate sounds
V1. None

Grimace - use if there is no verbal
(audible) response, i.e. if silent or intubated.
G5. Spontaneous normal facial/oro-motor
    activity
G4. Less than usual spontaneous ability
    or only response to touch stimuli
G3. Vigorous grimace to pain.
G2. Mild grimace to pain
G1. No response to pain
NA. Not applicable

Motor - Adult/child (or infant) according to
usual ability.
M6. Obeys commands (or normal
    spontaneous movements)
M5. Localise to painful stimuli (or
    withdraws to touch)
M4. Withdraws to painful stimuli
M3. Abnormal flexion to pain (decorticate)
M2. Abnormal extension to pain
    (decerebrate)
M1. No response to pain
NA. Not applicable

Figure 13.2 Neurological Assessment Chart. Note: the Neurological Assessment Chart includes an example of the modified Glasgow Coma Scale, originally developed at Birmingham Children's Hospital from the James adaptation of the scale. It is now being used by most members of the National Paediatric Neuroscience Benchmarking group (see Paediatric pearls).

regard to observations of behaviour, activity, appetite, gait, balance, alertness and/or speech. Likewise, if they are concerned with regard to the development

of a headache or vomiting, these concerns need to be respected.
• Review carefully the signs and symptoms that should alert parents to seek care.

• Reinforce the importance of head injury prevention (seat belts, bike helmets, stair gates, window locks, never leaving infants unattended on high places, supervision of play, road safety, car seats, etc.).

- Provide parents with written information to supplement verbal instructions and include a telephone number that can be accessed if parents are worried or unsure about symptoms.

➡ FOLLOW-UP

- Dependent on the extent of the injury: in many cases of benign head injury, no follow-up is required.

🔄 MEDICAL CONSULT/ SPECIALIST REFERRAL

- Any child who has sustained a significant head injury and/or any child who has experienced a loss of consciousness.
- Any child with neurological findings on physical examination.
- Any child in whom a child protection issue is suspected.

🔘 PAEDIATRIC PEARLS

- Parents play a vital role in identifying their child's *usual abilities*; this opinion is vital for an accurate neurological assessment and for detection of problems early in their course; take heed when they tell you that 'my child is not right'.
- Evaluation of the head-injured child needs to be thorough. The mechanism of injury will give clues to the potential extent of the injury.
- In trying to determine loss of consciousness in an unwitnessed fall, ask the parent whether crying was heard immediately after the fall or was there a 'bang' and then silence.

- Always check for possible internal injuries, as accidents can also result in injury to major organs. Primary brain injury can be further compromised by haemorrhage, hypoxia or shock.
- A haematoma can result from a relatively mild preceding head injury; be sure families are well informed with regard to symptoms requiring emergency follow-up.
- The possibility of child protection issues needs to be considered for all head injury presentations; this is especially important in children less than 2 years of age.
- Further information about the National Paediatric Neuroscience Benchmarking Group (or the modified coma assessment chart) can be obtained from Alison Warren, Sister, PICU, Birmingham Children's Hospital.

📑 BIBLIOGRAPHY

Beattie TF. Minor head injury. Arch Dis Child 1997; 77(1):82–85.

Coombs JB, Davis RL. A synopsis of the American Academy of Pediatrics' practice parameter on the management of minor closed head injury in children. Pediatr Rev 2000; 21(12):413–415.

Crouchman M. Head injury – how community paediatricians can help. Arch Dis Child 1990; 65(11):1286–1287.

Crouchman M, Rossiter L, Colaco T, et al. A practical outcome scale for paediatric head injury. Arch Dis Child 2001; 84(2):120–124.

Ferguson-Clarke L, Williams C. Neurological assessment in children. Paediatr Nurs 1998; 10(4):29–35.

James HE, Trauner DA. The Glasgow Coma Scale. In: James R, ed., Brain injuries in infants and children. Orlando: Grune and Stratton: 1985.

Jennett B. Epidemiology of head injury. Arch Dis Child 1998; 78(5):403–406.

Kemp AM. Investigating subdural haemorrhage in infants. Arch Dis Child 2002; 86(2):98–102.

Lam WH, MacKersie A. Paediatric head injury: incidence, aetiology and management. Paediatr Anaes 1999; 9(5):377–385.

Light L. Imaging the less seriously head injured child. Arch Dis Child 2001; 84(3):281.

Rogers M. Cycle helmets. Arch Dis Child 1993; 68(2):237–239.

Savitsky EA, Votey SR. Current controversies in the management of minor pediatric head injuries. Am J Emerg Med 2000; 18(1): 96–101.

Schutzman SA, Barnes P, Duhaime AC, et al. Evaluation and management of children younger than two years old with apparently minor head trauma: proposed guidelines. Pediatrics 2001; 107(5):983–993.

Tatman A. Development of a modified paediatric coma scale in intensive care clinical practice. Arch Dis Child 1997; 77(6):519–521.

Warren A. Paediatric coma scoring researched and benchmarked. Paediatr Nurs 2000; 12(3):14–18.

Warrington SA, Wright CM, Team AS. Accidents and resulting injuries in premobile infants: data from the ALSPAC Study. Arch Dis Child 2001; 85(2):104–107.

Wickham T, Abrahamson E. Head injuries in infants: the risks of bouncy chairs and car seats. Arch Dis Child 2002; 86(3):168–169.

Wilkins B. Head injury: abuse or accident? Arch Dis Child 1997; 76(5):393–397.

ACKNOWLEDGEMENT

The authors wish to acknowledge the expertise of Alison Warren and the National Neuroscience Benchmarking Group for the contribution of the Neurological Assessment Chart.

Genitourinary Problems and Sexual Health

14.1 URINARY TRACT INFECTION

Evelyn Robinson and Sue Vernon

📖 INTRODUCTION

- Urinary tract infections (UTI) are one of the most significant, common and serious bacterial infections of childhood. Whilst the true incidence of UTI remains uncertain, rates in Northern England suggest that 2.8% of boys and 8.2% of girls will have had a UTI by the age of 7 years. This rate increases to 3.6% of boys and 11.3% of girls by the age of 16 years. Anatomical defects in young children (e.g. obstructive anomalies and/or vesicoureteric reflux) and sexual activity in adolescents may increase incidence numbers. UTI may be recurrent, with a higher recurrence rate in girls, approximately one third of girls are likely to have a further UTI within a year of the first infection and some may have repeated UTIs.
- UTI causes considerable upset for the child and family and appropriate identification of children with urinary tract infections is critical because renal scarring from UTI may lead to subsequent end-stage renal disease. UTI may be associated with both renal abnormality and potential longterm problems (*at some time in later life*) including hypertension and possible renal failure (secondary to renal scarring).
- Diagnosis of a UTI may be difficult in young children and infants, who may have non-specific symptoms and/or in whom there is no obvious suspicion of a UTI.

🔬 PATHOPHYSIOLOGY

- The normal urinary tract is sterile, however bacterial contamination can occur from a variety of organisms. *Escherichia coli* (from the bowel) accounts for approximately 75% of all infections, while *Proteus* spp. are responsible for roughly 30% of UTIs among boys. Less common organisms implicated in urinary tract infection include *Klebsiella* and enterococcus.
- The gold standard for the diagnosis of a UTI is a positive urine culture; defined as pure bacterial growth (i.e. growth of a *single* organism) with a colony count greater than 10^5/ml, in an appropriately collected specimen (see Additional diagnostics).
- Pyelonephritis is an acute infection of the renal parenchyma. Most febrile infants with a positive urine culture have upper tract infection. Lower tract infections are acute infections limited to the bladder (i.e. no involvement of the kidneys). These are most common in older children and adolescents and are usually characterised by urinary symptoms and a lack of fever. However, differentiation between upper and lower urinary tract infections is difficult and no reliable method has been identified.
- UTIs may occur as 'silent' infections in sick infants, therefore a urine should always be cultured in this situation.
- UTIs may be the result of one (or more) of the following: urinary

tract abnormalities (e.g. vesico-ureteric reflux, neurogenic bladder, urethral obstruction); dysfunctional voiding patterns; sexual activity or bladder instrumentation (such as catheterisation).
- Renal parenchymal damage can be caused by a urinary tract infection combined with vesicoureteric reflux (VUR). It is important to note that permanent, irreversible kidney damage can happen within a short time; a child with a UTI and VUR may damage the renal parenchyma within 3 days.

🔙 HISTORY

- General appearance, appetite and activity level of infant or child (see Ch. 4). UTI among infants is often missed as the signs and symptoms are very non-specific (poor feeding, irritability, fever and vomiting, and/or failure to thrive).
- Fever.
- Urinary symptoms: urgency, frequency, painful urination, dribbling and incontinence in a previously continent child.
- Presence of suprapubic, abdominal and/or flank/back pain and nausea.
- Possible sources of urethral irritation including: bubble bath usage, wiping from back to front, non-cotton underwear, perfumed talc powder, threadworms and tight fitting clothes or underwear.
- History of constipation or recent diarrhoea.

- In adolescence it is important to provide privacy in order to obtain a sexual history and rule out the possibility of pregnancy (in addition to UTI).
- History of UTI, urinary tract abnormalities or unexplained fevers in the past.
- Family history of renal disease.

PHYSICAL EXAMINATION

- **General appearance**: this is especially important in young infants, and includes growth parameters, vital signs and blood pressure. Note that fever may be high (40°–40.5°). Any unexplained fever on physical examination should arouse suspicion of UTI.
- **Head and ear, nose and throat (ENT)**: exclude acute infection, including pharyngitis. Note children with UTI may have abdominal pain related to inflammation of the mesenteric nodes.
- **Cardiopulmonary**: exclude unexpected findings, as lower lobe pneumonia can present with fever and abdominal pain.
- **Abdomen**: may be slightly distended with/without suprapubic tenderness and flank pain/costovertebral (CVA) tenderness to percussion. Bowel sounds should be normal (peritoneal signs are not associated with UTI).
- **Genitourinary**: should be normal examination; erythema can be seen with urethral irritation and/or hygiene issues.

DIFFERENTIAL DIAGNOSIS

- Diagnosis of UTI is dependent on positive urine culture (see Pathophysiology). UTI should be considered in any febrile infant or pre-school child presenting with fever without localising source, even in the absence of signs and symptoms (see Sec. 15.1).
- With lower tract symptomatology, consider the possibility of urethral irritation, especially if history of bubble bath use, vulvovaginitis or sexually transmitted infection (STI). See Sections 14.3 and 14.5.
- With upper tract symptomatology, consider: gastroenteritis, pelvic

inflammatory disease or tubal-ovarian abscess; appendicitis or ovarian torsion.
- The possibility of child sexual abuse should likewise be considered if history or physical examination warrant.
- Whilst dipsticks are unreliable in establishing a diagnosis of UTI, sometimes they can be useful; blood and protein may be diagnostic of glomerular nephritis if a urine culture is negative.

MANAGEMENT

- **Additional diagnostics:** Urine culture with sensitivities is *mandatory* for any child with suspected UTI. Urinalysis/urine dipstick may provide additional information, *but they are not diagnostic of UTI*. *Always* collect a urine sample (in an age appropriate manner) and send for culture and sensitivity *prior* to starting antibiotics. Appropriate methods of sample collection include (ranked in order of suitability): (1) clean catch; (2) pad specimen of urine; (3) suprapubic aspiration (rarely necessary except in the very sick infant). *Bag collection and catheter specimens are not recommended*. All methods carry a risk of contamination, therefore urine should be meticulously collected and stored (refrigerated post collection for a maximum of 48 hours). Note that leucocyte esterase-nitrite sticks may be useful if positive, however they carry a significant risk of false negativity and should be used with caution. *They should not be relied upon to make a diagnosis*. If dipstix reveals the presence of blood and protein, *when urine culture is negative*, consider glomerular nephritis. Note that infants and children with a documented UTI will require additional follow-up diagnostics (see Follow-up).
- **Pharmacotherapeutics:** Infants and children suspected of having a UTI should be treated with antibiotics as soon as possible after a urine culture is collected (do not delay treatment). Treat with a current 'best guess' antibiotic according to local microbiology laboratory recommendations. Change antibiotic, if necessary, when culture sensitivities are available. At any age a sick or toxic

child may require hospitalisation and treatment with intravenous antibiotics
- **Patient education:** It is important to advise parents on UTI prevention: avoid use of bubble baths and soap in the genital area of little girls; wipe from front to back after using the toilet; increase intake of extra fluids; use cotton underwear; void frequently and avoid 'holding' urine for long periods (both during treatment and as part of good urinary health practices). In addition, discuss UTI prevention with the child. If there is avoidance of school toilets (bullying, etc.) the school may need contacting and alternative facilities provided. Among sexually active adolescent females, encourage voiding after intercourse. Review interventions to minimise constipation (see Sec. 12.2) and instructions for all medication use.

FOLLOW-UP

- Check urine culture result as soon available, change antibiotics if necessary.
- All children with a documented UTI will require further evaluation to rule out renal abnormality/damage (see Table 14.1). This should include dimercaptosuccinic acid (DMSA) scintography scan and renal ultrasound. An additional test may include a micturating cystourethrogram (MCUG) or radionuclide cystogram. Any child presenting with a repeat UTI may require further investigation according to age.
- Children under 4 years of age should be given antibiotic prophylaxis until all imaging is completed. Prophylaxis should also be extended to infants and children with an abnormal MCUG and those with recurrent UTI.
- In children between 1 and 4 with a previously normal DMSA and US scan (but no MCUG performed) an *index of high suspicion* should be adopted: urine should be cultured every 3 months until 4 years of age and whenever the child is unwell, re-referral is necessary for repeat DMSA/MCUG if another episode of UTI.
- Children with a UTI caused by *Proteus* bacilli will need additional

Table 14.1 Schedule of Follow-up Diagnostics

Age	Diagnostics	Follow-up
<1 year	• DMSA/renal US and MCUG	• If all tests normal no further follow-up needed unless repeat UTI • Specialist follow-up if abnormal results
1–4 years	• DMSA/renal US	• If normal consider child with an index of high suspicion (see follow-up above) • Specialist follow-up if abnormal results
Repeat UTI <4 years	• Repeat MCUG and if <3.5 years • Repeat DMSA if 3.5–4 years	• Specialist follow-up pending results
>4 years	• DMSA and renal US	• If normal results, discharge to primary care as UTI unlikely to scar kidneys after 4 years of age • Specialist follow-up if abnormal results

• Any child of any age with renal scarring will require BP monitoring for life
• Any child with VUR needs active monitoring (with or without prophylaxis) until VUR resolved

US = ultrasound; MCUG = micturating cystourethrogram; DMSA = dimercaptosuccinic acid.

investigation of abdominal X-ray (to exclude renal stones).

⇄ MEDICAL CONSULT/ SPECIALIST REFERRAL

• Any infant or child with a toxic appearance, high fever and vomiting or unclear diagnosis.
• Any child with abnormal findings after micturating cystourethrogram (MCUG), renal ultrasound or DMSA scan.
• Any child with recurrent UTI or those who remain symptomatic 2–3 days after initiation of antibiotic therapy.

PAEDIATRIC PEARLS

• Always consider the possibility of a UTI in a febrile infant or child without obvious cause.
• Consider urinary tract abnormality in any child presenting with UTI regardless of the child's age.
• The sequelae of a missed diagnosis (e.g. untreated pyelonephritis) can be devastating.
• Remember, a child presenting with a UTI at any age may have had a 'silent UTI' previously. Therefore *all* children should be investigated following a documented UTI, whatever their age.
• Signs of UTI in infants are very non-specific; sometimes the only complaints will be 'poor feeding' or the carer's report that 'my baby is just not right'; a urine sample should be cultured.

• Do not rely on dipstick testing (approximately 10% of febrile infants with a UTI will have false-negative screening tests).
• Consider blood cultures in any infant with suspected pyelonephritis (approximately 10% are bacteraemic).
• Rule out the possibility of UTI in a young child presenting with secondary enuresis (whether diurnal or nocturnal).
• If a definitive diagnosis is to be made accurately a urine sample needs meticulous collection and storage.

▤ BIBLIOGRAPHY

American Academy of Paediatrics. Practice parameter: the diagnosis, treatment and evaluation of the initial urinary tract infection in febrile infants and young children. Paediatrics 1999; 103:843–852.

Benador D, Benador N, Slosman D, Mermillod B, Girardin E. Are children at highest risk of renal sequelae after pyelonephritis? Lancet 1997; 349:17–19.

Blethyn AJ, Jenkins HR, Roberts R, et al. Radiological evidence of constipation in urinary tract infection. Arch Dis Child 1995; 73(6):534–535.

Coulthard M, Lambert H. Child with the urinary tract infection. In: Webb N, Postlethwaite R, eds, Clinical paediatric nephrology, 3rd edn. Oxford: Oxford University Press; 2003; chapter 11.

Coulthard M, Lambert H, Keir M. Occurrence of renal scars in children after their first referral for urinary tract infection. BMJ 1997; 315:918–919.

Jacobson S, Hansson S, Jakobsson B. Vesico-ureteric reflux: occurrence and long-term risks. Acta Paediatr Suppl 1999; 431:22–33.

Hellström A-L, Hanson E, Hansson S, Hjälmås K, Jodal U. Association between urinary symptoms at 7 years old and previous urinary tract infection. Archives of Disease in Childhood 1991; 66:232–234.

Koff S, Wagner T, Jayanthi V. The relationship among dysfunctional elimination syndromes, primary vesico-ureteral reflux and urinary tract infections in children. Journal of Urology 1998; 160:1019–1022.

Kumar RK, Turner GM, Coulthard MG. Don't count on urinary white cells to diagnose childhood urinary tract infection. BMJ 1996; 312:1359.

http://www.prodigy.nhs.uk/ Guidelines on childhood UTI (updated 2002).

Ransley PG, Risdon RA. Reflux and renal scarring. British Journal of Radiology 1978; 14(suppl 51):1–35.

Sharied N, Petts D. Dipstick examination for urinary tract infection. Arch Dis Child 2001; 84(5):451.

Steele R. The epidemiology and clinical presentation of urinary tract infections in children 2 years of age through adolescence. Pediatr Ann 1999; 28(10):653–659.

Stokland E, Hellström M, Jacobsson B, Jodal U, Sixt R. Evaluation of DMSA scintography and urography in assessing both acute and permanent renal damage in children. Acta Radiol 1998; 39:447–452.

Thayyvil-Sudhan S, Gupta S. Dipstick examination for urinary tract infections. Arch Dis Child 2000; 82(3):271–272.

Turner GM, Coulthard MG. Fever can cause pyuria in children. BMJ 1995; 311:924.

van der Voort J, Edwards A, Roberts R, Verrier Jones K. The struggle to diagnose UTI in children under two in primary care. Fam Pract 1997; 14(1):44–48.

Vernon S, Foo C, Coulthard M. How general practitioners manage children with urinary tract infection: an audit in the former Northern Region. British Journal of General Practice 1997; 47:297–300.

Vernon S, Redfearn A, Pedler SJ, Lambert HJ, Coulthard MG. Urine collection on sanitary towels. Lancet 1994; 344:612.

Vernon S, Coulthard M, Lambert H, Keir M, Matthews J. New renal scarring in children who at age 3 and 4 years had had normal scans with dimercaptosuccinic acid: follow up study. BMJ 1997; 315:905–908.

Wettergren B, Jodal U, Jonasson G. Epidemiology of bacteriuria during the first year of life. Acta Ped Scand 1985; 74:925–933.

COMMON PAEDIATRIC PROBLEMS

14.2 ENURESIS

Linda Smith and Cheryl Ward

📖 INTRODUCTION

- Enuresis is repeated involuntary urination, usually nocturnal, in individuals who are beyond the age when voluntary bladder control should be acquired.
- Primary enuresis is when the child has never been dry for extended periods (i.e. continence has never been achieved).
- Secondary enuresis is the onset of wetting after a continuous dry period of more than 1 year (i.e. recurrence of incontinence).
- It is thought that enuresis has a familial component. More specifically, 70% of enuretic children have a parent who was enuretic. If both parents were enuretic, there is a 77% chance of enuresis in the child. If one parent was enuretic, the likelihood is 45–47% and if neither parent was enuretic the probability drops to 15%.
- The genes associated with daytime wetting and urgency have been isolated on the human genome (they appear to be involved in gaining bladder control) but research in this field is in its infancy.
- The prevalence of enuresis among 5-year-old children is approximately 7% (boys) and 3% (girls). Enuresis persists, among 10-year-old boys and girls (respectively) for 3% and 2% of them. Primary nocturnal enuresis continues in approximately 1% of adults (less than 1% among females).
- Nocturnal enuresis is much more common than diurnal (daytime) wetting, which occurs in only 1% of 7–12 year olds. Nocturnal enuresis is 2–3 times more common in males than females, whereas daytime wetting is more common in females. There is a higher frequency of enuresis among children of lower socioeconomic groups and among black children.
- Children with enuresis describe themselves as anxious and often admit to sleep difficulties and/or nightmares. In addition, older children with enuresis (i.e. those from 6–11 years of age) tend to have highly strung temperaments.
- Embarrassment, poor self-esteem and reluctance to participate in overnight activities with peers are some of the complications of delayed continence. Behavioural problems associated with enuresis are much more likely to be a result of the enuresis rather than a cause.
- For the most part, primary enuresis is benign and self-limiting. Secondary enuresis is much more likely to be related to an underlying medical or surgical problem. The prognosis for enuretic children is very good (even without treatment); the spontaneous cure rate is approximately 15% per year.

🔬 PATHOPHYSIOLOGY

- The pathophysiology of enuresis appears to be multifactorial with several theories (and different mechanisms) probably playing a greater or lesser role in each child. For the most part, however, enuresis is primarily a problem of delayed/incomplete neuromaturation in which the bladder empties at a lower volume (that is often accompanied by a smaller functional bladder capacity). A bladder volume of approximately 300–350 ml is required to hold one night's urine output. More specifically, the enuretic child is unable to inhibit bladder contractions once the bladder has been distended beyond a certain volume and, therefore, he is unable to achieve age-appropriate bladder control.
- In some children it is thought that the hormone arginine vasopressin (secreted from the posterior pituitary gland to stimulate the reabsorption of water through the kidneys during sleep) can be under-produced. Consequently, urine production through the night is not reduced, large amounts of urine are created and the child is unable to inhibit bladder contractions.
- Extreme constipation can result in enuresis, as a loaded rectum and sigmoid colon can exert pressure on the bladder.
- Abnormalities of sleep (e.g. children with extremely deep sleep states) have been postulated as a factor in nocturnal enuresis. They have not, however, been proven to play a role despite historical information from mothers claiming their children fail to waken in the night when voiding. It has been suggested that enuretic children do receive messages to void but choose not to acknowledge them.
- Anxiety associated with potty training and dysfunctional parent–child relationships have also been suggested as potential aetiologies for enuresis. These have not been proven to play a role.
- Some children exhibit temporary regressive behaviour after the birth of a sibling and, therefore, will present with secondary enuresis.
- Daytime wetting can be related to excitement or engrossment in an occupation that results in unintentional leakage of urine.

⬅ HISTORY

- Toilet-training history (e.g. age at toilet training, age when daytime and night-time dryness achieved) if applicable.
- Onset of enuresis (to determine whether enuresis is primary or secondary).
- Occurrence of wetting (e.g. night-time and/or daytime) and how often.
- Number of dry nights/month and number of consecutive dry nights.
- Bladder empty at bedtime?
- Whether child self-awakens to full bladder or self-awakens to wet bed or does not awaken spontaneously.
- Evening fluid intake (amount and times).
- Toileting habits, frequency of voiding and stooling, bathing habits (e.g. use of bubble bath).
- Pattern of urination and urinary stream (dribbling, dysuria, hesitancy and urgency suggest possible structural defect).
- Associated symptoms (stool incontinence, weight loss, polydipsia, polyuria).

- History of other medical problems, including urinary tract infections, neurological problems, gait disturbances, night-time snoring, adenoidal hypertrophy and/or obstructive sleep apnoea.
- The family's attitude towards the enuresis (accepting, ashamed, aggravated, etc.).
- Effect of enuresis on child.
- What happens after wetting episode (Who changes bed? Who washes bedclothes? Where is change of clothes? What happens at school? etc.).
- Treatments (or punishments) tried thus far, with results.
- Family history of enuresis (and, if positive, is child aware of this).
- Developmental history (milestones, toilet-training methods, behavioural and/or school problems).
- Recent environmental stressors.
- Medications.

PHYSICAL EXAMINATION

- **General:** growth parameters, blood pressure and vital signs.
- **Head and ENT:** rule out tonsillar hypertrophy and/or obligate mouth breather (consider adenoidal hypertrophy).
- **Abdomen:** rule out masses, renal enlargement, palpable bladder and constipation.
- **Urine:** consider observation of urinary stream for ability to start/stop stream, characteristics of stream and presence of dribbling.
- **Genitalia:** rule out irritation, adhesions, rash and child protection issues.
- **Consider rectal examination** (if history positive for encopresis): observe for perianal sensation, anal sphincter tone and child protection issues.
- **Neurological:** deep tendon reflexes, gait, strength and tone of lower extremities, and spinal examination for bony defects and/or cutaneous signs of underlying defects.

DIFFERENTIAL DIAGNOSES

- A number of underlying conditions or diseases may present with enuresis. This is especially true in secondary enuresis, which is more likely to have an organic cause. It is important to rule out organic causes of enuresis as part of the initial work-up. Urinary tract infection, diabetes mellitus, diabetes insipidus, sickle cell disease, structural genitourinary abnormalities, neurological or spinal cord pathology, constipation, child protection issues and any condition causing polyuria (e.g. malignancies) can present with enuresis.

MANAGEMENT

Children with any form of organic enuresis will require management specific to the aetiology of the wetting. In addition, children with associated diurnal enuresis, diurnal frequency, constipation and/or encopresis need these treated first.

- **Additional diagnostics:** urinalysis (including glucose), urine culture and specific gravity (to rule out UTI). In the majority of cases this is all that is required. If there is a history of UTIs, additional diagnostics will be required (see Sec. 14.1). Likewise, if there are findings suggestive of neurological involvement, additional diagnostics will be required.
- **Pharmacotherapeutics:** medication therapy can be a valuable adjuvant to other strategies; a synthetic version of the hormone vasopressin (desmopressin, DDAVP or Desmotabs) can be used to reduce urine production overnight. The treatment is available in tablet or nasal spray and is given immediately prior to bedtime for 3–6 months. The dose is gradually reduced until the child is consistently dry. It is effective in 75% of cases but is not recommended for use in children under 5 years of age. Note however, that initiation of desmopressin therapy should not occur until organic causes of enuresis have been eliminated. Desmopressin is also helpful for older children who, on special occasions, wish to participate in a sleep over at a friends or other social occasion.
- **Behavioural intervention:**
  - Approaches should be practical in nature, based upon sound common sense and evidence-based practice. The goals are to cure the enuresis *and* protect the child's self-esteem; therefore, punishment and/or punitive action for bed-wetting are inappropriate.
  - Evaluate the child's home environment, including practical issues of getting to the toilet at night (e.g. is the route warm, adequately lit and without obstacles?). Children may be afraid of the dark and thus reluctant to get out of bed if they are cold (which can also exacerbate the enuresis). The availability of a potty and night-light in the bedroom can increase a child's confidence and encourage them to awaken and void.
  - Clarify the goal of getting up at night to use the toilet. The child should be assisted to assume some responsibility for becoming dry (*'We'll help you, but it is you that can solve this problem'*). Likewise, the child should take some responsibility for the morning clean-up (disposal of wet bedding/clothes in an agreed manner) and a shower or bath before school is important. Preservation of self-esteem is essential and, therefore, successful completion of these activities should be rewarded. In turn, the child subconsciously begins to take ownership for the enuresis.
  - Intake of caffeinated and carbonated drinks should be avoided at least 90 min before bedtime and the bladder should be emptied before bed. Encourage an adequate fluid intake during the day and avoid a 'just before bed' bolus of fluid. Extra fluids during the day will also reinforce the sensation of a full bladder and potentially increase awareness of the signals to void.
  - If after a 2-week period of intervention the child has not made significant progress (4–5 consecutive dry nights) parents should be allowed to discontinue intervention. Emphasis should shift to managing the practicalities of the enuresis (e.g. minimising laundry and mess by purchasing protective bedding and use of absorbent pants beneath nightwear). This 'treatment break' reduces the pressure on both parent and child (e.g. the annoyance of wet bedding is largely eliminated and no pressure on child to stay dry). The intervention can then be

Table 14.2 Behavioural Interventions for Non-organic Nocturnal Enuresis		
Intervention	Process	Comments
Parent awakening programme	• Parent agrees (at child's request) to awaken child before parent retires to bed • Sequence is practised during day and before bed (i.e. child lays on bed, closes eyes, pretends to be asleep and then imagines sensation of full bladder with subsequent rising, walking to toilet, voiding and returning to bed) • Hierarchy of prompts used by parent (e.g. calling, nudging, shaking child). There should be no leading or carrying child to toilet	• To be attempted only at child's request • Useful for children capable of getting up but who do not understand the importance ('every wet night is a night when he needed to get up') • Can be a valuable precursor to enuresis alarms • If child becomes angry or yells at parent, process stops and incident discussed in morning
Enuresis alarms	• Assess readiness/ability of child to awaken with parent awakening or use of an alarm clock • Allow child to choose type of alarm (sound, tactile or simple use of an alarm clock)	• Child must want alarm • Highest cure rate of any treatment modality; succeeds in 75% of children with low relapse rate • Desmopressin can be used as adjuvant for first 3 weeks to provide some success; then taper • Failures most commonly due to premature discontinuation of alarm or under-motivation of parent or child
Motivational therapy	• Use of star charts, calendar and/or reward system for each dry night • For the most part only successful when child has achieved a sustained period of dry nights • Critical that 'reward' is something that will motivate child; try to avoid use of food as reward. Better choices include a day out, trip to cinema, etc.	• Most children experience the occasional dry night that is typically received with rapture from a parent • While child enjoys the positive attention, he appreciates that nothing extraordinary was done to promote the dryness (simply that the bladder was able to hold the amount of urine excreted by the kidneys on this occasion) • When the cycle of wet nights continues, the child soon becomes demotivated
Bladder re-training	• Child needs an adequate fluid intake (1000 ml) between the hours of 8 a.m. and 4 p.m. • Goals are to promote regular, satisfactory filling of the bladder; increase detrusor tone; and reinforce the sensation of a full bladder • Children are encouraged to action the signal to void as they become aware of it (daytime and night-time); organise their time to facilitate arrival at the toilet dry; see 'self-control' as the key to successfully becoming dry • Evidence of progress should not be confined to 'dry nights' but by observing the volume of urine on the bedding • Children should be encouraged to change their perception of bed-wetting: 'to be dry is to be normal/expected'; 'to waken to void is normal/expected'; 'to sleep on when needing to void is not normal/expected'	• Most children drink much less, particularly while at This results in a decreased urine school. output and a bolus of fluid in the afternoon/evening (i.e. children slake thirst once at home) • Increased fluid intake during the day has the potential to regularly raise the child's awareness of the signal to void • Children with enuresis often delay passing urine and, as a result, small leakages are viewed as insignificant. The idea of 'self-control' is to raise the child's awareness of the consequences of his persistent delay in addressing the need to void • The child must be committed to attempts to cease voiding once wetness is experienced and to finish emptying the bladder in the toilet. Urine in the bed should gradually diminish in both volume and frequency until the child wakens to the signal to void • Parents and siblings often unintentionally condone enuresis because of their unequivocal love. There is an unwritten family rule that enuresis remains a 'family secret'. The child is thus excused of responsibility on the pretext of being soundly asleep
Relapse management	• Reinitiate whatever intervention was successful • Can attempt over-learning: after 1 month of success force child to awaken earlier (8 ounces of water just before bed, increased to 12 ounces, then 16 ounces)	• If >8 years of age, put child in charge of problem-solving relapse • If <8 years of age, can attempt parent awakening

re-introduced at regular intervals (e.g. school holidays) in anticipation that with maturity will come success.

• Regular counselling sessions with a health care professional who has a special interest in childhood continence allow the child to discuss the implications and practicalities of the enuresis. The child accepts responsibility for the disorder and the necessary learning. Note that this is dependent on the child's cognitive development, thought to be indicative from 8 years of age.

• Behavioural interventions for non-organic nocturnal enuresis are summarised in Table 14.2.

• **Patient education:**
  • Review with child and family behavioural interventions above.

  • Remind the child and family that they will conquer this. Stress with them that there should be no criticism: ridicule, punishment or demoralisation.

  • If the child is taking desmopressin, it is important to provide advice to avoid fluid overload (including during swimming) and to stop the medication during an episode of vomiting or diarrhoea. Concomittant use of desmopressin and tricyclic antidepressants should be avoided.

  • Review the rationale behind the interventions as well as the mechanisms related to the enuresis. If there is a heredity component, remind the child of this.

  • Enuresis resources for families: health visitor; GP; practice nurse or specialist nurse with a special interest in childhood continence; also, community hospital enuresis clinics and ERIC (Enuresis and Information Centre).

⇨ FOLLOW-UP

• Follow-up should be ongoing. Close family support is the key to concordance and successful management of enuresis.

⇄ MEDICAL CONSULT/ SPECIALIST REFERRAL

• Any child in whom an organic cause is suspected.
• Any child in whom there is a suspicion of sexual abuse.

- Any child in whom enuresis is persistent, unresolved and without an organic cause (consider behavioural referral to paediatric psychology, psychiatry or family therapy).

PAEDIATRIC PEARLS

- Concordance, good follow-up and close family support are key to successful management of enuresis.
- Families may expect instant results; careful discussion/explanation of normal bladder function and the rationale behind specific interventions often improves concordance with treatment.
- Rule out any organic cause before treatment is attempted.
- Child protection issues can present as enuresis.
- Adenoidal and tonsillar hypertrophy are associated with nocturnal enuresis; consider ENT referral if sleep-associated apnoea is a possibility.
- Often urinalysis and/or culture is only diagnostic required.
- Remember natural course of the symptoms (spontaneous cure rate of 15% per year). Balance the potential use of medication against the social and/or emotional impact of the enuresis on the child and family.
- Treatment breaks are invaluable in diffusing the pressure within a family. It is important to reinforce their usefulness as a 'period for timing realignment' rather than as an indication of 'failure' per se.

- Teenage children especially respond positively to management by a specialist nurse with an interest in childhood continence. Support for this group needs to be home-based, as they are extremely sensitive to the stigma of enuresis clinic attendance.
- Support, educate and encourage; support, educate and encourage; support, educate and encourage … .

BIBLIOGRAPHY

Devlin JB. Predicting treatment outcomes in nocturnal enuresis. Arch Dis Child 1990; 65:1158–1161.

Forsythe WI, Redmond A. Enuresis and spontaneous cure rate. Arch Dis Child 1974; 49:259–263.

Gandhi K. Diagnosis and management of nocturnal enuresis. Curr Opin Pediatr 1994; 6(2):194–197.

Garber K. Enuresis. J Pediatr Health Care 1996; 10(5):202–208.

Hicks MR, Clarke G. Top 100 nocturnal enuresis. GP Med 1999; August 30–31.

Howe A, Walker E. Behavioural management of toilet training, enuresis, and encopresis. Pediatr Clin North Am 1992; 39(3):413–432.

Levine MD. Disordered processes of elimination. In: Levine MD, ed., Developmental–behavioural pediatrics. Philadelphia: WB Saunders; 1983.

Mack A. Dry all night. Boston: Little Brown; 1989.

Moffat ME. Nocturnal enuresis: psychological implications of treatment and non-treatment. J Pediatr 1989; 114(4 Pt 2):697–704.

Moffat ME. Nocturnal enuresis: a review of the efficacy of treatments and practical advice for clinicians. J Dev Behav Pediatr 1997; 18(1):49–56.

Norgaard JP, Rittig S, Djurhuus JC. Nocturnal enuresis: an approach to treatment based on pathogenesis. J Pediatr 1989; 14(4 Pt 2):705–709.

Paterson H. Management of enuresis in children. Br J Nurs 1993; 2(8):418–424.

Pierce CM. Enuresis. In: Kaplan H, Friedman A, Sadock B, eds, Comprehensive textbook of psychiatry, 3rd edn. Baltimore: Williams & Wilkins; 1980.

Rappaport LA. The treatment of nocturnal enuresis (where we are now). Paediatrics 1993; 92(3):465.

Riley KE. Evaluation and management of primary nocturnal enuresis. J Am Acad Nurse Pract 1997; 9(1):33–39.

Rittig S. Diurnal variation in plasma levels and anti-diuretic hormone and urinary output in patients with enuresis and control subjects. Nephrol Urodyn 1997; 6:260–261.

Robson J. Diurnal enuresis. Pediatr Rev 1997; 18(12):407–412.

Rushton HG. Nocturnal enuresis: epidemiology, evaluation and currently available treatment options. J Pediatr 1989; 114(4 Pt 2):691–696.

Schmitt B. Nocturnal enuresis. Pediatr Rev 1997; 18(6):183–190.

Stark M. Assessment and management of the care of children with nocturnal enuresis: guidelines for primary care. Nurse Pract Forum 1994; 5(3):170–174.

Von Gontard A, Eiberg H, Hollman E, et al. Molecular genetics of nocturnal enuresis: linkage to a locus on chromosome 22. Scand J Urol Nephrol 1999; 202:76–78.

Wan J, Greenfield S. Enuresis and common voiding abnormalities. Pediatr Clin North Am 1997; 44:1117–1131.

14.3 VULVOVAGINITIS IN THE PREPUBESCENT CHILD

Dolsie Allen

INTRODUCTION

- Vulvovaginitis in the prepubescent child is a common gynaecological complaint seen in the paediatric population. Patients often present with complaints of vaginal pruritus with or without discharge, perineal discomfort and dysuria. Carers may site presence of discharge on patient's undergarments.
- Common causes (sexual abuse excepted) of vulvovaginitis in the prepubescent child are outlined in Table 14.3.

PATHOPHYSIOLOGY

- Several factors contribute to the prepubescent girl's vulnerability to this condition. Physiological factors include the presence of non-oestrogenised vaginal mucosa, a neutral vaginal pH and a relative lack of protective vaginal lactobacilli.

- In addition, developmental issues (e.g. the increasing desire for privacy and independence) can combine with often suboptimal hygiene to result in the common symptoms of vaginal itching and perineal discomfort.

⬅ HISTORY

- Onset and severity of symptoms.
- Typical bathing and hygiene routines (including degree of supervision).
- Medication use (including recent antibiotics).
- Use of bubble baths and bath products.
- Presence of discharge (mucoid or purulent, smell, quantity, colour and consistency).
- Presence of bloody drainage.
- Fever, dysuria, abdominal or pelvic pain.
- Rectal pruritus and irritation.
- Similar symptoms in family members.
- Possibility of sexual abuse and history of patient contacts if suspected.

📖 PHYSICAL EXAMINATION

- It is important to observe the child's affect and behaviour during the history and physical examination. Likewise, note the carer/child interaction and elicit the child's perception of the problem. Although a diagnosis of potential sexual abuse is less likely than other aetiologies, the possibility of abuse must be evaluated in any young girl presenting with vulvovaginitis. Findings associated with child sexual abuse are outlined in Table 14.4.

- For the majority of children who present with non-specific vulvovaginitis, coupled with little or no discharge, a brief examination of the external genitalia and rectal area may be all that is required. This includes a gentle, patient approach, careful explanation and consent from both child and parent. *Be sure to ask the carer what term(s) the child uses to identify/describe her genitals.*

- *Note that any child whose affect, behaviour, interactions with carer or history are unsettling, will require a head-to-toe inspection and physical examination.*

Table 14.3 Differential Causes of Vulvovaginitis

Aetiology	Consider
Non-specific origin	• Poor hygiene • Culture shows mixed flora colonic bacteria
Irritant	• Soaps, detergents, bath products • Foreign body (most often toilet paper) • Synthetic undergarments and tights • Masturbation, horseback riding
Infection	• Group A β-haemolytic streptococci (GABHS) • Bacterial vaginitis (adolescents) • *Candida albicans* (postpubescent)
Parasites	• Threadworm
Sexual abuse[a]	• Gonorrhoea • *Trichomonas* (possibly) • *Chlamydia trachomatis* • Herpes simplex • Condyloma acuminata

[a] Sexually transmitted infections are all extremely unusual organisms to document in the prepubescent population: thus, the possibility of sexual abuse must be investigated.

Table 14.4 Findings Associated with Child Sexual Abuse

Category	Possible findings
Subjective complaints	• Recurrent (or acute) abdominal pain • Dysuria, enuresis and/or frequent urinary tract infections • Chronic constipation • Painful defecation • Genital irritation/itching and/or anal bleeding • Perianal itching • Aberrant genital care practices
Behavioural changes	• Depression, withdrawn affect • Self-injury/harm (including suicidal ideation/attempts) • Eating disorders, conduct disorders, aggression and/or school problems • Sleep disturbances/nightmares • Promiscuous behaviour or inappropriate sexual behaviour • Alterations in parent/child relationship
Physical examination findings	• Hard and soft palate bruising • Anal and vulval erythema • Posterior hymen injuries • Mucosal injuries • Pregnancy

- Positions for examination include (1) placing the child on mother's lap (straddling her thighs); (2) a 'frog-legged position' (the child is supine with heels together); or (3) the 'knee-chest' position (the child is prone on the examination table with knees drawn up to the chest and buttocks in the air). See McCann et al. (1990) or McClain et al. (2000) for a more complete discussion of positioning.

- Labial traction technique (gentle traction of labia forward and laterally) allows for better visualisation of vaginal opening. Although the otoscope can be used as a light source, it is often easier to have both hands free by using an examination lamp to illuminate the area.

- Inspect genitalia for:
  - Perineal excoriation (often seen with threadworm infection, especially around anus).
  - Evidence of poor hygiene.
  - Vaginal discharge and bleeding: the type, amount and characteristics of the discharge can provide clues to its aetiology (Table 14.5). Note that normal physiological discharge in prepubescents is non-irritating, white–grey and odourless. Children presenting with significant or bloody discharge will most likely require an internal examination.

- Physical signs of sexual abuse and trauma: note that blatant physical signs are relatively uncommon; therefore, it is important to consider subjective complaints and behavioural changes (see Table 14.4). *Note that child protection procedures should be clearly outlined in all clinical settings. In addition, Appendix 4 outlines further resources related to child protection.*

⚗ DIFFERENTIAL DIAGNOSES

- There can be numerous aetiologies for the symptomatology of vulvovaginitis. In addition to those outlined in Table 14.3, consider UTI, rectal foreign body and normal physiological discharge. *Note that any possibility of sexual abuse presenting as vulvovaginitis must be meticulously and sensitively investigated by experienced professionals.*

✚ MANAGEMENT

The treatment of non-specific vulvovaginitis—which is by far the most frequently encountered cause in the prepubescent population—includes removal of any irritants, coupled with proper and regular hygiene. Retained foreign body involves removal (using ring forceps) and vaginal irrigation with warm saline.

- **Additional diagnostics:** if cause is not apparent (i.e. poor hygiene) consider:
  - urinalysis and urine culture/sensitivity
  - tape test for threadworm
  - wet prep slide with saline (looking for *Trichomonas*); consider 'whiff' test with potassium hydroxide (KOH)
  - all vaginal and rectal discharge should be cultured and sent to the laboratory for specific analysis (see Sec. 14.5)
  - X-rays are not usually beneficial, as most inserted items are not radio-opaque.
- **Pharmacotherapeutics:** aetiology-specific (Table 14.6).
- **Behavioural interventions:**
  - proper perineal hygiene (wiping front to back) with loose cotton undergarments (avoid nylon tights and leggings)

Table 14.5 Types of Vaginal Discharge in Prepubescent Girls

Type of discharge	Consider
Foul-smelling, bloody	• Retained foreign body (toilet roll is the most common object identified in this population, but any object is possible)
Copious discharge, foul smell	• Group A β-haemolytic streptococci (GABHS)
Grey, thin with fishy odour	• Bacterial vaginosis
Scant, varied in colour with concurrent signs of erythema	• Chemical or mechanical irritants
Non-irritating, white–grey and odourless	• Normal physiological discharge (seen at birth to 12 months before puberty)
Thick, adherent, largely odourless white curd that is combined with red, inflamed tissue	• Candidiasis

Table 14.6 Specific Drug Therapies Based on Culture Results

Specific organism	Medication
Group A β-haemolytic streptococcus (GABHS)	• Penicillin V (phenoxymethylpenicillin) 250–500 mg orally (four times daily) for 7 days
Candida vaginitis	• Several preparations available with variable course lengths (intravaginal creams or pessaries): • clotrimazole • econazole • miconazole
Sexually transmitted infections (STIs)	• See Section 14.5

- double rinsing of cotton under-garments
- warm water baths with avoidance of irritants (bubble baths, oils, sprays and powders)
- sleeping 'bare bottom' until irritation clears.
- **Patient education:**
  - review behavioural interventions (above) with parent and child
  - stress that in the majority of cases proper hygiene, avoidance of irritants and simple care measures are sufficient to address the condition (which should resolve rapidly).

⇨ FOLLOW-UP

- Usually not required; return visit or phone call if symptoms fail to resolve.

⇄ MEDICAL CONSULT/ SPECIALIST REFERRAL

- Any child with documented genitourinary anomalies.
- Any child with documented (or suspected) sexually transmitted infection (STI).
- Any child in whom there is a suspicion of sexual abuse.
- Any child with recurrent vaginal and/or rectal bleeding.
- Any child with a retained foreign body.

⊙ PAEDIATRIC PEARLS

- The most frequent cause of vulvovaginitis in prepubescent children is a 'non-specific' irritation.
- Children with a vaginal discharge are significantly more likely to have a specific documented diagnosis than those with only slight irritation.
- When a child presents complaining of itching, ask the child to 'show you where it itches most'. If she reaches around the back, it's most likely threadworm.
- Vaginal candidiasis is relatively uncommon after the nappy-wearing stage and before puberty unless recent antibiotic/steroid use, diabetes mellitus or immunodeficiency.
- Most retained foreign bodies are not radio-opaque; thus, X-rays are not recommended.

BIBLIOGRAPHY

Altchek A. Finding the cause of genital bleeding in pre-pubertal girls. Contemp Pediatr 1996; 13(8):80–92.

Baldwin DD, Landa HM. Common problems in pediatric gynecology. Urol Clin North Am 2000; 22:161–176.

Emans SJ. Vulvovaginitis in the child and adolescent. Pediatr Rev 1986; 8(1):12–19.

Garden AS. Paediatric gynaecology: an overview of current practice. Hospital Med 1998; 59(3):232–235.

Hawkins JW, Nichols DM, Haney JL. Protocols for nurse practitioners in gynecologic settings. New York: Tiresias Press; 1995.

Hill NC, Oppenheimer LW, Morton KE. The aetiology of bleeding in children. Br J Obstet Gynaec 1989; 96(4):467–470.

Hornor G, Ryan-Wenger N. Aberrant genital practices: an unrecognized form of sexual abuse. J Pediatr Health Care 1999; 13(1):12–17.

McCann J, Voris J, Simon M, Wells R. Comparison of genital examination techniques in pre-pubertal girls. Pediatrics 1990; 85(2):182–187.

McClain N, Giardet R, Lahoti S, Cheung K, Berger K, McNeese M. Evaluation of sexual abuse in the pediatric patient. J Pediatr Health Care 2000; 14(3):93–102.

Preminger M, Pokorny S. Vaginal discharge—a common pediatric complaint. Contemp Pediatr 1998; 15(4):115–122.

14.4 ADOLESCENT CONTRACEPTION

Gilly Andrews

INTRODUCTION

- The UK has one of the highest rates of teenage pregnancy in Western Europe (four times that of France and seven times that of the Netherlands). Half of those who have sex before the age of 16 do not use contraception and in 1997 there were 8.9 conceptions per 1000 girls under 16 in England, Scotland and Wales. In an attempt to improve these statistics the Social Exclusion Unit highlighted a number of strategies, including better sex and contraceptive education that will focus on young men as well as women.

- Adolescents under 16 years of age *can legally* be given contraceptive advice and treatment, although, strictly speaking, it's illegal for someone to have sexual intercourse with a girl under 16. Prosecutions are rare for underage sex if the couple are about the same age and both are consenting. Health professionals seeing a young woman under 16 years are legally obliged to discuss the value of parental support. However, if a girl refuses to involve her parents or guardian, contraception can be given provided the health care provider is satisfied that:
  - the adolescent, even though under 16, will understand the professional's advice
  - she cannot be persuaded to inform her parents or allow the health professional to inform them
  - she is very likely to begin or continue having sexual intercourse with or without contraceptive treatment
  - her physical and/or mental health are likely to suffer unless she receives contraceptive advice and treatment
  - it is in her best interest to proceed without parental consent.

- If the above criteria are met, the young woman is said to be 'Gillick Competent' and, therefore, she is able to receive contraceptive advice and treatment without parental involvement.

- Although delivery of contraceptive services should be limited to those health professionals with recognised family planning training (or at clinics that are specifically for young people, such as Brook Advisory Centres), the opportunity to discuss contraceptive options, provide contraceptive advice and reinforce healthy choices should be part of a consultation for other reasons (travel vaccines, acne, etc.).

HISTORY

- **Full medical history:** details of major illnesses; history of headaches and migraine (focal migraines are a contraindication to the combined pill); current medication use and details of smoking, alcohol intake and recreational drug use.

- **Family history:** health details of first-degree relatives is important, particularly with regard to venous thromboembolic events and coronary heart disease. If there is a positive family history, blood lipids and a clotting screen may be required if the young person wishes to take the contraceptive pill.

- **Gynaecological history:** age of menarche, usual cycle length, whether there is any abnormal bleeding (menorrhagia, intermenstrual or postcoital), dysmenorrhoea, dyspareunia, pelvic pain, abnormal vaginal discharge and any previous pregnancies.

- **Date of last menstrual period (and whether it was normal):** a pregnancy test should be performed if her period is late or the last period was different from normal.

- **Sexual history:** length of current relationship; number of partners over last year; current method of contraception (if any); other methods tried; currently having sex with more than one partner; history of vaginal or pelvic infections; and any abnormal discharge or other symptoms at present.

- **Contraception:** ask the adolescent what she already knows (and/or has heard) about different contraceptive methods; what her friends use and whether they have any problems. Her answers will uncover any misapprehensions and anxieties, enable advice to be targeted and more positive messages given.

- **Relationships:** discuss the relationship an adolescent has at home with parents and, more specifically, the degree to which parents are aware/unaware of her sexual activity.

PHYSICAL EXAMINATION

- Weight, blood pressure and body mass index (BMI) should be recorded.
- Young women requesting contraception need reassurance that they do not need a physical examination, unless they have pain, discharge or irregular bleeding (in which case a pelvic and speculum examination would be necessary). If a sexually transmitted infection (STI) is suspected (see Sec. 14.5), then ideally the woman should be referred to her local genitourinary medicine (GUM) clinic for swift diagnosis, treatment and contact tracing; most GUM clinics offer a 'fast track' service for the under-16s.
- Cervical cytology should not be performed on an asymptomatic woman until the age of 20, as the adolescent cervix is undergoing rapid changes which frequently cannot be distinguished from the changes of a low-grade abnormality.

DIFFERENTIAL DIAGNOSES

- Although a request for contraception is not an illness-related complaint per se (and, therefore, does not have a lengthy list of differential diagnoses), it is important to rule out the possibility of pregnancy and sexually transmitted infection.

MANAGEMENT

Individual methods of contraception and their suitability for adolescents are summarised in Table 14.7. Additional sources for more in-depth information are listed in the Further Reading list.

- **Additional diagnostics:** consider STI and cervical screening if history suggests increased risk (see Sec. 14.5).

- **Pharmacotherapeutics:** method-specific, (see Table 14.7).

- **Behavioural interventions:** see below.

- **Patient education:**
  - see Table 14.7
  - distinguish between 'safe sex' (i.e. sexual activities that carry minimal or no risk of spreading HIV) and 'safer sex' (i.e. sexual activities that reduce the risk of transmitting HIV but are not completely safe)
  - reinforce idea that any sexual activity that includes penetrative sex carries the risk of acquiring or spreading HIV
  - encourage adolescents to use the 'double Dutch' method of contraception (barrier methods to protect from sexually transmitted infections and an additional method, such as the pill, to prevent pregnancy).

FOLLOW-UP

- See Table 14.7.
- Follow-up includes confirmation that the adolescent remains happy with her contraceptive choice; correct use continues; and questions are answered.
- If using hormonal contraception, weight and blood pressure should be checked and enquiries made about any adverse effects experienced. Confirm that there have not been any changes in her medical and family history.

MEDICAL CONSULT/ SPECIALIST REFERRAL

- Concurrent or significant medical illnesses (e.g neurological, cardiac, haematological) and/or a past history of an illness where the diagnosis may have been uncertain, e.g. deep vein thrombosis.
- Suspected abuse—the adolescent must be informed that confidentiality will have to be broken.
- If a sexually transmitted infection is suspected.
- If the adolescent is pregnant: refer for antenatal care or for a termination of pregnancy.
- If abnormal pelvic pathology is suspected, a vaginal or abdominal ultrasound should be requested.

PAEDIATRIC PEARLS

- If the adolescent is adamant that parents should remain unaware of her sexual activity (and thus there is reluctance to use pills or condoms in case these are discovered at home), advise ways of broaching discussion with a parent; offer ideas for remembering to take pills regularly if they are to be hidden; and/or consider an injectable method which might be more suitable in this situation.
- The key to a successful consultation with adolescents is to ensure they have made an informed choice and are confident about their decision. This means helping them to understand the methods available and to weigh up the advantages, disadvantages and side-effects in relation to their own lifestyle and relationship.
- Careful teaching of the chosen method is vital and all information must be backed up with leaflets (excellent ones are available from the Family Planning Association). Adolescents should be given clinic times and phone numbers and encouraged to seek advice promptly should an unexpected problem arise.
- Young women often request a pregnancy test but, with careful questioning, what they really require is emergency contraception.
- Although it is preferable to see a young girl on her own, she will often find it more supportive to have a friend with her.

RESOURCES

Brook Advisory Centres (National Office tel: 0800-0185023): will provide details of local clinics nationwide that provide contraception, abortion advice, counselling and health information.

Family Planning Association (FPA): 2–12 Pentonville Road, London N1 9FP: tel: 0845-310-1334 (general helpline).

Sex Education Forum: National Children's Bureau, 8 Wakely Street, London EC1V 7QE: tel: 020-7843-6052. Fact sheets and publications.

Table 14.7 Methods of Contraception

Method	Advantages	Disadvantages	Patient education	Follow-up
Abstinence	• No risk of pregnancy • No risk of sexually transmitted infections (STIs) • No medication or products	• Requires self-esteem and ability to counter peer pressure	• Need encouragement to develop negotiating skills (can be rehearsed in role play/scenarios) • Mutual masturbation or massage are suitable alternatives	• Check still happy with method
Barrier methods: • condoms • diaphragms (with spermicide)	• Easily obtainable • Protection from STIs and human immunodeficiency virus (HIV) • Condoms (if used correctly) 98% effective. Men take responsibility for contraception • Can include spermicidal lubricant for extra protection	• Must be used every time • Can split if not used correctly or oil-based lubricants used • Putting on a condom or inserting a diaphragm can interrupt sex so may not be used every time • Diaphragms rarely used in this age group (users need to be able to feel their cervix)	• Should be taught how to put a condom on a plastic model (preferably in the dark!) • Need to be aware of how to obtain emergency contraception if necessary	• Encourage to always have a small supply available • Check being used correctly and no penetration occurs without a condom

Combined oral contraceptive pill (COC)	• Over 99% effective
	• Ideal method for young people
	• Many non-contraceptive benefits:
	  • regulates periods
	  • reduces dysmenorrhoea and menorrhagia
	  • protects against ovarian and endometrial cancer
	• Many different formulations
		• Must remember to take daily
		• Initial minor side-effects such as breast tenderness and nausea
		• Small risk of deep vein thrombosis
			• Must be started within first 5 days of period (additional method should be used for 1 week if started on any day after day 1)
			• Needs careful teaching about:
			  • ideas to remember daily pill
			  • what to do if late with pill
			  • interacting drugs
			  • what to do if vomiting or diarrhoea
				• After 3 months increase to 6-monthly if no problems
				• Check taking correctly and understands rules for missed pills
				• Remind of the need to use condoms in addition to the pill—particularly if starting a new relationship

Progestogen-only pill (POP)	• Suitable for those who have contraindications to the COC • Suitable if breast-feeding	• Not ideal for this age group as requires very reliable, regular pill taking	• Not generally suitable for those with a chaotic lifestyle, so importance of a regular routine to be stressed	• After 3 months increase to 6-monthly if no problems • Check taking correctly and understands rules for missed pills
Injections	• Over 99% effective • No anxiety about regular pill taking—ideal for those who are forgetful • No obvious reminder of contraception—useful if parents not aware of sexual activity • Only given every 12 weeks (Depo-Provera) or 8 weeks (Noristerat) • Periods usually much lighter—may have amenorrhoea	• Can get irregular bleeding • Amenorrhoea may cause parental anxiety if unaware of sexual activity • Possible weight gain • Periods may take 1 year to return to a regular pattern (important if wanting to become pregnant)	• Must be started in first 5 days of cycle with deep intramuscular injection • Explain irregular bleeding common in first few months • Emphasise importance of not being late for next injection	• Every 8 or 12 weeks depending on type used • Check bleeding pattern and knowledge of next injection date

Method			
Implants	• Over 99% effective • Ideal if forgetful about pills or cannot attend for repeat prescriptions • Lasts for 3 years • Rapid return of fertility when removed	• Irregular bleeding • Possibility of weight gain	• Implanon is a single rod inserted subdermally in the upper arm • Local anaesthetic used—may be some bruising and tenderness for a day or two	• 3 months then 6-monthly • Check bleeding pattern and any untoward side-effects
Intrauterine device (IUD) and intrauterine system	• Over 98–99% effective, depending on device used • Effective immediately after insertion • Can stay in for 3–8 years, depending on type inserted	• Rarely used in this age group unless in monogamous relationship due to increased risk of STIs and potential problems of insertion in a young adolescent • Can cause heavier and more painful periods	• Careful counselling about need for barrier contraception if new partner • Should be taught how to feel for threads	• After 6 weeks then 6-monthly if no problems • Can she feel threads? • Is she in same relationship? • Any pelvic pain or dyspareunia?
Emergency contraception	*Oral:* • Can be used up to 72 hours after unprotected sex, but more effective if taken earlier • Levonelle-2 available from pharmacists without prescription if over 16 years • Will prevent at least three out of four pregnancies that would occur if no emergency contraception taken *Copper IUD:* • Can be fitted up to 5 days after unprotected sex or within 5 days of earliest time of ovulation • Very effective (nearly 100%) • Offers ongoing contraception	*Oral:* • Rarely feel nauseated or sick *IUD:* • Consider testing for STIs and giving prophylactic antibiotics	• Emergency contraception is for emergencies only—other methods of contraception are more effective • Is continuing contraception needed? • Ensure adequate knowledge of other methods	• Must return for pregnancy test if period late • Re-attend for removal of IUD after period if not continuing with method • If continuing with IUD, follow-up required 6 weeks after insertion
Natural family planning	• No hormones used • No side-effects • Gives a greater awareness of her body	• Not recommended in this age group due to irregular cycle lengths and less predictable pattern of intercourse • Higher failure rate	• Enables information to be given regarding timing of maximum fertility • Needs careful teaching from a trained teacher	
Withdrawal	• No medication or products	• Requires self-control • High failure rate (pre-ejaculate contains sperm) • No protection from STIs	• Sex is frequently unplanned—encourage both sexes to carry condoms • Young men need to have the sexual finesse to withdraw in time	• Encourage to use a more effective method

BIBLIOGRAPHY

Andrews G. Women's sexual Health, 2nd edn. London: Baillière Tindall; 2001.

Belfield T. FPA contraceptive handbook: the essential reference guide for family planning and other health professionals, 3rd edn. London: FPA; 1999.

Contraceptive Education Service (CES). Young people: sexual attitudes and behaviour. Factsheet No. 7. London: Contraceptive Education Service; 1998.

Department of Health. Seeking consent: working with children. London: Department of Health; 2001. Available online: http://www.doh.gov.uk/consent

Garden AS. Paediatric gynaecology: an overview of current practice. Hospital Med 1998; 59(3):232–235.

Harrison T. Children and sexuality: perspectives in health care. London: Baillière Tindall; 1998.

National Health Service Cervical Screening Programme (NHSCSP). A national priority review. Sheffield: NHSCSP; 1999.

Office for National Statistics. Birth statistics. London: The Stationery Office; 1998.

Social Exclusion Unit. Teenage pregnancy. London: The Stationery Office; 1999.

Stevens-Simon C. Providing effective reproductive health care and prescribing contraceptives for adolescents. Pediatr Rev 1998; 19(12):409–417.

14.5 SEXUALLY TRANSMITTED INFECTIONS (STIs)

Dolsie Allen

INTRODUCTION

- Sexually transmitted infections (STIs) continue in epidemic proportions in the adolescent population. Within the UK, the number of diagnoses of gonorrhoea, genital chlamydia and genital warts has risen steadily over the last 5 years. As with previous years, rises were sharpest in teenage males and females.
- Gonorrhoea diagnoses in England have risen steadily from 1995 to 1999, with a total rise of 56%. Infection can often be asymptomatic, particularly in females. Serious complications include infertility and ectopic pregnancy.
- Chlamydia diagnoses have almost doubled since 1995 (from 29,286 to 51,863 cases in 1999). The rise occurred in all regions and both sexes, with the sharpest increase occurring in males and females under 20 years of age. Many cases of chlamydial infection are asymptomatic and thus go undiagnosed. Long-term complications can be severe, especially for females, where it can lead to pelvic inflammatory disease (PID), ectopic pregnancy and infertility.
- Genital warts in England have also risen steadily. Between 1995 and 1999, diagnoses of warts in 16–19-year-old males increased by 74%. The rise in females was also greatest among 16–19 year olds. Warts are caused by the human papilloma virus (HPV), with certain types of warts associated with cervical cancer.
- Using a detailed history and physical examination, a degree of 'risk' can be assigned based on the adolescent's sexual behaviour and presenting symptoms. Screening tests and treatment can then be initiated as history and examination dictates. Box 14.1 outlines indicators of increased risk of STI.
- Establishing a trusting environment is critical when interviewing the adolescent. Studies show that when adolescents are assured of confidentiality, they are much more likely to provide reliable information (see Ch. 3).

Box 14.1 Indicators of increased risk of sexually transmitted infection (STI)
• Early age of sexual intercourse
• Multiple sex partners
• Sexual abuse or rape
• Sex with homosexual or bisexual male
• History of past STI(s)
• Alcohol and drug use, intravenous (IV) drug use (self and partner)
• Prostitution
• Anal sex

PATHOPHYSIOLOGY

- Each pathogen has its own unique pathophysiology with regard to incubation time, mode of transmission, communicability and mechanisms of infection. However, for the most part, all STIs are transmissible via genital mucosal exposure to semen, blood, vaginal secretions and vesicular fluids.
- Adolescent females are particularly at risk of acquiring STIs due to columnar epithelium extending into the exocervical surface area.
- In general, bacterial STIs tend to have relatively short incubation periods and are usually easy to cure (once diagnosed). Conversely, viral STIs often have longer incubation periods and, although many symptoms can be treated, the disease itself is most often not curable.

HISTORY

- Date of last menstrual period.
- Current medications.

- Information regarding current symptoms: onset and frequency (constant, intermittent and relationship to menses) of symptoms; colour, consistency and odour of drainage; presence of bleeding; postcoital symptoms.

- Information regarding associated symptoms: fever and chills; abdominal and pelvic pain; joint pain and myalgia; nausea, vomiting and diarrhoea; dysuria and haematuria; genital itching, swelling and/or burning; ulcerations and sores; presence of rashes.

- **Social history:** age of first sexual activity; frequency of sexual contacts; number of sexual partners; last sexual intercourse; sexual preferences; known contact with STI risk; partner symptoms; drug, alcohol and tobacco use.

- **Past medical history:** previous STI/PID; pregnancy history; methods of contraception (oral and barrier); recent antibiotic use.

- **Personal hygiene:**
  - females: tampon use; douches, menstrual towels (if douche, when was last douche?).
  - males: time of last void.

PHYSICAL EXAMINATION

- **Initial examination:** it is important to observe the adolescent's overall appearance, affect and interpersonal communication, as these can sometimes provide clues to risky behaviour (e.g. drug/alcohol use, homelessness, etc.).

- **Skin:** rashes, lesions, ulceration.

- **Head and ENT:** erythema, leucoplakia, ulcers, thrush, cervical lymphadenopathy.

- **Abdomen:** organomegaly, tenderness (suprapubic, rebound), flank pain or costovertebral angle (CVA) tenderness.

- **STI specific findings:** these are outlined in Table 14.8.

- **External genitalia (female):** erythema, vaginal discharge, ulcerations, warts, urethral discharge, trauma, inflammation of Bartholin's and Skene's glands; inguinal lymphadenopathy.

- **External genitalia (male):** inguinal lymphadenopathy or hernia; ulcerations of scrotum; assessment of scrotal content (masses, tenderness); inspect epididymis for size, induration, tenderness; palpation of spermatic cord (tenderness); inspection and milking of urethral opening (discharge); inspect penile head with foreskin retracted (lesions, ulcerations, masses, warts).

- **Internal genitalia (female):**
  - Speculum examination: inspect vaginal walls for discharge, lesions, ulcerations, warts, foreign bodies. Check cervix for oedema, erythema, friability and discharge.
  - Bimanual examination: assess for cervical motion tenderness, adnexal tenderness and masses, uterine size, position and tenderness.

- **Perianal/rectum:** inspect for lesions, discharges, bleeding, ulcerations and/or warts.

DIFFERENTIAL DIAGNOSES

- STIs as outlined in Table 14.8; also consider physiological leucorrhoea, *Candida albicans*, contact dermatitis (e.g. latex allergy), urinary tract infection, retained foreign body (e.g. tampon, condom, diaphragm or other), HIV and the possibility of sexual abuse.

MANAGEMENT

- **Additional diagnostics:** (consider) urinalysis, urine culture with sensitivities, full blood count (FBC), pregnancy testing, wet mounts (saline and KOH), Venereal Disease Research Laboratories (VDRL), cervical smear, HIV testing, serological hepatitis testing, screening of partner (notification, examination and treatment) in addition to organism-specific diagnostics (Table 14.8).

- **Pharmacotherapeutics:** Organism-specific (Table 14.9).

- **Behavioural intervention:**
  - Abstinence from intercourse until patient and partner fully complete therapy and treatment. Should intercourse occur, *strongly* advise

condom use with spermicidal cream as barrier method.

- Avoid tampon use during treatment of STIs.
- Stress hygiene, cotton undergarments, no douching.
- During herpes simplex outbreak, use warm water poured over perineal area to facilitate voiding and lessen pain. For severe dysuria during herpes outbreak; suggest voiding while seated in a bathtub of warm water.
- After cleaning genital area, keep lesions as dry as possible. Suggest drying area with a hair dryer set at a cool temperature.
- Strongly advise condom usage with virucidal cream once genital symptoms resolve and always in presence of genital warts.
- Metronidazole—avoid all alcoholic beverages and medicines containing alcohol. May also affect the efficacy of combined oral contraceptives and, therefore, a barrier method of contraception should be recommended for use for the remainder of the cycle.
- Doxycycline—increases photosensitivity. Use sunscreen.

- **Patient education:**
  - Strongly advise and counsel patient regarding additional testing for HIV and hepatitis. Recommended for all patients with documented STI; sexual contact with known infected individual; intravenous (IV) drug use by patient or partner; sexual contact with homosexual or bisexual male; rape victims; and sexual contact without condoms.
  - Stress importance of patient and partner completing all medications concurrently.
  - Review 'safe and safer' sex protection practices with patient and partner.
  - Syphilis: counsel patient with regard to *Jarisch–Herxheimer* reaction (development of fever, malaise, chills and worsening of symptoms for 6–12 hours after injection; occurs in 50% of cases and persists for 24 hours).
  - Discuss with patient and partner the importance of avoiding STIs with regards to future fertility status.

Table 14.8 Sexually Transmitted Infection (STI) Physical Examination Findings and Organism-Specific Diagnostics

Infection	Incubation	Patient complaints	Examination findings	Additional diagnostics
Chlamydia trachomatis	• 7–21 days	• Females: pelvic pain, watery, purulent drainage, postcoital bleeding. *Note that 80% may be asymptomatic* • Males: dysuria with scant grey discharge and/or scrotal pain. *Note that 50% may be asymptomatic*	• Females: mucopurulent vaginal drainage; friable cervix, +ve chandelier sign, bartholinitis, salpingitis and pelvic inflammatory disease (PID) • Males: urethritis, scant grey discharge	• Endocervical swab for cells (not just drainage); *note that specimen collection technique important* • Chlamydia antigen swab • Direct immunofluorescent monoclonal antibody (Micro-trak) • Concomitant screening for gonorrhoea • Culture is gold standard diagnostic required for legal documentation in abuse cases
Neisseria gonorrhoeae	• 3–7 days	• Females: labial pain and swelling, purulent vaginal drainage, sore throat. *Note that 50% may be asymptomatic* • Males: scrotal pain, white creamy discharge, painful urination. *Note that 10% may be asymptomatic*	• Females: Bartholin's and/or Skene's abscess, purulent vaginal drainage, inflamed vulva, mucopurulent cervicitis, urethritis, joint pain with rash • Males: penile discharge, urethritis, joint pain with rash	• Endocervical swab for cells • Pharyngeal, rectal and urethral swabs (as indicated) • Thayer–Martin culture or DNA GenProbe • Screen for Chlamydia • Blood cultures with disseminated disease (i.e. if rash present)
Trichomonas vaginalis	• 7–30 days	• Females: dysuria, vaginal pruritus, frothy green vaginal drainage, foul odour • Males: dysuria, penile drainage. *Note: 15–50% may be asymptomatic*	• Females: friable, 'strawberry cervix', green, frothy foul smelling drainage • Males: urethral drainage	• Obtain sample of drainage with cotton swab • Saline wet mount—view motile trichomads • Endocervical swabs for gonorrhoea and Chlamydia • Lateral vaginal wall with pH > 5
Bacterial vaginosis (Gardnerella)	• Diffuse organisms often found. Not exclusively sexually transmitted (organisms can be part of normal flora)	• Females: watery vaginal drainage with fishy odour (worsens after intercourse), dysuria, pelvic discomfort	• Females: little or no vaginal or vulval erythema, thin watery discharge, +ve 'whiff' test	• Obtain sample of drainage with cotton swab • Saline wet mount—view 'clue' cells • 'Whiff' test (10% potassium hydroxide solution reveals 'fishy odour' when dropped onto swab) • Endocervical swabs for gonorrhoea and Chlamydia • Lateral vaginal wall with pH > 5
Herpes simplex (HSV-2)	• 2–14 days (long latency period)	• Painful genital ulcerations, vesicles and sores • Dysuria, urinary retention • Fever and malaise • Tender inguinal nodes	• Tender inguinal lymphadenopathy (speculum examination may be impossible) • Multiple clear, fluid-filled vesicles over external genitalia, rectal and perineal areas • Crusting of some ulceration with eroded base • Fever • Distension of suprapubic area	• Diagnosis upon clinical inspection • Viral culture of ruptured vesicle on genitalia or cervix • Swab of ulcer base • Cervical smear • Venereal Disease Research Laboratories (VDRL)

Organism	Incubation	Clinical features	Diagnosis
Human papilloma virus (HPV) Condylomata acuminata (genital warts)	• 90 days to several years (highly variable)	• Warty growth on genitals; in males it may partially obstruct urinary meatus • Genital itching or burning • Genital bleeding of 'wart' • May be asymptomatic • Papillomatous lesion noted on vaginal areas, penis and/or perineal areas • Lesion is soft, pink, flesh-coloured • Cervical smear, noting koilocytes	• Visual inspection • Inspection may be aided by application of 3% acetic acid, which may reveal flat, discreet lesions • Cervical smear to detect cellular changes and/or presence of koilocytes • Proctoscopic anal inspection for warts • Cutaneous biopsy of lesions for definitive diagnosis • VDRL • Evaluate for concurrent existence of other STIs
Treponema pallidum (primary syphilis)	• 3–90 days	• Often asymptomatic • Painless solitary sore noted on external genitalia or oral area • Chancre lesion is non-tender with 'punched-in' centre and indurated border • Non-tender lymphadenopathy • Chancre heals spontaneously in 3–10 weeks	• Definitive diagnosis via direct, dark-field microscopy to document *T. pallidum* • VDRL (non-treponemal) test may be negative for up to 10 weeks • Initial non-reactive VDRL: should be repeated in 1 week, 1 month and 3 months when lesion is suspicious for syphilis and dark-field exam is unavailable • Direct fluorescent antibody test (DFA-TP) • Rule out concomitant STIs
Treponema pallidum (secondary syphilis)	• 30–90 days	• Warty growth on genitalia • Generalised rash (especially on palms and soles of feet) • Headache and malaise • Genital condylomata • Copper-coloured, maculopapular rash • Anaemia, alopecia, oral mucous patches • Generalised lymphadenopathy	• VDRL • *Treponema pallidum* haemagglutination (TPHA) • Enzyme-linked immunosorbent assay (ELISA) methods • Rule out concomitant STIs • Note that a +ve VDRL in the absence of syphilis is termed a biological false positive (BFP). A BFP must always be proven not to represent syphilis • BFP may be caused by glandular fever, coagulation disorders, Lyme disease, malaria, viral pneumonia and lupus

Note: Avoid doxycycline and tetracycline in children under the age of 12 years and pregnant women.

Table 14.9 Sexually Transmitted Infection (STI) Pharmacotherapeutics and Follow-up

Infection	Drug of choice	Alternative choice	Follow-up
Chlamydia trachomatis	• Doxycycline 100 mg PO BID for 7 days or Azithromycin 1 g PO once (do not use if pregnant)	• Erythromycin 500 mg PO four times daily for 7 days or Erythromycin 500 mg PO twice daily for 14 days (first choice in pregnancy)	• If no response to treatment or possibility of reinfection • Gonorrhoea cultures if not done previously • VDRL if not done previously • Consider test of cure 3 weeks after completion of treatment with erythromycin
Neisseria gonorrhoeae	• Cefriaxone 250 mg IM once plus doxycycline 100 mg PO twice daily for 7 days or Azithromycin 1 g PO once	• Amoxicillin 3 g PO once plus Probenecid 1 g PO once plus treatment for chlamydia	• Test of cure is recommended at least 72 hours after completed treatment • Chlamydia swab if not tested/treated previously • VDRL if not done previously
Trichomonas vaginalis	• Metronidazole 2 g PO once • Counsel regarding no alcohol during treatment	• Metronidazole 200–400 mg PO twice daily for 7 days	• None necessary unless symptoms persist or recur after treatment
Bacterial vaginosis (Gardnerella)	• Metronidazole 2 g PO once or metronidazole gel 0.75% one application intravaginally once daily for 5 days (unlicensed use)	• Clindamycin cream 2% one applicator intravaginally each evening for 7 nights or Metronidazole 400–500 mg PO twice daily for 7 days	• None necessary unless symptoms persist or recur after treatment
Herpes simplex (HSV-2)	• Aciclovir 200 mg PO five times daily for 5 days	• Aciclovir cream 5% topically five times daily for 5 days	• As symptoms dictate • Follow-up secondary bacterial infections of HSV lesions • If suspected ocular lesions referral indicated • Follow cervical smear testing • VDRL if none done previously
Human papilloma virus (HPV) Condylomata acuminata (genital warts)	• Podophyllum resin (15%) applied weekly. Allow to remain on lesions for 6 hours then wash off. Protect surrounding skin • Note: contraindicated in pregnancy, breast-feeding and children • Liquid nitrogen treatments appropriate substitute	• Podophyllotoxin (Warticon) 0.15%: apply to area twice daily for 3 consecutive days. Treatment may be repeated at weekly intervals • Contraindicated in pregnancy, breast-feeding and children • Cryosurgery is acceptable alternative	• Follow weekly for 4–8 weeks during treatment • Re-treat If warts recur • Follow cervical smear every 6 months until normal • VDRL if not done previously
Treponema pallidum (primary, secondary or early latent syphilis)	• Procaine penicillin 600,000 units (Jenacillin A) IM once daily for 10–14 days or benzylpenicillin benzathine 2.4 g IM weekly for 2 weeks • Penicillin allergy: doxycycline 200 mg twice a day for 14 days • Parenteral treatment refused: amoxicillin 500 mg four times a day plus probenecid four times a day (Doherty et al., 2002)	• Erythromycin 500 mg PO four times daily for 14 days or doxycycline 100 mg PO BID for 14 days	• Serology tests for syphilis should be done at 3-, 6- and 12-months intervals • Falling titre should be demonstrated if treatment is adequate
Treponema pallidum (secondary syphilis)	As above	• Erythromycin 500 mg PO four times daily for 21 days or doxycycline 100 mg PO twice daily for 21 days	• As above

Note: Re-evaluate outpatient follow-up and symptomatology of pelvic inflammatory disease (PID) within 24 hours—sooner, if symptoms fail to improve. Re-examine (pelvic and bimanual examinations) after treatment course completed and review culture results.
BID = twice a day; IM = intramuscularly; PO = orally; VDRL = Venereal Disease Research Laboratories.

⇨ FOLLOW-UP

- See Table 14.9.

⇄ MEDICAL CONSULT/ SPECIALIST REFERRAL

- Any patient with the following documented STIs is to be referred to an NHS Health Advisor for contact tracing (and concurrent treatment) of current and/or recent sexual contacts: chlamydia, genital herpes, gonorrhoea, syphilis, condylomata acuminata.
- Any child or adolescent in whom there is a suspicion of sexual abuse and assault. This includes children with documented gonorrhoea, genital herpes, *Chlamydia trachomatis* and/or syphilis infections.
- Any patient that is pregnant.
- Any patient with seizure disorders requiring metronidazole due to a potential interaction with anticonvulsant medications (phenytoin, phenobarbital) and has been associated with epilepiform seizures (rare).
- Any patient with suspected herpetic ocular lesions.
- Condylomata acuminata patients who are pregnant and/or have abnormal cervical smears, cervical lesions or lesions on rectal mucosa. These patients are likely to require biopsy of the lesion(s).

- Any child or adolescent with a gravely ill appearance or one requiring a more extensive evaluation.

♂ PAEDIATRIC PEARLS

- Any patient who presents with genital ulcerations or lesions needs a VDRL to be screened for syphilis.
- Always treat patient's partner(s).
- When treating chlamydia, always provide treatment for assumed concurrent gonorrhoea infection.
- Positive VDRL is syphilis unless proven otherwise.
- 1% of positive VDRLs are false-positives due to possible glandular fever, lupus, malaria, Lyme disease and coagulation disorders.
- All patients with human papilloma virus (HPV) require a cervical smear.
- Doxycycline and tetracycline are contraindicated in children <12 years of age. Likewise, do not use with pregnant women.
- Avoid metronidazole in pregnancy, breast-feeding and in patients with renal compromise.
- If possible choose medications that cure in one dose to avoid patient error.
- When one STI is documented, always search for additional infections. Likewise, the possibility of sexual abuse needs to be considered as a potential aetiology when an adolescent is being treated for a STI.
- Always consider pregnancy testing when dealing with sexually active adolescents.

▤ BIBLIOGRAPHY

Adelman W, Joffe A. The adolescent male genital examination: what's normal and what's not. Contemp Pediatr 1999; 16(7):76–92.

Andrews G. Women's sexual health, 2nd edn. London: Baillière Tindall; 2001.

Clayton B, Krowchuk D. Skin findings and STDs. Contemp Pediatr 1997; 14(9):119–137.

Doherty L, Fenton KA, Jones J, et al. Syphilis: old problem, new strategy. BMJ 2002; 325(7356):153–156.

Fenstermacher K, Hudson B. Practice guidelines for family nurse practitioners. Philadelphia: WB Saunders; 1997:281–284.

Garden AS. Paediatric gynaecology: an overview of current practice. Hospital Med 1998; 59(3):232–235.

Hawkins JW, Nichols DM, Haney JS. Protocols for nurse practitioners in gynecologic settings, 5th edn. New York: Tiresias Press; 1995.

Lappa S, Moscicki A. The pediatrician and the sexually active adolescent. Pediatr Clin North Am 1997; 44(6):1405–1445.

Pimenta J, Catchpole M, Gray M, et al. Evidence based health policy report: screening for genital chlamydial infection. BMJ 2000; 321(7261):629–631.

Public Health Laboratory Service (PHLS). Clinical effectiveness group: UK national guidelines. London: AGUM; 2000.

Taylor-Robinson D. *Chlamydia trachomatis* and sexually transmitted disease. BMJ 1994; 308:150–151.

14.6 PAINFUL MALE GENITALIA

Peter Wilson

▢ INTRODUCTION

- The three major areas of the male genitalia to consider are the penis, scrotum/testes and inguinal regions.
- Problems arising with the male genitalia are often age-dependent.

- In children, the major penile complications are trauma, infection and phimosis. The major scrotal problems are testicular torsion (which is the only true testicular surgical emergency), trauma, varicocele, hydrocele, orchitis and epididymitis.

The major inguinal problems are hernias.
- Urinary tract infections and viral illnesses (e.g. orchitis) may cause painful genitalia. In addition, an unexplained discharge is always suspicious and a careful history

should be taken to rule out child protection issues and/or sexually transmitted infections.

PATHOPHYSIOLOGY

- The *penis* consists of the shaft and the glans. The urinary meatus should open at the tip of the glans. If it does not, and opens along the base of the penis, it is known as a hypospadias. This can be associated with other genital or renal abnormalities. The foreskin at birth is completely adherent to the glans. It becomes progressively more retractile through childhood, so that by 6–12 years of age it is fully retractile. Phimosis occurs where the foreskin cannot be retracted. This can be either physiological (the foreskin has not completed its normal separation from the glans) or pathological (the foreskin can no longer be retracted, despite it having been previously retractable). This is most commonly due to scarring from inflammation or infection. Paraphimosis occurs when the foreskin has been retracted but cannot be returned to normal. This is most commonly due to trauma from forceful retraction of the foreskin. It results in a swollen tight foreskin that causes congested (and therefore decreased) blood flow to the glans. If left untreated it could result in a necrotic glans.
- The *scrotum* and its contents can be divided into four sections: scrotum, testes, spermatic cord and epididymis. The testes are each encased in a fascial sheath called the tunica albuginea. Two-thirds of a testicle's volume is made up of the seminiferous tubules. Therefore, small testes normally indicate decreased/absent spermatogenesis. The left testicle is normally lower than the right. There is an appendix testis, found at the superior pole of the testis, in 90% of males. In younger children the testes may be retracted due to a strong cremasteric reflex. The epididymis is found along the posterolateral wall of the testis, and is made up of many efferent ducts joining the testis and the spermatic cord. It attaches the testes to the scrotal wall. The appendix

epididymis is attached to the head of the epididymis. The spermatic cord contains blood vessels, nerves, the vas deferens and the cremasteric muscle. The blood vessels are made up by the pampiniform plexus, which runs down the spermatic cord around the vas deferens. When abnormally dilated, they form a varicocele, which can be felt as a 'bag of worms'. The vas deferens carries the sperm from the testes. They can be absent, as in cystic fibrosis, or unilateral, as in ipsilateral renal agenesis. It is normally felt as a smooth rubbery tube.
- The *inguinal region* consists of the external inguinal ring, inguinal ligament (which runs from the anterior superior iliac spine to the symphysis pubis) and the internal inguinal ring. The forming testes pass through the inguinal canal in a fibrous sheath called the processus vaginalis. This sheath normally disappears once the testes have entered the scrotum. If it does not, this patent processus vaginalis can result in fluid (hydrocele) or omentum (inguinal hernia) entering the scrotum.
- Figure 14.1 outlines male genital structures.

HISTORY

- Location, onset, duration and type of pain (i.e. penile, scrotal or testicular pain).
- Additional symptoms (e.g. fever, urinary symptoms, nausea, vomiting, etc.).
- History of trauma and its relationship to the pain.
- Sexual history.
- Recent infection and/or viral illness.
- Past medical history.
- Other genitourinary problems (e.g. undescended testicle, bladder or renal problems, urinary tract infections).
- Family history of genitourinary problems.
- Home management and treatment used previously (including results).
- Table 14.10 outlines important historical information specific to common causes of painful male genitalia.

PHYSICAL EXAMINATION

- Examining a child with painful genitalia can be very distressing for

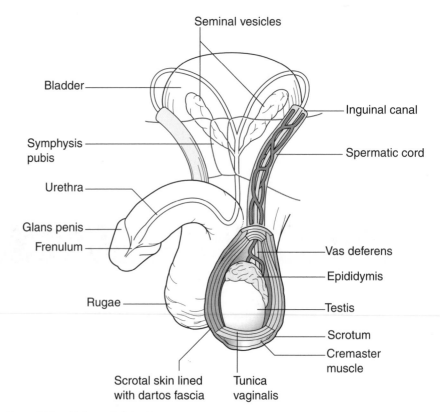

Figure 14.1 Male genital structures.

Table 14.10 History, Physical Examination Findings, Diagnostics and Management of Common Causes of Painful Male Genitals

Problem	History	Physical examination	Additional diagnostics	Management	Comments
Balanitis	• Malodorous discharge • May complain of ulcers and erosion • May have history of irritation (chemical irritant or hair caught around coronal sulcus) • May have history of unprotected sexual intercourse indicative of STI (urethritis and urethral discharge) • Complaints of urinary frequency and/or dysuria • Fever not uncommon	• Inflammation and erythema of the glans and prepuce • May have discharge with oedema of glans • Syphilis will cause erosion and multiocular pustules • Anaerobic infection will result in erosion and ulceration • Candidal infection will have glazed appearance with satellite pustules	• Routine culture and sensitivity with sexually transmitted infection (STI) cultures if appropriate. (Include dark-field staining to rule out *Treponema pallidum*) • Gram stain	• Frequent warm water (no soap) bathing of penile head • If superficial; topical antibiotic ointment, if cellulitis, systemic antibiotics • If STI-related, treat partner	• In young boys and men with recurrent episodes, circumcision is often recommended; circumcision not indicated for a single episode • Swimming pools do not cause • Stress good penile hygiene • If STI-related, discuss issues surrounding unprotected intercourse • If bubble bath is used in bath water, discontinue (eliminate potential irritants) • Can be associated with a phimosis as the urine collects under the foreskin, creating an ideal breeding ground for pathogens
Epididymitis	• Complaints of pain (mild) worsening over several days • Complaints of urinary frequency and/or dysuria • Fever not uncommon	• Fever • Tender, swollen, erythematous scrotum	• Urine dipstick for haematuria and/or urine microscopy • Consider Doppler ultrasound of the testes/scrotum to rule out testicular torsion	• Antibiotics required	• If pain resolves and then returns a few days later, consider traumatic epididymitis • Previous history of viral illness (especially mumps) or urinary tract infection suggests epididymo-orchitis or urethritis • Renal ultrasound and micturating cystourethrogram necessary for confirmed cases of epididymitis (rule out renal pathology) • History of neurogenic bladder or congenital renal abnormality (hydronephrosis, duplex ureters, etc.) is associated with increased risk of epididymitis
Henoch–Schönlein purpura (HSP)	• History of purpura (classic of HSP), arthralgia, colicky abdominal pain	• Purpura on extensor surfaces and buttocks • Haematuria	• Urine dipstick for haematuria • Full blood count (FBC) • Clotting screen	• Medical management and supportive care	• FBC and clotting screen are normal
Hydrocele	• Complaints of acute scrotal swelling (can be marked) that is painless • More obvious when patient lying for a long time	• Painless scrotal swelling • Swelling transilluminates • Can get 'above' swelling during examination of testes/scrotum • Enlarges with crying	• Not usually indicated • Transillumination	• Supportive care • Reassurance regarding self-resolving nature of hydrocele • Analgesics if mild discomfort	
Infection	• Complaints of penile pain • May have symptoms indicative of STI or urinary tract infection • May have history of preceding viral illness (especially mumps) or urinary tract complaints	• STIs with discharge and/or lesions • May have normal examination	• Haematuria • Penile discharge	• Antibiotics (dependent on organism and sensitivities) • May be required for as long as 6 weeks	• Urinary symptoms in addition to penile or scrotal pain suggest epididymo-orchitis or urethritis
Inguinal hernia	• Swelling of groin area • Intermittent scrotal pain (reducible inguinal hernia). If severe scrotal pain, hernia may be incarcerated	• Inguinal swelling • Cannot get 'above' swelling during examination of scrotum • Mass does not transilluminate • If hernia present, check reducibility • If strangulated: skin is red and painful	• Not usually indicated • Doppler ultrasound if diagnosis unclear	• Will require surgical reduction (which is urgent if hernia is strangulated) if manual reduction unsuccessful	• Manual reduction includes pain relief, opiates and gentle pressure • Surgery is an attempt to prevent bowel ischaemia and necrosis

(continued)

Table 14.10 continued

Problem	History	Physical examination	Additional diagnostics	Management	Comments
Penile trauma	• Pain associated with trauma (saddle-type injury or blunt abdominal trauma) • May complain of 'bloody urine'	• Abdominal and/or pelvic tenderness • Frank haematuria (urethral traumas)	• Urine dipstick for haematuria; if positive, urethral trauma likely • Consider retrograde urethrogram • Consider computed tomography (CT) scan of abdomen and pelvis (if extensive injuries)	• Repair of urethra • Mild analgesics for benign injury	• Potentially very serious, especially if mechanism of injury is that of falling astride a bar (may result in transection of the urethra) • If haematuria and/or pain does not settle quickly (especially if associated with micturation), refer immediately • Never insert urethral catheter (suprapubic only) • Important to establish whether bladder trauma or urethral transection when frank haematuria present
Phimosis	• Inability to retract foreskin • History of previous infection, inflammation or trauma associated with attempts to retract foreskin	• Thickened edge of foreskin • Unable to retract foreskin	• None usually required	• Ongoing hygiene • If severe and recurrent infections, circumcision may be necessary	• Important to educate parents about normal expectations regarding foreskin retraction and importance of hygiene
Paraphimosis	• Foreskin unable to be pushed over glans • Painful penis that is associated with a swollen glans and retracted foreskin	• Swollen, congested glans	• None	• Manual reduction of glans • Will require anaesthesia (penile block)	
Scrotal trauma	• History of trauma	• Painful scrotum • May have swelling and redness	• Consider Doppler	• Mild trauma should settle • Safety counselling • If ruptured or torsed testicle surgery likely required	• Pain should settle within 1–2 hours; if persist may be due to rupture or torsed testicle
Testicular torsion	• Severe scrotal pain of abrupt onset • Nausea and vomiting	• Tender, swollen, erythematous scrotum • High riding testicle and absent cremasteric reflex • Affected testis is larger and more tender than unaffected	• Consider Doppler ultrasound of the testes/scrotum (Doppler will indicate decreased arterial blood flow if testicular torsion)	• Surgery required for de-torsion (immediate)	• Testicle removed if unviable • Presence of cremasteric reflex makes testicular torsion unlikely • History of undescended testicle increases risk of testicular torsion and tumours
Testicular appendiceal torsion	• Complaints of pain (mild) worsening over several days	• Painful, red scrotum • Bluish discoloration of the superior aspect of the testis indicative of appendiceal torsion	• Consider Doppler ultrasound of the testes/scrotum	• Will require immediate surgical intervention	
Tumour	• Can present as painless mass (most common) or with pain (likely due to bleeding within tumour) • Often incidental finding	• Painless unilateral mass/testicular swelling	• Numerous (tumour markers, testicular ultrasound, biopsy, etc.)	• Surgery with or without chemo or radiation therapy (dependent on tumour)	• History of undescended testicle increases risk of testicular tumours and torsion
Varicocele	• Painless • Often incidental finding • May have history of dull ache or 'dragging' sensation	• Hypotrophic left testicle indicates decreased spermatogenesis • Spermatic cord feels like 'a bag of worms' • Small varicocele may present as thickened spermatic cord • More commonly occurs on the left • Size decreases when supine, increases with Valsalva manoeuvre	• Doppler ultrasound of the testes/scrotum (assessing testis size) • Semen analysis (determine degree of spermatogenesis)	• Large varicocele (with small testis) will likely require surgery	• Important to determine testicular function • If size of mass is unchanged when supine, consider lipoma of spermatic cord

both him and his parents. A chaperone should always be present, and the examination should be done in a relaxed and warm room. This not only allows the child to feel safe but also prevents the cremasteric reflex from retracting the testicles, which would make the examination very difficult. Table 14.10 outlines important examination findings for the more common causes of painful male genitalia.

- Perform a thorough general examination as testicular tumours and infections will likely manifest systemic findings (e.g. lymphadenopathy, vital sign changes). Determine the child's sexual maturity by using the Tanner staging technique (Sec. 12.7).

- **Abdomen/inguinal:** rule out masses, swelling (including renal swelling) and/or hepatosplenomegaly. Palpate the inguinal canal and external inguinal ring to rule out a mass (hernia or hydrocele). If there is a mass, and superior edge can be palpated, it is probably a hydrocele (which will also transilluminate). If superior edge cannot be determined and there is no transillumination, it is most likely a hernia. Ask patient to cough to check for any herniation of abdominal contents.

- **Penis/perineum:** inspect for warts, bacterial and/or fungal infection. Examine the penile meatus for discharge, redness, warts and hypospadias. In cases of trauma, the meatus should be inspected for frank haematuria. In uncircumcised males, the foreskin should be examined for phimosis and retracted so that the glans can be inspected for signs of infection or ulceration (syphilis, herpes, trauma). Do not retract the foreskin in children under 3 or 4 years of age as the foreskin might still be adherent to the glans. After the age of 5 years inability to retract the foreskin is known as phimosis. In children where there is the possibility of child protection issues, a superficial examination of the perineum and anus can be performed initially (with follow-up later on). A rectal examination should never be undertaken in these circumstances.

- **Scrotum:** initiate the cremasteric reflex before the scrotum and testes are examined (stroke the inner thigh to cause elevation of the testis on the same side). If present, then the presence of testicular torsion is highly unlikely. Inspect the scrotum for any evidence of erythema or discoloration of the skin (especially a bluish discoloration at the superior aspect of the testis, which is highly suggestive of an appendiceal torsion), oedema of the scrotal wall and the presence of any swellings. Unilateral swelling without pain or erythema suggests a hydrocele. Erythema, oedema and pain may be present in torsion and epididymitis. The presence of a high-riding testis and the lack of a cremasteric reflex would suggest it was a torsion rather than epididymitis. Palpate the testis and epididymis (normal side first) for any lumps, swellings and testicle size comparisons. It is important to palpate both testicles. If they rise into the inguinal canal they should be able to be palpated there. Alternatively, to prevent them from rising into the canal, ask the boy to sit cross-legged on the examination table (with testes hanging between folded legs). This usually kinks off the canal enough to prevent the testicles from retracting (especially in response to cold). The spermatic cord is palpated for the presence of a varicocele, which feels like a 'bag of worms'. The vas deferens carries the sperm from the testes. They can be absent, as in cystic fibrosis, or unilateral, as in ipsilateral renal agenesis. It is normally felt as a smooth rubbery tube.

⚛ DIFFERENTIAL DIAGNOSES

- The differential diagnoses of painful male genitalia have a developmental component (Table 14.11). Whereas paraphimosis can occur at any age, other problems are more common during certain ages. If a sexually transmitted infection (STI) is suspected, see Section 14.5.
- Common causes of painful male genitalia are outlined in Table 14.10.

✚ MANAGEMENT

- **Additional diagnostics:** aetiology-specific (Table 14.10); note that Doppler ultrasound is the most useful diagnostic tool in ruling out testicular torsion. A full blood count (FBC), urine microscopy and swab of genital discharge are also useful for many potential diagnoses.

- **Pharmacotherapeutics:** aetiology-specific; consider pain relief or if an infection is present, appropriate antimicrobials. Note that antibiotic choice is dependent on the organism isolated and its sensitivities. Antibiotics may be required for as long as 6 weeks.

- **Behavioural interventions:**
  - good genital hygiene
  - no retraction of the foreskin in young boys.

- **Patient education:**
  - Discuss the child's problem (diagnosis, management, prognosis and prevention).
  - Stress with parents (and children) the importance of good genital

Table 14.11	Causes of Painful Male Genitalia by Age Group
Age group	Consider
Newborn	**Penile:** congenital abnormalities such as hypospadias **Scrotal:** testicular torsion, trauma, hydrocele, inguinal hernia
Toddlers	**Penile:** balanitis **Scrotal:** Epididymo-orchitis, inguinal hernia, idiopathic scrotal oedema, Henoch–Schönlein purpura
5–10 years	**Penile:** urethritis, balanitis, phimosis, paraphimosis **Scrotal:** torsion of appendix, orchitis
Adolescents	**Penile:** sexually transmitted diseases, warts, paraphimosis **Scrotal:** testicular torsion, tumours, torsion testicular appendix, epididymitis, spermatoceles, varicoceles

hygiene and instruct them *not* to retract the foreskin in young boys (including the perils of phimosis).

- Outline the expected course the problem will take, signs and symptoms of problems and when/where to return.
- Reassure (if appropriate) the child and family regarding the impact the diagnosis will have on future genitourinary functioning. This includes the implications for subsequent fertility and sexual functioning (if appropriate).
- Encourage families to speak with their sons (and daughters) about STIs and their prevention. Likewise, adolescents should be counselled regarding the importance of STI prevention and barrier methods of contraception.
- Adolescent males should be instructed on testicular self-examination and encouraged to check their testicles routinely.

➡ FOLLOW-UP

- Aetiology-specific.
- Any infections (phimosis and/or paraphimosis) are likely to benefit from a follow-up home visit to assist with ongoing education of child and family.

⇄ MEDICAL CONSULT/ SPECIALIST REFERRAL

- Any child with acute scrotal pain should be referred immediately, as failure to act may result in necrosis of a testis.
- Any child with phimosis and paraphimosis.
- Any child with penile trauma who has frank haematuria.
- Any child with an inguinal hernia. If not incarcerated, an urgent outpatient appointment can be made. If incarcerated, immediate referral to a specialist is required.

♂ PAEDIATRIC PEARLS

- Examination of a child's genitalia can be extremely traumatic. They should feel relaxed and safe before any attempt is made to examine them.
- Acute scrotal pain is a medical emergency, as the only treatment for testicular torsion is immediate surgery.
- In children with epididymitis, always consider non-accidental injury.
- Never catheterise a child with penile trauma and frank haematuria.
- An embarrassed child may refer pain to abdomen; be sure to specifically enquire about painful genitalia and

thoroughly examine the penis, scrotum, testicles and inguinal area.
- Observation of the child lying on the couch (before the physical examination) will assist in assessing the degree of pain experienced.
- The relationship of any potential trauma to the genital pain is very important.
- Painless scrotal swelling is likely to be a hydrocele.
- A sexual history is essential in any adolescent with genital pain (rule out STI).

▤ BIBLIOGRAPHY

Adelman WP, Joffe A. The adolescent male genital examination: what's normal and what's not. Contemp Pediatr 1999; 16(7):76–92.

Bown MR, Cartwright PC, Snow BW. Common office problems in pediatric urology and gynecology. Pediatr Clin N Am 1997; 44:1091–1100.

Davenport M. Acute problems of the scrotum. BMJ 1996; 312:435–437.

Kass EJ, Lundak B. The acute scrotum. Pediatr Clin N Amer 1997; 44:1251–1266.

Kilham H, Isaacs I. General surgery. In: Kilham H, Isaacs I, eds, The New Children's Hospital Handbook. Melbourne: Children's Hospital; 1999:320–323.

Wilson-Storey D. Scrotal swellings in the under 5's. Arch Dis Child 1987; 62:50–52.

CHAPTER 15

Infectious Diseases and Haematology

15.1 ACUTE FEVER (<7 DAYS DURATION)

Katie Barnes

📖 INTRODUCTION

- Fever is a common complaint in paediatric practice, accounting for 10–20% of illness-related visits and 20–30% of after-hours calls. A large percentage of children with fever are <3 years old as they can average 4–6 infectious illnesses/year. The majority of illnesses presenting with fever are of viral aetiology, benign and self-limiting; however, assessment and decision making (especially in children <36 months of age with marked fevers) can be complicated.
- There are three categories of fever (Table 15.1).
- Fever without localising source (FWLS) can be a marker for serious bacterial illness (SBI) which includes: meningitis, bacteraemia, osteomyelitis, septic arthritis, pneumonia, bacterial gastroenteritis and serious skin/soft tissue infections. The risk of serious bacterial illness decreases with age;

those at greatest risk are neonates, infants under 3 months old and children from 3 months to 36 months of age. However, a missed diagnosis can result in significant sequelae.
- Occult bacteraemia (OB) complicates assessment and diagnosis as it often presents as a mild illness in conjunction with an upper respiratory tract infection (URTI), otitis media or urinary tract infection (UTI).
- Age influences the bacterial pathogens most likely to be involved in SBI/OB (Table 15.2). Likewise, selected physical examination findings have developmental dimensions:
  - infants and children with a UTI often present with very non-specific findings (poor feeding/appetite, irritability)
  - meningeal signs may not be present in children <16 months of age
  - infants <90 days of age may not mount a fever response despite acute infection.

- Objectives of the assessment and management of the acutely febrile child are:
  - differentiation of children who are seriously ill (e.g. at increased risk of serious bacterial illness or occult bacteraemia) from those that are not
  - identification of a focal infection from the history, physical examination and laboratory tests
  - implementation of management strategies that diminish the risk of secondary complications (sequelae from missed diagnosis or sequelae from diagnostic work-up, hospitalisation and/or use of antibiotics).

FEVER, AGE AND RISK OF SERIOUS BACTERIAL ILLNESS

- Age, appearance and degree of temperature elevation are the key components for establishing an individual child's risk of serious bacterial illness or occult bacteraemia when there is no localising source of infection. In general, the higher the temperature and the younger the age, the greater the risk (Table 15.2).
- Neonates and infants <3 months of age with rectal temperature ≥38°C are considered at *high risk* and require more aggressive assessment and management. Likewise, children 3–36 months with fever ≥39°C, that *do not* meet low-risk criteria (Box 15.1) are considered at increased risk and should be considered for more aggressive assessment and management.

Table 15.1	Categories of Fever
Category	*Description*
Acute fever *with* localising signs and symptoms	• Fever <7 days duration with diagnosis easily established from history and physical examination; laboratory tests usually not indicated (e.g. varicella or roseola)
Acute fever *without* localising source/ signs and symptoms (FWLS)	• Febrile episode that is <7 days in duration; history and physical examination do not establish the diagnosis, but laboratory tests might
Pyrexia of unknown origin (PUO)	• Fever lasting >7 days; history, physical examination and preliminary laboratory tests fail to reveal a source

Table 15.2   A Developmental Perspective of Bacterial Pathogens in Infants and Young Children

Age and fever	Bacterial pathogens	Prevalence of serious bacterial illness (SBI) and occult bacteraemia (OB)[a]
• 0–90 days • Temperature ≥ 38°C	• Group B streptococcus[b] • *Escherichia coli* • *Salmonella* spp. • *Streptococcus pneumoniae* • *Haemophilus influenzae* type B[c] • *Staphylococcus aureus*[c] • *Listeria monocytogenes*[c] • *Enterococcus*[c]	• SBI approx. 5–9% • OB approx. 3–4%
• 91 days to 36 months • Temperature ≥ 39°C	• *S. pneumoniae*[d] • *Neisseria meningitidis* • *Salmonella* spp.[c] • *Staphylococcus pyrogenes*[c] • *Staph. aureus*[c] • *E. coli*[c] • *Klebsiella pneumoniae*[c]	• OB[e] approx. 3–5%
• >36 months • Temperature ≥ 39°C	• *Staph. pyrogenes* • *E. coli* • *Staph. aureus* • *N. meningitidis*[c]	• Localised findings are generally reliable

[a] Prevalence rates may be overstated as much of the data were collected prior to widespread *H. influenzae* type B vaccination.

[b] Most common cause of SBI in young infants: approx. 73% of cases of SBI attributable to group B streptococcus.

[c] Uncommon.

[d] Responsible for approx. 70–90% of cases of occult bacteraemia in this age group.

[e] Occult bacteraemia most common in this age group because of declining maternal antibodies, bacterial colonisation of nasopharynx and increased contact with other ill children.

Sources: Avner, 1997; Baraff, 1993; Nizet, 1994.

Box 15.1.   Low-risk criteria for infants 3–36 months of age

- Non-toxic appearance (engagable without signs of irritability, lethargy, poor perfusion, poor feeding or cyanosis)

- Previously well infant/child (full term, no peri/postnatal complications, no history of antibiotic use or underlying illness) with good social situation (including telephone and responsible carer living within a reasonable distance from A&E department)

- No focal findings on physical examination (otitis media excepted)

- Laboratory values:
  - white blood cell (WBC) count of 5000–15,000 × 10⁹/l with band forms <500 × 10⁹/l
  - urine sediment with <10 WBCs/hpf (white blood cells/high-power field) and negative for leucocyte esterase and nitrite on urine dipstick
  - stool (if diarrhoea present) with <5 WBC/hpf

Controversy exists with regard to the WBC cut-off; a lower full blood count (FBC) treatment threshold (15,000 × 10⁹/l) increases sensitivity for occult bacteraemia (OB) but lowers the ability to correctly predict. A higher FBC threshold (20,000 × 10⁹/l) decreases sensitivity but improves ability to correctly predict and probably results in less empirical treatment.

- Children from 3 to 36 months with fever ≥39°C that are considered to be at *decreased risk* for serious bacterial infection are those that meet all of the low-risk criteria (Box 15.1).
- Children >36 months with fever ≥39°C are less likely to present with serious bacterial infection (meningococcal septicaemia excluded) as their immune systems are better equipped to localise and mount a response. Although these children still require thorough assessment, in the absence of a toxic appearance, careful watching is a mainstay of treatment.
- Note that *all* children with temperature ≥40°C require careful assessment for a serious bacterial infection.
- Consider the possibility of pelvic inflammatory disease in febrile, ill-appearing adolescents with a history of sexual activity.

PATHOPHYSIOLOGY

- The specific pathophysiology of an acute fever is related to the inciting aetiology. Physiological processes of temperature elevation are discussed in Section 15.4.

HISTORY

- Parent/carer's perception of the child's well-being: playing, feeding, interacting.
- Duration, height and pattern of fever (the greater the temperature, the greater the risk).
- Temperature-taking method and parental confidence in reading result.
- Additional symptoms are: rash, vomiting, diarrhoea, dysuria, abdominal/throat/ear pain, change in activity levels, weight loss, URTI symptoms, lethargy, photophobia and headache.
- Immunisation status.
- Underlying illnesses (especially immunocompromise).
- Recent medication use (including antibiotics and antipyretics).
- Exposure to other children/family members with ill health (day care/nursery attendance?).
- Recent travel.
- Exposure to pets or bites (animal and insect).

PHYSICAL EXAMINATION

- Effect of fever on vital signs should be noted. Heart increases approx. 10 beats/min for each 0.5°C rise above 37°C. Tachycardia disproportionate to the degree of temperature elevation may be indicative of sepsis or dehydration. Tachypnoea is a potential sign of respiratory involvement but may also represent metabolic acidosis (secondary to sepsis or shock).
- Observation of infant/child is *key*. Note weight, hydration status,

level of activity (feeding/playing), interactiveness/engagability, tone of cry and response to stimuli (positive and negative). Repeat observations often and after fever relief.

- **Skin:** look carefully for rashes inside and out (i.e. careful look in the mouth and head to toe).
- **Head and ear, nose and throat (ENT):** careful assessment of anterior fontanelle tympanic membrane, oropharynx and head/neck nodes.
- **Cardiopulmonary:** evaluate for the presence of murmurs (physiological flow murmurs are commonly heard secondary to the increased metabolic rate of fever) and any adventitious sounds in the chest. It is important to assess for signs of shock (pulse rate and capillary refill). Tachypnoea is a potential sign of respiratory involvement but may also represent metabolic acidosis.
- **Abdomen:** check for tenderness and hepatosplenomegaly; consider rectal examination if severe abdominal pain, abscess or appendicitis are suspected.
- **Musculoskeletal:** no redness, swelling, tenderness or decreased range of motion of any joints.
- **Neurological:** level of engagability/interactiveness.
- **Genitourinary:** consider pelvic examination in adolescents if history suggests pelvic inflammatory disease.

🔎 DIFFERENTIAL DIAGNOSES

- *Numerous:* Head and neck infections (dental abscess, otitis media, sinusitis, gingivostomatitis, herpangina); upper and lower respiratory tract infections (RSV, influenza, adenovirus, epiglottitis, pneumonia, bronchiolitis, TB); gastroenteritis (bacterial and viral) and appendicitis; genitourinary problems (UTI, pyelonephritis, pelvic inflammatory disease); skin and/or musculoskeletal infections (cellulitis, osteomyelitis, septic arthritis) meningitis, bacteraemia, immunisation reaction and numerous viral infections

(enteroviruses, roseola, Epstein–Barr infection).
- See also aetiology-specific sections and Section 15.4.

✚ MANAGEMENT

- For all infants and children *with* fever source, management is aetiology-specific.
- For children with FWLS management is outlined in Table 15.3. Note that the management of febrile infants from 3 to 6 months of age is controversial. Consequently, there is debate regarding routine sepsis evaluation and empirical use of antibiotics in well-appearing (or low-risk) infants.
- Use of paracetamol and ibuprofen for fever ≤38–39°C is controversial (especially among healthy children), as slight temperature elevations are considered an adaptive/protective response. However, the physiological processes that accompany fever can put some children (those with cardiopulmonary disease, metabolic disorders and/or neurological problems) at increased risk. Antipyretics have a significant role to play for these children and should likewise, be considered for relief of associated discomfort and malaise among all children with higher temperatures. Thus, the use of antipyretics in fever management remains an individual one.
- Important components in the management of young infants and children with FWLS include a positive relationship with the family; clear and specific patient education/ anticipatory guidance; and a competent carer with prompt access to treatment if child's condition deteriorates.

➡ FOLLOW-UP

- Telephone contact is reassuring for many parents, especially with first-time febrile episodes; otherwise, if fever resolves spontaneously with return to usual state of health, no further follow-up is necessary.

⇄ MEDICAL CONSULT/ SPECIALIST REFERRAL

- All infants <6 months of age with fever >38°C or any child with fever >40°C.
- *Immediate* referral for any child who appears gravely ill or who manifests signs of shock.
- Any child with a suspected serious bacterial illness (meningococcal septicaemia, bacteraemia, osteomyelitis, septic arthritis, pneumonia, bacterial gastroenteritis and serious skin/soft tissue infections).
- Any child who is immunocompromised and presents with a temperature >38°C.

🔍 PAEDIATRIC PEARLS

- In most cases, a temperature reported by a reliable parent or carer should be considered accurate; in addition, the presence of fever cannot be excluded in an infant who has been treated with antipyretics within the last 4–6 hours.
- The management of low-risk infants from 3 to 6 months of age continues to be controversial with regard to diagnostic aggressiveness and routine antibiotic use.
- If a full blood count (FBC) is easily available, it can be important in the decision-making process.
- The possibility of a UTI is often overlooked as a potential cause of FWLS in infants and young children. Clinical findings with UTI among this group are very non-specific and thus, it should always be considered in the differential (see Sec. 14.1). It is imperative that a diagnosis of UTI is not missed.
- If bundling is suspected as the cause of fever in neonate/infant, unwrap and recheck temperature in 15–30 min.
- Aspirin should *not* be used as an antipyretic due to the risk of Reye's syndrome.
- The management of the acutely febrile infant and child is a very common but very calculated process; the key to an accurate and timely diagnosis is careful history, thorough examination, astute observation of child and partnership between family and health care providers.

Table 15.3 Management of Acute Fever without Localising Source (FWLS)

Age and temperature	Additional diagnostics	Pharmacotherapeutics	Management — Behavioural interventions	Patient education	Comments
0–3 months of age with temperature ⩾ 38°C	• Full sepsis work-up with likely hospitalisation	• Intravenous antibiotics or intramuscular ceftriaxone likely until culture results available	• Careful assessment of vital signs, feeding, activity and temperature monitoring	• Parental support/ anticipatory guidance through hospitalisation and diagnostics	• Controversy exists regarding neonates and infants considered to be 'low risk'; less aggressive treatment has been advocated
3–36 months of age with temperature ⩾ 39°C	• Dependent on risk assessment and appearance; consider full blood count (FBC), urinalysis/culture, lumbar puncture and throat, blood and/or stool cultures	• Antibiotics not usually indicated without source • Consider paracetamol, 10 mg/kg, 4–6 hourly as needed or ibuprofen, 5 mg/kg, 6–8 hourly (max = 30 mg/kg/day) as needed • Use of aspirin is contraindicated	• Monitor for deterioration in condition • Adequate rest, hydration and nutrition	• Review temperature taking, fever management, behavioural interventions, signs and symptoms of deteriorating condition • Discuss plan for return to school, day-care or nursery • Clearly outline situations in which care should be sought immediately	• Important to consider age, appearance, temperature and white blood cell (WBC) count in clinical decision • The likelihood of SBI/OB (serious bacterial illness/ occult bacteraemia) increases with higher temperatures, marked leucocytes and younger age • Management (diagnostics of choice, use of empirical antibiotics and routine hospitalisation) is controversial; largely setting-dependent (acute or primary care)
3–36 months of age with temperature ⩽ 39°C	• Not usually indicated	• Antipyretics not routinely necessary • Dosage as above	• As above	• As above	• Collaboration between family, nurse practitioner (NP) and general practitioner (GP) is vital
>36 months of age with temperature ⩾ 40.5°C	• Careful consideration • Dependent on age, appearance and temperature; consider FBC, urinalysis/culture, throat, blood and/or stool cultures	• Empirical use of antibiotics not recommended • Consider antipyretics for comfort; dosage as above, although paracetamol can be increased to 15 mg/kg and ibuprofen to 10 mg/kg • No aspirin	• Closer follow-up and monitoring during acute/ febrile phase of illness	• As above	• Source for fever often becomes apparent; adjust management accordingly

BIBLIOGRAPHY

Avner J. Occult bacteremia: How great the risk? Contemp Pediatr 1997; 14(4):53–65.

Baker M. Evaluation and management of infants with fever. Pediatr Clin N Am 1999; 46(6):1061–1072.

Baker M. The efficacy of routine outpatient management without antibiotics of fever in selected infants. Pediatrics 1999; 103(3):627–631.

Baraff L. Management of infants and children 3 to 36 months of age with fever without source. Pediatr Ann 1993; 22(8):497–504.

Baraff L. Practice guidelines for the management of infants and children 0–36 months of age with fever without source. Pediatrics 1993; 92(1):1–12.

Baraff L. Management of fever without source in infants and children. Ann Emerg Med 2000; 36(6):602–614.

Browne GJ, Ryan J, McIntyre P. Evaluation of a protocol for selective empiric treatment of fever without localising signs. Arch Dis Child 1997; 76(2):129–133.

Jaskiewicz J. Febrile infants at low risk for serious bacterial infection: an appraisal of the Rochester criteria and implications for management. Pediatrics 1994; 94(3):390–396.

Lewis-Abney K, Ross-Smith E. Managing fever of unknown source in infants and children. J Pediatr Health Care 1996; 10(3):135–138.

Lopez JA. Managing fever in infants and toddlers: toward a standard of care. Postgrad Med 1997; 101(2):241–242.

McCarthy P. Fever. Pediatr Rev 1998; 19(12):401–407.

Nizet V, Vinci RJ, Lovejoy FH. Fever in children. Pediatr Rev 1994; 15(4):127–134.

Prober C. Managing the febrile infant: no rules are golden. Contemp Pediatr 1999; 16(6):48–55.

Wilson D. Assessing and managing the febrile child. Nurse Practr 1995; 20(11 part 1): 59–73.

15.2 GLANDULAR FEVER (EPSTEIN–BARR INFECTION)

Debra Sharu

INTRODUCTION

- Glandular fever (infectious mononucleosis) is usually a mild, self-limiting illness that is characteristically associated with the classic symptom triad of prolonged fever, pharyngitis and lymphadenopathy.
- While the vast majority (approx. 90%) of cases are caused by Epstein–Barr virus (EBV), cytomegalovirus (CMV), adenovirus, human herpes 6 virus (HHV-6) and others have been implicated in the clinical syndrome of prolonged fever, pharyngitis and lympadenopathy.
- EBV is a member of the herpes virus family, and one of the most common human viruses, infecting the majority of the world's population at some time during their lives.
- Susceptibility to EBV begins as soon as maternal antibody protection disappears. Children often become infected with EBV and are either symptom-free or have symptoms that are indistinguishable from other mild, brief, childhood illnesses. EBV infection in adolescence or young adulthood causes glandular fever 35–50% of the time. The majority of

all cases involve individuals between 15 and 30 years of age.
- The duration of the illness varies, with the uncomplicated disease course lasting 3–4 weeks.
- As almost all body organs can be involved, Epstein–Barr infection is considered to be the 'great impersonator', often mimicking a variety of illnesses.
- Complications are uncommon, but include splenic rupture, agranulocytosis, thrombocytopenia, orchitis, myocarditis, haemolytic anaemia and chronic EBV infection. Dehydration can develop in very young children with glandular fever if oral intake is severely compromised. Very rarely, EBV has been implicated in fatal disseminated disease or B-cell lymphoma and its role as a causative agent in chronic fatigue syndrome remains controversial.

PATHOPHYSIOLOGY

- Primarily a disease of the lymphoid tissue and peripheral blood, EBV infects and then reproduces in the salivary glands with subsequent infection and spread via B lymphocytes and the lymphoreticular system.

Cellular immune responses are critical in limiting EBV replication and spread.
- EBV remains in the body for life, replicating in a subset of B lymphocytes. Direct contact with the host's saliva is the main mode of transmission; hence the term kissing disease. Acquisition of the virus through air or blood does not normally occur.
- The incubation period ranges from 2 to 7 weeks following exposure with variable lengths of viral shedding after onset of symptoms (months to years). No special isolation precautions are recommended, as EBV is frequently found in the saliva of healthy people. Given the intermittent shedding of the virus, it is almost impossible to prevent transmission.

HISTORY

- Onset, pattern and duration of symptoms (fatigue, malaise, anorexia, fever, headache, sore throat, 'swollen glands' and sore/swollen eyes or lids).
- Presence and pattern of fever (common complaint, may reach 39–40°C, last 1–2 weeks and have variable patterns).

217

- Presence of prodrome (malaise, chills, anorexia) 2–5 days prior to onset of other symptoms.
- Presence of other symptoms (rash, abdominal pain, jaundice).
- Known exposures to others with glandular fever.
- Extent to which pharyngitis is preventing oral intake.
- Indications of potential complications (rare, but include cranial nerve palsies, encephalitis, upper airway obstruction, splenic rupture, and distortion of size, shape and spatial orientation of objects).

PHYSICAL EXAMINATION

- Assessment of the patient's general appearance, vital signs and level of hydration.
- Observation of the skin for colour and exanthems (approx. 5% of patients will have a rash that is variable in presentation: macular, petechial, scarlatiniform, urticarial or erythema multiforme-type).
- **Head and ENT:** rule out periorbital pain and/or oedema (observed in about 30% of cases); obstruction of the airway from enlarged tonsils or lymphoid tissue (often exudative pharyngitis with palatal petechiae).
- Assessment of lymphadenopathy (particularly the cervical chains).
- **Cardiopulmonary:** routine heart and lung examination.
- **Abdomen:** careful palpation of abdomen may reveal splenomegaly (50–75% of cases), hepatomegaly (approx. 20% of cases) and generalised, mild abdominal tenderness (probably related to mesenteric lymphadenopathy). Rule out costovertebral angle (CVA) tenderness.
- **Neurological:** routine assessment to rule out CNS involvement.

DIFFERENTIAL DIAGNOSES

- Differential diagnoses are numerous, as EBV imitates many diseases. Additional aetiologies to be considered are streptococcal pharyngitis (distinguished from other types of pharyngitis by posterior cervical adenopathy and splenomegaly); toxoplasma infection; other viral

syndromes (adenovirus, CMV, rubella and HHV-6); hepatitis A; HIV; malignancy (including leukaemia).

⊕ MANAGEMENT

- **Additional diagnostics:** suspicion of EBV infection derived from patient's age and presentation. For a more definitive diagnosis consider:
  - FBC (may reveal elevated WBC count, lymphocytosis and >10% atypical lymphocytes).
  - Throat swab/rapid strep test can be used to identify group A β-haemolytic streptococci (GABHS) infection.
  - Heterophil antibody test (e.g. Monospot or Paul–Bunnell test will identify 90% of cases in those >4 years of age if symptoms present for at least 2 weeks (high rate of false-negative results if done early in the disease process). If original test is negative and symptoms persist, repeat.
  - EBV serology (EBV immunoglobulin G (IgG) and immunoglobulin M (IgM) viral capsid antigen, nuclear antigen and early antigen) useful in combination with heterophil antibody test (especially if initial Monospot is negative). Important to consider checking in children <4 years of age and those with atypical, persistent or severe illness with negative heterophil test. (Note: these tests involve greater expense, careful interpretation and likely medical consultation.)
  - PCR (polymerase chain reaction) EBV antigen detection (expensive and not readily available). Only necessary in severe cases where identification is essential for diagnostic purposes.
- **Pharmacotherapeutics:**
  - Treatment is supportive and aimed at relieving discomfort; therefore, paracetamol, ibuprofen and salt water gargles or lozenges may be helpful. Aspirin use should be avoided, as there is a potential association with Reye's syndrome, aspirin usage and acute EBV infection.
  - Patients with streptococcal pharyngitis (GABHS) can be treated with erythromycin or phenoxymethylpenicillin (penicillin V). Note that amoxicillin (amoxycillin) is contraindicated.

- Corticosteroids have been used when there is risk of impending airway obstruction and severe life-threatening EBV infection.
- Efficacy of aciclovir (acyclovir) has not been established and is not recommended.
- **Behavioural interventions:**
  - A realistic schedule ought to be planned based on the patient's condition. Adequate food intake should be maintained and fluids increased to guard against dehydration.
  - Contact sports need to be avoided for at least a month or until splenomegaly subsides.
  - Patient isolation is not necessary, but good handwashing and prevention of fomite spread should be encouraged in order to avoid infecting others.
- **Patient education:**
  - Carers and patients need to be aware that there is currently no treatment which can eradicate the virus; management is symptomatic; adequate nutrition, hydration and rest are key factors in recovery. Emphasise and reassure them regarding the self-limiting nature of the illness.
  - Advise on the expected duration/course of the illness (which is usually uneventful and lasts 1–4 weeks).
  - Stress that although complications are rare, advice should be sought if there is no improvement in symptoms after 1–2 weeks or if symptoms deteriorate.
  - Warn parents that recovery is often biphasic (symptoms sometimes worsen briefly after a period of improvement).

⇨ FOLLOW-UP

- Not routinely required in uncomplicated cases, but consider phone contact every 2 weeks until symptoms resolve.

⇄ MEDICAL CONSULT/ SPECIALIST REFERRAL

- Patients with complications (CNS involvement, splenic rupture/marked

abdominal pain, jaundice, potential upper airway obstruction).
- Patients with persistent symptoms for more than 2 weeks (without any improvement) or those patients whose condition deteriorates warrant discussion with a collaborating physician.

PAEDIATRIC PEARLS

- Positive GABHS infection does not rule out EBV infection, as 5–25% of patients with EBV glandular fever will have concomitant GABHS.
- Negative Monospot does not automatically rule out EBV infection; simultaneous evaluation of EBV serology is likely to improve diagnostic

efficiency, especially if initial Monospot is negative.
- 90–100% of patients treated with ampicillin- or amoxicillin-containing products will develop a pruritic, maculopapular rash 7–10 days after first dose.
- If complaints of abdominal pain are marked, consider possible splenic rupture (1 in 1000 cases, more common in males, half are spontaneous).
- Recovery is often biphasic (worsening of symptoms after period of improvement).
- Positive Monospot is not diagnostic of active EBV disease, as heterophil antibodies can persist for months.
- Atypical lymphocytosis (>10%) is also a feature of CMV, toxoplasmosis,

HHV-6, rubella and hepatitis A, and HIV infections.

BIBLIOGRAPHY

Cozad J. Infectious mononucleosis. Nurse Pract 1996; 2:13, 14–16, 23, 27–28.
Godshall SE, Kirchner JT. Infectious mononucleosis: complexities of a common syndrome. Postgrad Med 2000; 107(7): 175–179, 183–184, 186.
Hickey SM, Strasburger VC. What every pediatrician should know about infectious mononucleosis in adolescents. Pediatr Clin N Am 1997; 44(6):1541–1556.
Peter J, Ray CG. Infectious mononucleosis. Pediatr Rev 1998; 19(8):276–279.
Tosato G. Epstein–Barr virus as an agent of haematological disease. Baillières Clin Haematol 1995; 8(1):165–199.

15.3 LYMPHADENOPATHY

Karen Selwood

INTRODUCTION

- Lymph node enlargement in children is relatively common. Forty-five percent of children and 34% of neonates have palpable head and neck nodes due to steady increases in lymphoid tissue after birth and during early childhood in response to environmental antigens.
- Regional lymphadenopathy is lymph node enlargement in one drainage area, whereas generalised lymphadenopathy is enlargement of two or more non-contiguous areas.
- Regional lymphadenopathy is most commonly caused by an ongoing infective process in areas that drain nodes; generalised lymphadenopathy usually represents a systemic (and often more significant) disease process.
- Although rare, lymphoma is an important cause not to be forgotten.

PATHOPHYSIOLOGY

- Lymph nodes are found in the head and neck, axillae, mediastinum, near the abdominal great vessels, in the

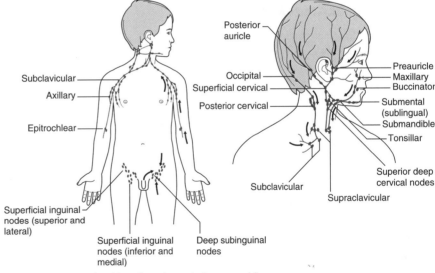

Figure 15.1 Superficial lymph nodes with direction of flow.

inguinal regions and the large vascular trunks of the extremities (Fig. 15.1). Presenting symptoms of lymphadenopathy will depend on which nodes are enlarged (e.g. infection in the throat, cervical nodes will be enlarged).
- Enlarged nodes can be classified as nodes larger than 1.0 cm with two

exceptions: epitrochlear nodes greater than 5 mm and inguinal nodes greater than 15 mm may be abnormal. Nodes become enlarged due to lymphocytic proliferation in response to infection or malignancy.
- Specific pathophysiology is aetiology-dependent, with processes numerous and varied.

HISTORY

- Onset, duration, location and degree of tenderness of enlarged node(s).
- Illness prior to the enlargement of node(s) and presence/absence of fever.
- Rate of lymph node enlargement.
- Associated rashes or other symptoms of illness (vomiting, diarrhoea, URTI).
- Recent foreign travel.
- Exposure to pets (especially cats).
- Weight loss, cough, dyspnoea, fever and/or night sweats, pallor, pruritus, myalgia/arthralgia or any other systemic complaints. As these symptoms are uncommon in children (as opposed to adults), their presence is worrying.
- Presence of any risk factors (HIV infection, history of TB/TB exposure or contact with anyone who is ill).
- History of bleeding.
- Treatment/management, thus far, for this episode of lymphadenopathy (or others in past)?
- Dental problems.
- Current medications (phenytoin, allopurinol, hydralazine, carbamazepine).

PHYSICAL EXAMINATION

- Important to determine whether the node(s) is enlarged or not. Examination should be done with both hands (from behind and in front of the child) comparing nodal chains bilaterally. Nodes may be tender, so take care to obtain the child's confidence before examination begins. All lymph nodes need to be examined to establish whether the child has general or local enlargement; with localised enlargement examine appropriate drainage area (see Fig. 15.1).
- Note location, size and characteristics (consistency, mobility, tenderness and temperature) of node. Roll node(s) under fingertips to appreciate these characteristics and consider marking opposite edges to allow specific measurement of the diameter. This will assist in future monitoring of node(s) for further enlargement. It is very important to note if node is matted or appears tethered to underlying fascia as it is a worrying sign of lymphoma.
- **Skin:** note any infective lesions, exanthematous rashes and/or scratches (especially from cats). Likewise, note any soft tissue inflammation of the areas surrounding the nodes (consider especially areas which individual nodes drain). Any signs of anaemia and/or petechiae need to be identified, as they may indicate bone marrow disease.
- **Head and ENT:** A full ear, nose and throat examination looking for possible aetiologies for the nodal enlargement. Nasal discharge, obstruction or depression of the soft palate may indicate an infection or malignancy.
- **Cardiopulmonary:** careful auscultation of the chest, as a mediastinal mass may cause difficulty breathing or a non-productive cough.
- **Abdomen:** examine for tenderness (especially with generalised lymphadenopathy, as mesenteric nodes deep within the abdominal cavity may be enlarged and tender); enlarged liver, spleen and/or presence of masses.
- **Musculoskeletal and neurological:** routine examination, looking for abnormalities which may provide clues to lymphadenopathy.

DIFFERENTIAL DIAGNOSES

- Aetiologies are numerous and varied. It is helpful to consider causes of generalised and regionalised presentations separately, although note that there can be overlap (Tables 15.4 and 15.5).
- See also Sections 15.1 and 15.4.

MANAGEMENT

The management of lymphadenopathy associated with other illnesses is aetiology-specific. Table 15.6 outlines

Table 15.4	Differential Diagnosis of Generalised Lymphadenopathy	
Aetiology		Consider
Infectious	Systemic viral	CMV, HIV, EBV (glandular fever), varicella zoster, mumps, rubella, measles, enterovirus infection, herpes simplex, adenovirus
	Fungal	Histoplasmosis, blastomycosis, coccidioidomycosis
	Bacterial	Syphilis, brucellosis, yersiniosis, cat-scratch disease (rare), mycobacteria
	Parasitic	Malaria, leishmaniasis, toxoplasmosis
Neoplastic		Lymphoma, leukaemia, neuroblastoma or rhabdomyosarcoma
Autoimmune/connective tissue (rare)		SLE, JRA, sarcoidosis
Drug reactions (rare)		Phenytoin, carbamazepine, isoniazid
Other (rare)		Kawasaki disease, X-linked lymphoproliferative disease

CMV = cytomegalovirus; EBV = Epstein–Barr virus; HIV = human immunodeficiency virus; JRA = juvenile rheumatoid arthritis; SLE = systemic lupus erythematosus.

Table 15.5	Differential Diagnoses of Regional Lymphadenopathy
Involved node(s)	Consider
Anterior/posterior cervical	URTI (usually bilateral), herpes infection, dental abscess, mumps, streptococcal pharyngitis, facial impetigo, lymphoma (rare), cat-scratch disease (rare), atypical mycobacterium infection (rare), toxoplasmosis, Rosai–Dorfman disease (rare)
Occipital	Scalp infection (impetigo, tinea capitis, head lice)
Pre/post-auricular	Acute otitis media, otitis externa
Supraclavicular	Hodgkin's disease
Axillary	Infection/trauma of axilla (insect bites, folliculitis), cat-scratch disease (rare)
Epitrochlear	Infection of hand and lower arm, cat-scratch disease (rare)
Inguinal	Infection of lower extremities and external genitalia (genital herpes, syphilis), cat-scratch disease (rare)

URTI = upper respiratory tract infection.

Table 15.6 Management of lymphadenopathy

Finding	Additional diagnostics	Pharmacotherapeutics	Behavioural interventions	Patient education	Follow-up
Localised lymphadenopathy with fever (suspected bacterial infection of the lymph node)	• A swab for culture and sensitivity of any infected area may be of benefit • Can consider FBC	• Consider treatment with antibiotics to cover streptococci and staphylococci: ○ amoxicillin ○ flucloxacillin • Treat fever with antipyretics: ○ paracetamol ○ or ibuprofen	• Warm compresses may encourage lymph drainage and provide symptomatic relief	• Clarify medication dosages, administration and timing • Review behavioural interventions • Reinforce importance of seeking assistance immediately if difficulty swallowing and/or breathing • Explain the importance of seeking assistance immediately if enlargement of node is accompanied by symptoms/appearance of increased illness • Warn parents that the infected node(s) may get slightly larger (without other signs of increased illness) during first 24 hours of antibiotics but should start to shrink after that	• Reassess by visit or telephone after 72 hours • If nodes fail to resolve after 2–3 weeks refer for further evaluation • If node worrying (non-mobile, matted and firm) refer sooner
Localised lymphadenopathy without fever	• None necessary if no obvious cause and no evidence of systemic disease • FBC and ESR may be useful • Serum assays for glandular fever may be helpful (EBV and CMV)	• May attempt antibiotic trial if cause thought to be infective • Use paracetamol or ibuprofen for analgesia if nodes are tender (doses as above)	• Document size and characteristics; then observe for 2–3 weeks • Warm compresses as above	• Reassure parents and explain rationale for careful observation • Discuss 'next steps' that will be taken if there is no resolution • Review medication administration and dosing • Teach parents how to monitor for signs of increased inflammation	• Reassess weekly for changes in node • If continued enlargement over period of observation and/or no diminution after 5 weeks, refer for further testing • If node worrying, refer sooner
Generalised lymphadenopathy	• Numerous; as this may represent more serious disease, diagnostics are likely to be extensive (see Table 15.4) • FBC with differential white count and chest X-ray often form part of initial work-up	• Aetiology-dependent	• Referral likely, especially if nodal biopsy required	• Parental and patient support with careful explanation of procedures, evaluation process, referral process	• In the absence of obvious aetiology, referral for further work-up is likely

CMV = cytomegalovirus; EBV = Epstein–Barr virus; ESR = erythrocyte sedimentation rate; FBC = full blood count.

the initial management of lymphadenopathy not initially attributable to other disease processes.

⇨ FOLLOW-UP

- With spontaneous resolution, no follow-up is needed.
- For nodes that require observation (prior to further investigation or treatment), observe weekly or biweekly for changes.

⇦ MEDICAL CONSULT/ SPECIALIST REFERRAL

- Any child with unexplained generalised lymphadenopathy accompanied by constitutional symptoms of weight loss, persistent fever and/or night sweats, enlarged liver or spleen, anaemia or bleeding.
- A child with progressive enlargement over 2–3 weeks with no diminution in lymph node masses after 5–6 weeks or lack of complete resolution by 10 weeks.
- Any child with an enlargement of mediastinal, supraclavicular or abdominal nodes and/or node(s) that are firm, non-mobile and matted.
- A child in whom there is suspicion of malignancy or underlying autoimmune disease.

♂ PAEDIATRIC PEARLS

- Watchful follow-up is key to further diagnostics/additional evaluation; most episodes are not an emergency and in the initial stages require only careful watching with minimal intervention.
- Cervical nodes that are soft, small, mobile and without signs of inflammation (or underlying cause) can initially be measured and watched for several weeks; it is the firm, matted and non-mobile nodes that require urgent referral.
- Lymphatic hypertrophy during growth spurts can be confused for lymphadenopathy.
- Persistent fever or signs of toxicity may be indicative of septicaemia.
- *Staphylococcus aureus* and *Streptococcus pyogenes* are a significant cause of unilateral, bacterial infection of lymph node.
- Local signs of inflammation in acute bacterial lymph infection sometimes increase during the first 24 hours of antibiotics (without other signs of toxicity) but should rapidly improve after that.
- Persistence of lymphadenopathy will depend on eradication of the inciting agent/process. However, it is not uncommon (especially with systemic viral infections) for nodal enlargement to gradually subside over several months; likewise, nodal involvement may persist after benign viral infections.
- Spontaneous drainage of a node with formation of fistula may indicate infection with mycobacterium.

▤ BIBLIOGRAPHY

Filston HC. Common lumps and bumps of the head and neck in infants and children. Pediatr Ann 1989; 18(3):180–186.

Ghirardelli ML, Jemos V, Gobbi PG. Diagnostic approach to lymph node enlargement. Haematologica 1999; 84(3):242–247.

Kelly CS, Kelly RE. Lymphadenopathy in children. Pediatr Clin North Am 1998; 45(4):875–888.

Kenney K. Lymphadenopathy. In: Fox FA, ed., Primary health care. New York: Mosby Year Book; 1997.

Margileth AM. Sorting out the causes of lymphadenopathy. Contemp Pediatr 1995; 12(1):23–40.

Margileth AM. Lymphadenopathy: when to diagnose and treat. Contemp Pediatr 1995; 12(2):71–91.

Morland B. Lymphadenopathy. Arch Dis Child 1995; 73(5):476–479.

Perkins SL, Segal GH, Kjeldsberg CR. Work-up of lymphadenopathy in children. Sem Diagnost Pathol 1995; 12(4):284–287.

15.4 PYREXIA OF UNKNOWN ORIGIN (PROLONGED FEVER OF >7 DAYS DURATION)

Monica Hopkins

▥ INTRODUCTION

- Prolonged pyrexia or pyrexia of unknown origin (PUO) is rare. It is commonly defined as a febrile illness (>38.5°C) for more than 1–2 weeks, without discernible cause despite careful evaluation based on history and physical examination. The major causes of a prolonged fever in this country are infection, connective tissue disease and malignancy.

- Body temperature depends on many factors and there is considerable variance in the normal range (lowest early in the morning and highest in late afternoon and early evening). Rectal temperatures are about 0.6°C higher than oral temperatures and younger children have a normal range that runs about 0.5°C higher than older children. Consequently, normal rectal temperatures in young children can fluctuate between 36.2 and 38°C with oral fluctuations 36.0–37.4°C. Normal temperatures represent only the mean: 50% of healthy children will run outside these routinely.

- Low-grade temperatures in a child straight after school or an activity can be discounted due to rise in metabolic rate and time of the day; the same goes for low temperatures straight after eating. Over-wrapping of babies can prevent natural heat loss, and so give falsely high readings; it is essential that these anomalies (in addition to errors in temperature measurement) are ruled out.

PATHOPHYSIOLOGY

- The specific pathophysiology of PUO is related to its inciting aetiology; however, the physiological processes of temperature elevation are well known.
- Body temperature is regulated by thermosensitive neurones in the anterior hypothalamus. Fever is a resetting of the hypothalamic set point that is manifested in a controlled increase of body temperature. It is symptomatic of an underlying process or condition that has stimulated inflammation, with the aim of decreasing microbial growth and/or increasing the inflammatory response to tissue injury.
- Regardless of the cause, the body's thermostat is reset in response to stimulation by *endogenous* (cytokines, stimulated leucocytes, prostaglandins, antigen/antibody complexes and steroid metabolites) or *exogenous* (microbial endotoxins) pyrogens.
- Higher temperatures are maintained through a combination of *physiological* (redirection of blood from cutaneous vasculature, variation of sweat production and extracellular fluid volume regulation) and *behavioural* responses (bundling up, shivering, moving to warmer environment) and will continue until the hypothalamic thermostat is reset to its normal level.
- Paracetamol acts directly on the hypothalamus to produce heat reduction, whereas ibuprofen is a prostaglandin inhibitor that mediates the effect of endogenous pyrogens in the hypothalamus (thereby decreasing their effect on the set point). Antipyretics have no effect on interleukin-1 (cytokine involved in the proliferation of helper T cells) and, therefore, do not significantly affect the body's ability to fight infection.
- In neonates, the pyrexic response is immature and resetting of the

thermoregulatory centre may not occur despite the presence of an infection. Consequently, the neonate may be septic and afebrile or even hypothermic.

HISTORY

- Detailed fever history (including time of onset, peak temperature, time of peak, relationship of fever to activities and time of day, motivation for checking temperature, clinical symptoms/activity at time of fever and pattern of spikes/normalisations).
- Method of temperature-taking (ear, skin, rectal) and perceived confidence in reading results.
- Other associated signs and symptoms (careful review of systems: rashes, ENT complaints, gastrointestinal symptoms, any signs or symptoms of infection, etc.).
- Development of any other symptoms with temporal components (since onset of fever).
- Travel history (recent foreign travel or contact with travellers).
- Exposure to animals and/or history of eating non-food items (sand, dirt, grass) or any recent change in activity, appetite or temperament.
- Recent ingestion of raw meat, fish, unpasteurised milk or contaminated water.
- Medication use (including non-prescription drugs and eye drops) and immunisation history.
- Note any other medications that are currently held in the home that may have been accidentally ingested.
- Past medical history (including contact with ill individuals, history of 'fevers' in family, impaired linear growth or weight gain, physical and cognitive development and general growth patterns).
- Family history (chronic disease, inflammatory or autoimmune disorders).

PHYSICAL EXAMINATION

- **Observe general appearance:** (vital signs, growth parameters, activity levels, colour) and parent–child interaction. Note that pulse rate

elevated out of proportion to the temperature rise is suggestive of non-infectious disease, dehydration or toxin exposure (rather than an organism). While bradycardia (despite fever) suggests drug fever, typhus, brucellosis, leptospirosis or defect in cardiac conduction (potentially related to acute rheumatic fever, Lyme disease, viral myocarditis or infective endocarditis).
- **Careful examination of skin:** hydration status, lesions, rashes, bite/tick marks, petechiae, trauma or infection.
- **Head and ENT:** condition of hair, oral lesions, conjunctivitis, sinus tenderness/nasal discharge, pharyngitis, and lymphadenopathy.
- **Cardiopulmonary:** adventitious lung sounds and murmurs.
- **Abdomen:** distension, tenderness, hepato-splenomegaly.
- **Careful musculoskeletal assessment:** palpation/manipulation of all joints/bones (osteomyelitis and septic arthritis due to *S. pnemoniae* can present with prolonged fevers).
- **Routine neurological assessment or milestone development in infants:** assessing for gross abnormalities which may be indicative of CNS dysfunction.

DIFFERENTIAL DIAGNOSES

- The list of differential diagnoses associated with PUO is exhaustive; however, some factors commonly occur. Therefore, it is useful to consider the three most probable causes of PUO: infection, connective tissue disorder and malignancy (in that order). These can be further subdivided as in Table 15.7 but the order in each column does not necessarily indicate likelihood of cause.
- Note that fungal sepsis is unusual in immunocompetent children; therefore, if found, the child's immune status should be investigated.
- There may also be further infectious possibilities in children recently returned from travel abroad, and specialist advice should always be sought regarding common infections for the countries from which they have returned.

Table 15.7 Differential Causes of Prolonged Fever

Infectious aetiologies	Connective tissue/immune-related problems	Other
Bacterial • Sinusitis • Osteomyelitis • Abscess (dental, liver, pelvic perinephric, subdiaphragmatic) • Bacterial endocarditis • Tuberculosis • Brucellosis, leptospirosis, salmonellosis	• Juvenile rheumatoid arthritis • Systemic lupus erythematosus • Polyarteritis	• Malignancy • Kawasaki syndrome • Drug fever • Thryrotoxicosis • Pancreatitis • Periodic fever • Serum sickness • Familial dysautonomia
Viral • Cytomegalovirus • Hepatitis • Infectious mononucleosis		
Fungal • Systemic candidiasis • Histoplasmosis • Blastomycosis		
Parasitic • Toxoplasmosis • Malaria (history of foreign travel) • Visceral larva migrans (history of foreign travel)		

✚ MANAGEMENT

- **Additional diagnostics:** In the absence of any potential source for the fever, the following should be considered (setting-dependent and often with medical consultation):
  - Full blood count (FBC): with film and differential.
  - Urinalysis and urine culture.
  - Stool and throat cultures.
  - Blood cultures and baseline viral screen (including EBV, CMV, hepatitis, Coxsackie and possibly HIV).
  - C-reactive protein (CRP), erythrocyte sedimentation rate (ESR), Monospot and EBV serology.
  - Liver function test (LFT): considering the possibility of hepatitis.
  - Chest X-ray.
  - Mantoux test.
  - Lumbar puncture.
  - Agglutination tests for typhoid, paratyphoid, brucella and leptospirosis.
  - Repeat viral antibody screen after 10 days.
  - Isotope bone scan can exclude low-grade osteomyelitis, whereas an echocardiogram (ECG) can rule out endocarditis. Note that these would be considered secondary investigations to be done when there is sound evidence of problems in these systems or nothing found in the preliminary investigations.
  - Further studies to investigate the possibility of connective tissue or autoimmune disease and malignancy should be considered if consistently abnormal FBC, persistently high ESR, low leucocyte alkaline phosphatase level, hypergammaglobulinaemia, abnormal antibodies in serum and/or + ANA (antinuclear antibody).
- **Pharmacotherapeutics:**
  - Aetiology-dependent.
  - Empirical treatment of fever (especially among healthy children with fevers <39°C) is controversial, as slight temperature elevations are considered an adaptive/protective response. However, the physiological processes that accompany fever can put some children (those with cardiopulmonary disease, metabolic disorders and/or neurological problems) at increased risk. Antipyretics have a significant role to play for these children and should likewise be considered for relief of associated discomfort and malaise among all children with higher temperatures. Thus, the use of antipyretics in fever management remains an individual one.

- **Behavioural interventions:**
  - The most obvious interventions here are rest, fluids and good nutritional intake. These can be trite if delivered to the parent without any suggestions on how to deal with a possibly malaised child who is uncomfortable doing anything. The rest should really be dictated by the child; children will restrict their own activity if given the opportunity of a low-stimulation environment and a comfortable place to rest in view of the family and/or company.
  - Diet: in small quantities and often, of high carbohydrate foods and nibbles of protein are about the most a parent can hope for. In their absence, high carbohydrate drinks (not coke but perhaps fruit-based products) may be useful as well as milk shakes and ice cream or frozen yoghurt. Brightly coloured vessels and fun-shaped food may entice children and should be preferred over drinks and foods high in artificial colours and sweeteners.
  - Despite the need to allow children to rest and convalesce, their bodies (especially if a virus has infected them) do need some daily activity and fresh air in order to build themselves up for a possibly protracted illness.

- **Patient education:**
  - Parent education can start right at the moment of the first meeting, as one should explain all procedures and answer all questions as to their relevance and possible consequences.
  - It is vital to be able to assess parent temperature-taking technique and correct any misunderstandings or misinterpretations of instructions. It is also important that parents understand something of normal temperature regulations in children and the natural highs and lows in a daily temperature at different ages to avoid incorrect documentation of data at home.
  - Parents should be encouraged to keep a diary of the progression of the situation from when they leave your care (if unresolved) until their next follow-up appointment. The instructions on how this should be

constructed and exactly what data you are particularly interested in should be made explicit, perhaps even with a drawn table for clarity.

- Reinforce behavioural interventions as above. Note that not everyone is completely clear about high carbohydrate foods and protein; try to work with examples from the child's normal diet after consultation with parents. It may be possible to issue leaflets from your dietetic department on tips for home.

- Possible patterns of progression should be discussed in explaining levels of deterioration that parents must report back promptly. Relevant phone numbers and contact names should be issued with strict instructions to use them at any time of day or night, especially in the young child.

⇨ FOLLOW-UP

- All children that were not satisfactorily diagnosed on the initial visit require a follow-up visit for parental support, reassessment and review of test results. Complete documentation of the PUO work-up is important should there be a recurrence or failure to resolve. Even if the illness proves to be self-limiting and the child gradually recovers, it is useful to have a follow-up appointment to discharge the child and record no late effects. A referral to a GP and health visitor will be advantageous at this point for future reference.

- If the child's condition deteriorates, obviously rapid access is essential and the parents should have relevant phone numbers and contact names before they leave your care.

- Should the child's condition continue along the same path, then a 1-week appointment should be sufficient to systematically re-evaluate the child and to have some results from your baseline investigations as well as to have allowed time for consultation with medical colleagues.

⇄ MEDICAL CONSULT/ SPECIALIST REFERRAL

- Consultation is warranted in cases where there is little evidence of an obvious cause for the fever. Likewise, any system abnormality found in conjunction with the fever (and not indicative of a more routine infection) should always be referred on.

- Abnormalities associated with haematological screening, musculoskeletal examination or respiratory assessment (physical or radiological) should be referred promptly, as immediate reassessment may be necessary. Positive results on investigations for the more serious or rare infections (Table 15.7) should also be quickly consulted about.

⊙ PAEDIATRIC PEARLS

- PUO often represents an atypical presentation of a common illness rather than a typical presentation of an uncommon disease.

- Consider PUO as pyrexia of *undiscovered* origin (rather than *unknown* origin); therefore, a systematic approach is required with frequent rethinking and re-evaluation of historical, clinical and laboratory data.

- Although 7 days is typically used as a guideline for PUO referral, *do not* postpone consultation if there is earlier

concern regarding illness severity or diagnostic uncertainty; these children can be worrying.

- Non-pharmacological cooling measures are only truly effective when the hypothalamic set point has been reduced (via antipyretics or removal of pyrogen stimulation). Until this point, cooling measures will be met by bodily attempts to maintain the fever, which can result in a core temperature rise even when skin temperatures appear reduced. The temperatures of children who receive only non-pharmacological cooling measures should be monitored carefully.

- The speed of fever decline, in response to pharmacological agents, does not distinguish serious bacterial infections from less-worrying viral ones.

- Never make assumptions about the level of understanding between yourself and parents or children about descriptions of symptoms, definitions of high fever and duration of symptoms; check and recheck details of history so you are clear in the pattern of onset and aggravating factors.

⊟ BIBLIOGRAPHY

Gutman SJ. Evaluating febrile children. Can Family Phys 1999; 45:1687–1688.
McCarthy PL. Fever. Pediatr Rev 1998; 19(12):401–408.
Miller ML, Szer I, Yogev R, et al. Fever of unknown origin. Pediatr Clin North Am 1995; 42(5):999–1015.
O'Callaghan C, Stephenson T. Pocket paediatrics. Edinburgh: Churchill Livingstone; 1999.
Park JW. Fever without source in children; recommendations for outpatient care in those up to 3. Postgrad Med 2000; 107(2):259–266.
Wilson D. Assessing and managing the febrile child. Nurse Pract 1995; 20(11):59–60, 68–74.

15.5 ROSEOLA

Sigrid Watt

▢ INTRODUCTION

- Roseola, also known as exanthem subitum, exanthemous fever and 3-day

rash, is one of the lesser known acute diseases of infants and young children.

- It is an acute, self-limiting viral infection, affecting infants and children

from 2 months to 4 years old. The peak incidence is from 7 to 13 months of age and it is uncommon before 3 months or after 3 years of age.

Although cases of roseola occur throughout the year, they are often clustered in the spring and early summer.

- Roseola is characterised by a high fever (that lasts 3–5 days) and a blanching maculopapular rash that appears after, or just before, the child's temperature returns to normal; the rash typically lasts for 1–2 days. Note that while the fever is significant, the child does not appear extremely ill, with behaviour that varies from playful to slightly irritable. Mild cough, coryza and lymphadenopathy are common concurrent symptoms.
- Most 4 year olds are seropositive; therefore, it is likely that there are subclinical cases of roseola infection that do not present with the characteristic history of fever and rash.

PATHOPHYSIOLOGY

- The major causative agent appears to be the human herpes virus type 6 (HHV-6), which was first linked with roseola in 1988. HHV-6 is a herpesvirus similar to cytomegalovirus and Epstein–Barr virus (EBV). However, numerous other viruses have been associated with roseola-like illnesses (e.g. Coxsackie virus, adenovirus, parainfluenza virus and measles vaccine virus).
- The specific pathophysiology is not well understood; however, the typical arrival of the rash as the fever is disappearing may represent virus neutralisation in the skin.
- Humans are the only known reservoir and the mode of transmission is thought to be through the respiratory tract.
- The incubation period is not certain, but it is likely to be between 7 and 17 days. The child is probably infectious during the febrile phase of the illness and may be contagious even before the fever begins.

HISTORY

- General activity, appetite and behaviour.
- Onset, duration and height of the fever. Note that the fever is often

markedly elevated (38.9–40.5°C) and commonly lasts 3–5 days.
- Temporal relationship of fever to rash (i.e. which came first?).
- Recent medication use (especially oral antibiotics).
- Additional symptomatology.
- Exposure to others with similar symptomatology.
- Immunisation status.
- See also Section 15.1.

PHYSICAL EXAMINATION

- **General appearance:** generally non-toxic and essentially well-appearing, although once the rash appears child may be less playful.
- **Head and ENT:** eyelid oedema is common as are mild pharyngitis, posterior cervical and postauricular lymphadenopathy.
- **Cardiopulmonary:** normal examination with the exception of elevated heart and respiratory rates if child is febrile at the time of examination.
- **Skin:** if the rash is present, there will be a faintly erythematous, macular or maculopapular rubelliform exanthem with a mainly central distribution. The rash appears just before, or shortly after, the child's temperature returns to normal. It often presents initially on the trunk, nape of the neck and behind the earlobes; subsequently (and rapidly), it spreads distally but usually spares the face.

DIFFERENTIAL DIAGNOSES

- Other diagnoses to be considered include other communicable diseases, in particular measles (very important to rule this out), rubella, enterovirus infection or other viral exanthems; urinary tract infection; bacterial sepsis; and, if a febrile convulsion has occurred or the rash is atypical, meningococcal meningitis. It is also important to consider the possibility of an antibiotic-associated rash.

MANAGEMENT

- **Additional diagnostics:** the diagnosis of roseola is largely a clinical one,

based on the typical history of fever followed by maculopapular rash when the fever subsides. No specific tests are available to diagnose roseola; however, depending on the clinical presentation, an FBC may be considered. This often reveals an initial leucocytosis (first 24 hours of fever) followed by leukopenia and a relative lymphocytosis (up to 90%). In addition, a urinalysis and urine culture may be considered as part of an evaluation of acute fever without localising source. These should be negative.

- **Pharmacotherapeutics:** treatment is supportive and aimed at symptom relief (paracetamol or ibuprofen).
- **Behavioural interventions:** oral fluids, adequate nutrition, rest and light clothing to enhance heat loss.
- **Patient education:**
  - Review with parents the benign, self-limiting nature of the illness and the expected clinical course (i.e. fever for 3–4 days, followed by a rash that normally disappears within 1–2 days). It is important that parents understand the importance of an adequate fluid intake, especially during the febrile phase of the illness.
  - Reassure parents about their ability to manage the illness with antipyretics, fluids and extra rest. Discuss with them the difference between roseola and measles or rubella (i.e. in roseola a rash on the face is uncommon and it appears *after* the fever subsides). Remind them that the vast majority of infants and children recover without sequelae.
  - If the child has experienced a febrile seizure during the acute phase of the illness, the parents will require additional explanations and reassurance (see Sec. 13.4). It is important to tell parents that the seizure is due to the fever and not the roseola. Five to ten per cent of children with roseola may experience a seizure during the febrile phase of the illness.
  - Discuss carefully with parents events that would be considered 'unexpected' in roseola and instruct them that they should seek care immediately for symptoms such

as decreasing alertness, an ill appearance, onset of vomiting, a rash that looks like black pinpoints that do not blanch, etc. Inform parents that the child can return to daycare or nursery once the child is afebrile.

FOLLOW-UP

- Complications are uncommon and, therefore, follow-up is not routinely necessary. However, given the height of the fever, parents may be extremely anxious and often appreciate telephone follow-up, especially during the febrile phase.

MEDICAL CONSULT/ SPECIALIST REFERRAL

- Any child with a toxic appearance.
- Any child in whom the diagnosis is uncertain.
- Any child who experiences a complication (e.g. febrile seizures, thrombocytopenic purpura, etc.).
- Any child with signs of meningeal irritation.

PAEDIATRIC PEARLS

- The temporal characteristics of the fever and rash are very important in diagnosing roseola; do not make the mistake of labelling a viral exanthem in a pre-school child 'roseola' if the rash did not appear as the fever was subsiding.
- Eyelid oedema and fever are commonly the symptoms prompting parents to seek care before the onset of the rash; be sure to warn parents that it is likely that the maculopapular rash will follow.
- A child with an acute bacterial infection and an antibiotic-associated rash can be confused with roseola; i.e. the rash appears 48 hours after the start of the antibiotic when the child's temperature is back to normal.
- Parents may describe the rash as 'bumpy', due to the slightly papular feel of it; this is especially relevant among children with darker skin tones, as the faint erythema is not very apparent.

BIBLIOGRAPHY

Breese-Hall C. Herpesvirus 6: new light on an old childhood exanthem. Contemp Pediatr 1996; 13(1):45–57.

Caserta MT, Mock DJ, Dewhurst S. Human herpesvirus 6. Clin Infect Dis 2001; 33(6):829–833.

Frieden IJ. Childhood exanthems. Curr Opin Pediatr 1995; 7(4):411–414.

Hall CB, Long CE, Schnabel KC. Human-herpes-6 infection in children: prospective evaluation for complications and reactivation. New Engl J Med 1994; 331(7):432.

Jones CA, Isaacs D. Human herpesvirus-6 infections. Arch Dis Child 1996; 74(2):98–100.

Leach CT. Human herpesvirus-6 and -7 infections in children: agents of roseola and other syndromes. Curr Opin Pediatr 2000; 12(3):269–274.

Lusso P, Gallo RC. Human herpesvirus 6. Baillières Clin Haematol 1995; 8(1):201–223.

Mancini AJ. Exanthems in childhood: an update. Pediatr Ann 1998; 27(3):163–170.

Stoeckle MY. The spectrum of human herpesvirus 6 infection: from roseola infantum to adult disease. Ann Rev Med 2000; 51:423–430.

Yamanishi K, Okuno T, Shiraki K. Identification of human herpesvirus-6 as a causal agent for exanthem subitum. Lancet 1988; 1:1065.

15.6 VARICELLA (CHICKENPOX)

Debra Sharu

INTRODUCTION

- Varicella is a viral infection caused by an antigenic strain of the herpes virus, varicella zoster virus (VZV). It is most frequently seen in school-age children but may occur at any age. The predominant feature is a pruritic vesicular rash that develops in crops. Chickenpox (varicella zoster) is the primary infection in a non-immune host, whereas shingles (herpes zoster) is the reactivation infection.
- A highly infectious disease, VZV is most commonly spread by direct contact with vesicular fluid or through airborne respiratory secretions. Contact exposure to individuals with shingles may also transmit the virus to an unprotected host. It is estimated that approximately 96% of susceptible persons in a household will acquire the disease if exposed to an infected family member and that 95% of the population have had varicella by the time adulthood is reached. The greatest number of cases occur in the late autumn, winter and spring.
- Varicella is contagious 1–2 days before the onset of the rash and until all blisters have crusted over (approx. 5–7 days). It develops within 10–21 days after exposure to an infected person (mean incubation is 14–16 days). Once the individual has recovered, immunity is generally acquired, but subsequent exposure may result in an outbreak of zoster or shingles (especially among those with impaired cell-mediated responses). A vaccine is available for children 12 months of age or older; however, it is not licensed for children for use in the UK. It (varicella-zoster vaccine) is only available on a named-patient basis from SmithKline Beecham.

HISTORY

- Recent exposure to chickenpox.
- Prior knowledge of having the disease.
- Onset, configuration and pattern of rash.

- Prodrome such as headache, malaise, poor appetite and low-grade fever.
- Current management of symptoms (oral intake if mucus involved).
- Associated symptoms, potential complications and/or other medical problems (brief review of systems, especially respiratory symptoms, CNS or sensory organs).
- *Very important* to determine if the patient or other household contacts are immunocompromised, as this would put them at substantially increased risk.

PHYSICAL EXAMINATION

- Fever may range from low grade to a marked elevation (39–40°C). Often there is a direct correlation between the extent of the rash and pyrexia; the more severe the rash, the higher the fever.
- **Skin:** examine for crops of lesions that appear in stages over a 3–4-day period. Initially pink, maculopapular spots (most often on the head or trunk) quickly progress to clear vesicles on an erythematous base, then to cloudy vesicles which have developed a crust within 6–10 hours. There can be just a few lesions to more than 500 lesions involving mucous membranes (mouth, throat and genitalia). *Note:* lesions can easily become infected with group A streptococcus or *Staphylococcus aureus* being the most common pathogens. Important to check lesions for development of secondary skin infections that have the potential to progress to cellulitis and toxic shock syndromes if not treated early.
- **Head and ENT:** careful inspection as there commonly can be a concurrent acute otitis media, marked oral involvement and development of ocular lesions.
- **Lymph:** can present with localised or generalised lymphadenopathy (especially with extensive disease).
- **Cardiopulmonary:** careful assessment for respiratory complications, which include pneumonia.
- **Assessment for additional complications (rare):** acute cerebellar ataxia (typically presents 1–2 weeks post-onset), thrombocytopenia,

disseminated intravascular coagulation (DIC), encephalitis, pancreatitis, arthritis, nephritis, osteomyelitis and Reye's syndrome.

DIFFERENTIAL DIAGNOSES

- Includes insect bites, folliculitis, impetigo, drug eruptions, contact dermatitis, scabies, herpes simplex, secondary syphilis and enterovirus infections (hand, foot and mouth disease or Coxsackie virus) and non-accidental injury (cigarette burns).

MANAGEMENT

- **Additional diagnostics:** rarely required, as the typical rash (occurring in crops of macules, papules and vesicles) is distinctive. In cases where virus identification is required, Tzanck smears, viral culture or acute and convalescent antibody titres can be used.
- **Pharmacotherapeutics:** consider
  - Paracetamol for fever relief and comfort; *aspirin should never be given.*
  - Antihistamines for relief of itching (e.g. chlorphenamine).
  - Topical lotions (e.g. calamine). If kept cool in the refrigerator will help control the itching. *Do not use* any topical preparations that contain antihistamines (e.g. diphenhydramine) or steroids.
  - Oral aciclovir: use is largely limited to *immunocompromised children* (if given within 24 hours of rash onset). It is effective in reducing the duration of illness, number of vesicles and intensity of pruritus. It can occasionally be considered for secondary cases (especially adolescents) in households if initiated <24 hours after rash onset; (1 month to 2 years: 20 mg/kg, max = 800 mg, four times daily for 5 days; 2–5 years: 400 mg, four times daily for 5 days; >6 years: 800 mg, four times daily for 5 days; >12 years: 800 mg, five times daily for 7 days).
  - *Note: advice should be sought immediately for infants, children and adolescents considered to be immunocompromised (systemic steroids in preceding 3 months; significant doses of inhaled steroids;*

those with congenital or acquired immune deficiencies).

- **Behavioural interventions:**
  - Lukewarm baths with baking soda (2 or 3 tablespoons) or ground oatmeal (1 cup/bath) provide relief from itching. Consider putting oatmeal into an old sock and holding sock over bath tap (letting bathwater run through the oatmeal).
  - Scarring is caused by premature removal of crusts or secondary infection of lesions; keep nails short, hands clean and *do not pick scabs, allow them to fall off on their own.* Cotton socks or mittens on infants' hands will limit scratching. Daytime activities that distract the child will also be helpful.
  - Lightweight cotton clothing with daily change decreases irritation and risk of skin infection.
  - Children with sores in their mouth are often reluctant to eat or drink. Dehydration can be prevented by encouraging the child to take cold, clear liquids, and soft bland foods such as ice cream, ice lollies and soup. Avoid spicy, hot, citrus-based or carbonated drinks.
  - If child is reluctant to void because of genital lesions, void while in warm bathwater.
- **Patient education:**
  - Explain to parents that for healthy children varicella is a benign disease from which they recover completely. However, complications can occur rarely and help/advice should be sought *immediately* for infected lesions, dehydration (or refusal of fluids), behavioural changes (confusion or excessive drowsiness), CNS symptoms (severe headache, stiff neck, decreased level of consciousness, unsteady gait), respiratory distress, redness of the eye or eye pain, and/or deteriorating condition.
  - Reassure parents that their child can go back to school approximately 5–7 days after onset of rash. This will coincide with the crusting over of the lesions. Exposure of pregnant women, infants and immunocompromised individuals should be avoided.

- Instruct parents to seek advice *immediately* for significant vomiting (with or without altered level of consciousness).

⇨ FOLLOW-UP

- For healthy children with an uncomplicated course, no follow-up is necessary.

⊘ MEDICAL CONSULT/ SPECIALIST REFERRAL

- Immediate referral for high-risk groups (infants less than 4 weeks of age, pregnant adolescents, immunocompromised individuals).
- Any child that develops complications (pneumonia, ocular or CNS involvement, etc.).
- Any child presenting with significant vomiting (with or without altered level of consciousness).

⊙ PAEDIATRIC PEARLS

- Crops of lesions in different stages of development are the hallmark of varicella infection.

- Fever can be marked (40.5°C) and, in general, the higher the fever the more extensive the rash.
- Lesions on mucous membranes will form shallow ulcer rather than typical 'crust'.
- Important to treat secondary skin infections promptly; young children with involvement may require hospitalisation.
- Parents are often quite anxious as lesions seem to appear 'before their very eyes'—let them know that the eruption of lesions typically lasts 3–4 days.
- Children with eczema are not at particular risk, as eczema herpeticum is caused by herpes simplex virus (not varicella zoster). The rash may be slightly more severe but these children can be treated as those without eczema, although topical steroids should be discontinued during the course of chickenpox.
- Although development of cerebral ataxia is rare, it can occur 2–3 weeks after symptoms resolve; investigate neurological complaints after varicella infection promptly.

☰ BIBLIOGRAPHY

Brody MB, Moyer D. Varicella-zoster virus infection: the complex prevention–treatment picture. Postgrad Med 1997; 102(1):187–190, 192–194.

Centers for Disease Control and Prevention. Facts about chicken pox (varicella). Available online: http://www.cdc.gov/od/oc/media/fact/chickenp.htm

Kesson AM. Acyclovir for the prevention and treatment of varicella zoster in children, adolescents and pregnancy. J Paediatr Child Health 1996; 32(2):11–17.

McKendrick MW. Acyclovir for childhood chickenpox. Cost is unjustified. BMJ 1995; 310(6972):108–109.

Ogilvie MM. Anti-viral prophylaxis and treatment in chickenpox: a review prepared for the UK Advisory Group on Chickenpox on behalf of the British Society for the Study of Infection. J Infect 1998; 36(Suppl 1):31–38.

Storr J. Chickenpox. Prof Nurse 1997; 12(12):869–871.

Tarlow MJ, Walters S. Chickenpox in childhood: a review prepared for the UK Advisory Group on Chickenpox on behalf of the British Society for the Study of Infection. J Infect 1998; 36(Suppl 1):39–47.

COMMON PAEDIATRIC PROBLEMS

15.7 PARVOVIRUS B19 INFECTION (FIFTH DISEASE, ERYTHEMA INFECTIOSUM)

Diane Scott

📖 INTRODUCTION

- Parvovirus B19 (human parvovirus) has been isolated as the causative agent for erythema infectiosum or fifth disease, so named because it was the fifth disease to be described with similar rashes (the others being measles, rubella, scarlet fever and roseola).
- It most commonly presents as an erythematous, macular, papular rash in a patient that otherwise is afebrile and well-appearing.
- Parvovirus B19 infection appears to be ubiquitous worldwide, with school-aged children most frequently

affected (highest incidence is among children 5–15 years of age). Up to 30% of school-aged children have evidence of previous B19 infection—presence of B19-specific immunoglobulin G (IgG)—which rises to approximately 50–60% by adulthood.

- Given the ever-present nature of the pathogen, community outbreaks are common (most frequently in late winter or early spring); however, infection is possible throughout the year.
- For the most part, parvovirus infection is a benign, self-limited illness that resolves spontaneously without long-term clinical sequelae. However, B19

infection can result in transient aplastic crisis (TAC) among children with hereditary haemolytic anaemias (e.g. sickle cell disease, spherocytosis and thalassaemia) or marked immunosuppression.

- In addition, B19 infection among pregnant women has been linked to fetal infection and subsequent pregnancy loss (hydrops fetalis and spontaneous abortion). The risk is greatest for non-immune women infected via household exposure during the first 20 weeks of pregnancy, although fetal infection is not inevitably fatal (approx. 3–9% risk of fetal death).

- Some patients with B19 infection develop joint complaints (arthralgias and arthritis of the hands, knees and feet have both been reported), although adults are affected more often than children. Symptoms typically begin 1 week after the viral prodrome and coincide with the development of B19-specific antibodies, suggesting a role for immune complex formation.

PATHOPHYSIOLOGY

- Humans are the only know reservoir of parvovirus B19. The virus replicates in the red blood cell precursors of the bone marrow (thus the association with TAC in susceptible individuals).
- Transmission is via respiratory secretions (including aerosolised large droplets and nasal secretions). In addition, the virus is transmissible in blood and blood products during the viraemic stage (although transmission is rare). The incubation period ranges from 6 to 14 days, with patients only infective until the rash (i.e. the 'slapped cheeks') appears (usually 17–18 days after exposure).
- The natural history of the disease has a typical pattern of three phases: (1) the prodromal phase of non-specific symptoms (lasting 1–4 days), including those usually associated with a mild upper respiratory tract infection (low-grade fever, headache, malaise, conjunctivitis and pharyngitis); this is followed by (2) an asymptomatic phase of 4–7 days; after which (3) there is onset (approximately 17–18 days after exposure) of the typical 'slapped cheek' rash (fiery, red exanthem of the cheeks which spreads to the body). The body rash is typically a discrete, maculopapular rash involving the trunk and extremities (including the extensor surfaces of the limbs), which progresses into a lacy, reticulated rash. This last stage of the rash may persist for 1–3 weeks (and can involve the palms and soles of the feet). In addition, it is characterised by periods of flare and remission, often triggered by environmental changes (elevated temperatures, exercise, warm baths, stress and sun exposure). However, the child remains largely well, active and playful throughout (despite the rash).

HISTORY

- Onset of illness and progression of the illness with particular attention to the spread and pattern of the rash.
- Additional signs and symptoms (joint pain, arthropathy or other complaints).
- History of possible exposures (daycare/nursery attendance, community outbreaks in school or after-school clubs) and immunisation history.
- History to determine possibility of exposure of susceptible individuals (pregnant women, children with haemolytic anaemia).
- Management of rash and symptoms at home (creams, medicines, etc.).

PHYSICAL EXAMINATION

- General appearance of the child, including careful inspection of the skin for rashes (especially the fiery, red, maculopapular lesions that coalesce to give the appearance of 'slapped' cheeks). The lesions are usually warm, non-tender and may be pruritic with the circumoral region usually spared. Likewise, examine for other lesions, including progression on to the lacy, reticulated rash involving the body.
- Routine head/ENT and abdominal exam (to exclude other aetiologies/illnesses).
- Careful inspection of joints for signs of arthralgia and arthritis.

DIFFERENTIAL DIAGNOSES

- Additional aetiologies that should be considered include rubella, measles, enteroviral infection and drug reaction. In the older child with a rash and arthritis, consider the possibility of juvenile rheumatoid arthritis (JRA), systemic lupus erythematosus (SLE) and other connective tissue disorders.

MANAGEMENT

- **Additional diagnostics:** rarely indicated, as the diagnosis is dependent on recognition of the typical signs and symptoms. However, B19-specific antibodies can be measured and the virus can also be isolated from the plasma (although difficult to grow). Note that B19-specific IgM is diagnostic of parvovirus infection and B19-specific IgG antibodies are indicative of past infection as they persist for years (IgM levels start to fall 30–60 days after onset of illness). Both groups of immunoglobulins are detectable after approximately 3–7 days of illness. There are also B19-specific enzyme-linked immunosorbent assay (ELISA) and radioimmunoassay tests for B19.
- **Pharmacotherapeutics:** No specific antiviral treatment; care (if required) is supportive and includes paracetamol or a non-steroidal anti-inflammatory drug (NSAID) such as ibuprofen for symptomatic relief.
- **Behavioural interventions:**
  - Good handwashing and correct disposal of tissues containing secretions should be encouraged/stressed.
  - Pregnant women exposed to children with infectious B19 should seek guidance from their health care provider.
  - Routine isolation is unnecessary, as the disease is no longer contagious once the rash appears. However, contact with susceptible children or adults should be avoided (hereditary haemolytic anaemias, immuno-compromised and pregnant women). Consequently, children at increased risk from B19 infection should be observed for complications related to TAC.
- **Patient education:**
  - review behavioural interventions (above), including use of paracetamol or ibuprofen if necessary
  - discuss and reassure parents about the benign and self-limiting nature of the illness
  - warn parents that the rash tends to fluctuate over the next 1–3 weeks, especially with exposure to sunlight, heat (including a hot bath), exercise and stress

- let parents know that children can return to school (or nursery) once the rash has appeared if they are feeling well.

FOLLOW-UP

- Generally not indicated if symptomatology resolves.

MEDICAL CONSULT/ SPECIALIST REFERRAL

- Any child with joint involvement and/or a gravely ill appearance.
- Any child in whom doubt exists with regard to the diagnosis or the disease does not follow the expected course.
- Any child considered to be at increased risk of sequelae after B19 infection (or exposure); i.e. immunocompromised children or

those with hereditary haemolytic anaemias.

PAEDIATRIC PEARLS

- Although the typical appearance of the parvovirus rash is 'slapped cheeks' and a lacy reticulated rash, occasionally there can be an atypical appearance which includes papules, vesicles or purpura and involves the palms and soles.
- Children with B19 infection appear well and happy despite the rash; if not, consider another aetiology.
- The appearing/disappearing nature of the rash can be disturbing for parents; be sure to warn them of this possibility.
- Although there is a risk of fetal loss among pregnant women exposed to B19 during the first 20 weeks of pregnancy, this risk is relatively small.

Exposed women should be encouraged to discuss this with their individual midwife/GP/consultant. However, children who are *aplastic* following B19 infection are highly infectious and pregnant health care workers should not be in contact with these children.

BIBLIOGRAPHY

Adams D, Ware R. Parvovirus B19: How much should you worry? Contemp Pediatr 1996; 13(4):85–96.

Chong P. Prevention of occupationally acquired infections among health care workers. Pediatr Rev 1998; 19(7):219–230.

Gildea JH. Human parvovirus B19: flushed in face though healthy (fifth disease and more). Pediatr Nurs 1998; 24(4):325–329.

Jones SH, Jenista JA. Fifth disease: role for nurses in pediatric practice. Pediatr Nurs 1990; 16(2):148–151.

Ware R. Human parvovirus infection. J Pediatr 1989; 114:343–348.

15.8 MENINGITIS

Suzanne Garbarino-Danson

INTRODUCTION

- Meningitis is an inflammation of the meninges usually caused by bacteria, viruses or fungi; uncommonly, meningitis can be caused by protozoa or parasites.
- A high index of suspicion is vital so that meningitis is diagnosed and treated promptly. The goals of early identification and management are to minimise subsequent morbidity and mortality.
- Viral meningitis is more commonly seen than bacterial meningitis. Enterovirus infections (e.g. coxsackievirus, echovirus and numerous other strains) account for approximately 85% of cases. Enterovirus infections tend to occur in outbreaks, most commonly in the summer and early autumn.
- Bacterial meningitis is more serious, with a greater likelihood of acute

complications, long-term sequelae and/or death. Causative agents of bacterial meningitis have a developmental component, with some organisms more common in different age groups (Table 15.8). Bacterial meningitis predominantly affects children under 24 months old, especially those from 4 to 12 months of age. The highest mortality rate is among children from birth to 4 years of age. During the first 2 months of life, newborns have passive protection from maternal antibodies but are susceptible to group B streptococci infection (most common causative agent in the neonatal period). *Haemophilus influenzae* type B (Hib) was the most common cause of bacterial meningitis until widespread immunisation uptake significantly reduced the incidence of Hib meningitis and other invasive Hib infections.

- Fungal meningitis is usually associated with an underlying immune system compromise (e.g. multiple antibiotic courses, cental lines, etc., including premature birth. However, approximately one-quarter of patients with cryptococcal meningitis do not have an underlying immune deficiency.
- The incidence of tuberculous meningitis has paralleled the rise of tuberculosis (TB) throughout the world. TB meningitis occurs in approximately 1 in 300 cases of primary TB infection, although this number rises to 50% if the patient has miliary TB (increased with HIV infection).

PATHOPHYSIOLOGY

- Meningitis is almost always the result of haematogenic spread of a pathogen that enters the central nervous

Table 15.8   Presentation, Organisms and Antibiotic Therapy in Childhood Meningitis

Age	Signs/symptoms	Common organisms	Antibiotic therapy
Birth to 3 months	• Fever • Seizures • Anorexia • Vomiting, diarrhoea • Bulging fontanelle • Irritability, inconsolability • High-pitched cry • Apnoea • Paradoxical irritability • Lethargy • Altered sleep patterns • Petechial rash • Non-specific complaints	• Group B streptococci • Escherichia coli • Listeria monocytogenes • Haemophilus influenzae	• Ampicillin and gentamicin[a] (neonates) • Ceftriaxone • Cefotaxime • Ampicillin and chloramphenicol
4 months to 2 years	• Fever • Vomiting, diarrhoea • Irritability/lethargy • Decreased level of consciousness • Altered sleep patterns • Petechial rash • Possible nuchal rigidity	• H. influenzae • Neisseria meningitidis • Streptococcus pneumoniae • Mycobacterium tuberculosis • Enteroviruses	• Ceftriaxone • Cefotaxime • Ampicillin and chloramphenicol • Isoniazid, rifampicin, pyrazinamide and streptomycin
2–12 years	• Fever, irritability • Headache, stiff neck • Photophobia • Ataxia • Vomiting • Petechial rash • Kernig and/or Brudzinski's signs	• S. pneumoniae • N. meningitidis • Group A streptococci • Enteroviruses	• Ceftriaxone • Cefotaxime • Benzylpenicillin • Supportive care

[a]Not to be used in neonates with jaundice, hypoalbuminaemia or acidosis.

system (CNS) from the bloodstream. Consequently, septicaemia often accompanies meningitis.

- The membranes of the brain and/or spinal cord subsequently become inflamed, with a corresponding increase in white blood cells and exudate. There is an increase in intracranial pressure as the brain becomes swollen and hyperaemic. Bacterial meningitis can also cause the brain to be covered in a thick exudate, which obstructs the passage of cerebrospinal fluid (CSF) and can result in brain abscess, subdural effusions and thrombosis of the meningeal veins.
- Meningococcal septicaemia can lead to complications such as disseminated intravascular coagulation (DIC) and shock.

⇐ HISTORY

- Subjective information gathered includes information outlined in Chapter 4.
- Information specific to bacterial meningitis includes duration of illness;

presence of nausea and vomiting; complaints of headache, backache, neck pain and/or nuchal rigidity; photophobia; fever; rash and unusual drowsiness or lethargy.
- Information specific to viral meningitis includes presence of early symptoms/ prodrome (e.g. headache, fever, poor appetite and malaise) and duration of symptoms. Note that viral meningitis is characterised by a more gradual onset and shorter overall course.
- Information related to fungal meningitis includes potential exposure to pigeon or bird droppings (crytococcus) and presence of symptoms such as headache and vomiting gradually increasing over days to weeks.
- Infants often display very non-specific symptoms and, therefore, subjective information related to activity levels, eating, playfulness, fever and presence of an unusual cry, 'floppiness', crying when moved or handled and change in fontanelle (i.e. bulging or hardening) should be elicited.
- Immunisation status, possibility of immunocompromise and close

contacts who are unwell should also be ascertained.

🕮 PHYSICAL EXAMINATION

- A complete physical examination with careful assessment of the neurological system (including assessment for increased intracranial pressure and decreased level of consciousness).
- Signs of meningism include Kernig's sign (pain elicited with extension of the knee when the hip is flexed) and Brudzinski's sign (spontaneous flexion of the lower limbs following passive flexion of the neck). Alternatively, the patient can be asked to 'kiss their knees' in the supine position with the hips flexed or knees raised. Amongst infants, assessment of nucchal rigidity can be made by dropping a toy or asking the parent to walk across the room and observing the infant's ability to follow. Note that negative Kernig's and Brudzinski's signs do not indicate the absence of meningitis.
- Inspect the skin and mucous membranes carefully, checking for any rashes (which, if discovered, should be assessed for blanching: see Sec. 9.1).

- **Cardiovascular:** careful assessment for signs of septicaemia and shock.

❓ DIFFERENTIAL DIAGNOSES

- The differential diagnoses list is extensive. Consider poisonings, other viral or bacterial illness, migraines, septicaemia, bacteraemia, gastroenteritis, encephalitis, epilepsy and CNS malignancy.

➕ MANAGEMENT

- **Additional diagnostics:** laboratory tests are used to help narrow the differential diagnoses list and confirm the diagnosis. Consequently, numerous tests are often considered: full blood count, urea and electrolytes, blood culture, throat swab, urinalysis and culture. If TB meningitis is suspected, a Heaf test should be conducted. A lumbar puncture (LP) is the primary diagnostic procedure for meningitis. The CSF is examined for appearance (in meningitis it can be cloudy or turbid); white blood cell count (increased in meningitis, >500 polymorphs/mm^3) protein (increased in meningitis); and glucose (reduced in meningitis). A Gram stain and culture are also performed. Note that an LP should *not* be performed if the child has any decreased level of consciousness or if there is a suspicion of increased intracranial pressure (coning may result); a normal CT scan does not exclude the possibility of increased intracranial pressure (ICP).
- **Pharmacotherapeutics:** antibiotic therapy is based upon the pathogen identified or suspected of causing the infection (Table 15.8). Note that close contacts may be given antibiotic prophylaxis when deemed appropriate by the public health department.
- **Behavioural interventions:** these are largely supportive and include attention to the ABC's (airway, breathing and circulation) as a priority. Additional management includes adequate fluid and nutritional intake (with support if required), rest and monitoring for complications.

- **Patient education:**
  - Discuss with families the cause of the meningitis and the likelihood of a full recovery (if appropriate). If prophylaxis is to be instituted (this is determined by the local public health department), families should understand the rationale behind it. Outline the supportive care necessary and the signs and symptoms of complications that families should watch for.
  - A plan for adequate and appropriate monitoring and follow-up should be negotiated.

➡️ FOLLOW-UP

- Follow-up is dependent on clinical condition and aetiology of the infection. It is likely that telephone follow-up (as the minimum) should be considered. All children with confirmed cases of meningitis will require evaluation for neurological sequelae.

⇄ MEDICAL CONSULT/ SPECIALIST REFERRAL

- Any child with a gravely ill appearance.
- Any child in whom the diagnosis of meningitis is suspected and/or any child in whom the diagnosis is not clear.

🔎 PAEDIATRIC PEARLS

- In viral meningitis, the headache often improves after LP; many think this is diagnostic.
- Do not confuse meningitis (e.g. inflammation of the meninges resulting from many causes) with meningococcal septicaemia (i.e. septicaemia caused by *Neisseria meningitidis*).
- A high index of suspicion for meningitis is required, especially with infants and small children in whom the presentation may be very non-specific. Many times there is a vague history with parents reporting 'that my baby is just not right'. Although parents may not be able to articulate what is wrong, be sure to heed their concerns.

- Notify the public health department for all cases of suspected and/or confirmed meningitis.
- Ten per cent of children with tuberculous meningitis will not react to TB skin testing; if meningitis is suspected, therapy should be instigated.
- If no aetiology is discovered after a lumbar puncture and yet the child is not responding to therapy, repeat the LP in 36–48 hours.
- Meningococcal disease with septicaemia has a poorer prognosis than meningitis alone.

📖 BIBLIOGRAPHY

Atkinson PJ, Sharland M, Maguire H. Predominant enteroviral serotypes causing meningitis. Arch Dis Child 1998; 78(4):373–374.

Bedford H, de Louvois J, Halket S, et al. Meningitis in infancy in England and Wales: follow up at age 5 years. BMJ 2001; 323(7312):533–536.

Davies D. The causes of meningitis and meningoccocal disease. Nurs Times 1996; 92(6):22–27.

Fortnum HM, Davis AC. Epidemiology of bacterial meningitis. Arch Dis Child 1993; 68(6):763–767.

Goossens H, Sprenger MJ. Community acquired infections and bacterial resistance. BMJ 1998; 317(7159): 654–657.

Gunn A. Meningitis: public health issues. Nurs Times 1996; 92(6):27–29.

Jones R, Finlay F, Crouch V, et al. Meningitis and meningococcal septicaemia. Arch Dis Child 2000; 82(5):428.

Kumar R, Singh SN, Kohli N. A diagnostic rule for tuberculous meningitis. Arch Dis Child 1999; 81(3):221–224.

Newton RW. Tuberculous meningitis. Arch Dis Child 1994; 70(5):364–366.

Peate I. Meningitis: causes, symptoms, signs and nursing management. Br J Nurs 1999; 8(19):1290–1298.

Public Health Laboratory Service. PHLS meningococcal infection fact sheet; 2000. Available on line: www.phls.co.uk/ advice/mening.htm

Richardson MP, Reid A, Tarlow MJ, et al. Hearing loss during bacterial meningitis. Arch Dis Child 1997; 76(2):134–138.

Strawser J. Pediatric bacterial meningitis in the emergency department. J Emerg Nurs 1997; 23(4):310–315.

Wubbel L, McCracken GH. Management of bacterial meningitis. Pediatr Rev 1998; 19(3):78–84.

COMMON PAEDIATRIC PROBLEMS

15.9 BRUISING IN THE HEALTHY CHILD

Nan D. McIntosh

📖 INTRODUCTION

- Bruising is the visible result of extravasation of blood into the skin. Petechiae are characterised as flat, non-blanching, red/purple/black macules 1–3 mm, whereas bruising (ecchymoses) is larger and occasionally palpable. Both petechiae and ecchymoses are considered to be purpuric lesions.
- Bruising on shins, elbows or knees is commonly seen (especially among toddlers and teenagers). The majority can be explained by active play (trauma); however, it can also result from a low platelet count (thrombocytopenia) or a clotting mechanism defect. Unexplained bleeding or bruising (in an otherwise healthy child) that is excessive (or disproportionate to the injury/trauma sustained) *must be investigated*.
- Clotting abnormalities can be associated with a wide range of signs and symptoms but are most commonly caused by systemic disease, familial disorders and/or drug-related reactions.

🔬 PATHOPHYSIOLOGY

- Blood clotting is a critical defence mechanism that helps protect the integrity of the vascular system in association with inflammatory and general repair responses. Platelets (thrombocytes) are a mainstay of coagulation; disc-shaped cells without a nucleus, their role is fundamental in clotting.
- Platelets and plasma proteins play an essential role in the haemostatic mechanism and, in practice, are inextricably connected. When blood vessels are damaged, the haemostatic response is localised, immediate and controlled. Three basic mechanisms prevent bleeding from small blood vessels:
  - vascular spasm results in smooth muscle contraction (vasoconstriction) to slow blood flow
  - platelet recruitment from the circulation to the damaged endothelial cell barrier forms an occlusive platelet plug (a result of platelet adhesion and aggregation)
  - activation of the coagulation cascade (intrinsic and extrinsic pathways), commonly referred to as blood clotting factors.
- Any process that disrupts normal function (thrombocytopenia, coagulation disorder or extrinsic factors such as infection or trauma) will result in bleeding/bruising.

↩ HISTORY

- Bleeding/bruising episode(s) of recent onset or long-standing duration.
- Recent infections (e.g. sore throat or viral illness) with time frame.
- Associated nausea, vomiting, dark stools, fever, abdominal, joint pain or other signs of systemic illness. *Note*: blood abnormalities may be caused by systemic disease rather than specific blood disease, e.g. infection or malignancy.
- Excessive bleeding with previous dental treatment or surgical procedures.
- Family history of 'bleeding problems' (heavy menses, easy bleeding/bruising) in other family members.
- Observe reactions to questions and interactions by family members to ascertain relationships (although unfamiliar surroundings may cause difficulty in articulating concerns).
- History of drug/medication use: aspirin or warfarin therapy and non-steroidal anti-inflammatory drugs (NSAIDs) may trigger an undiscovered, mild inherited disorder, whereas loratadine and cetirizine have rare reports of associated purpura.

👁 PHYSICAL EXAMINATION

- **Appearance:** observe general appearance (ill or well), posture, movement and parent–child interaction; consider whether bleeding is limited to skin or extends to muscles, joints and viscera. Be especially aware of children who are becoming unwell, as this may be an early manifestation of meningococcal septicaemia.
- **Skin:** assessment of the severity and distribution of bruising/petechiae is vital. Consequently, inspect from head to toe, noting size, distribution, colour and pattern of all purpuric lesions. Petechiae may be most evident around pressure points, e.g. around ankles, resulting from elastic top on socks, around eyes, neck and upper trunk. Match history to presentation of bruising and note that Henoch–Schönlein purpura often presents with lesions on the ankles and buttocks.
- **Head and ENT:** may reveal retinal or conjunctival haemorrhage, blood blisters in the mouth and dried blood in nostrils. Do not use a spatula or carry out this examination in a distraught child as it may result in further bleeding.
- **Cardiopulmonary:** careful examination to rule out adventitious sounds and/or pathological murmurs.
- **Abdomen:** examination of liver, spleen and lymph glands is essential (see Sec. 15.3). Generalised lymphadenopathy and hepatosplenomegaly virtually excludes the diagnosis of idiopathic thrombocytopenic purpura (ITP) but should lead you to suspect systemic infection or acute leukaemia.

🔎 DIFFERENTIAL DIAGNOSES

- Numerous, but presenting symptomatology can provide clues as to aetiology (Table 15.9).

Table 15.9 Differential Diagnosis of Bruising/Bleeding

Presenting signs/symptoms	Consider

• Easy bruising and/or bleeding
• Bleeding from mucous membranes (mouth or nose)
• Excessive bleeding after minor trauma
• Spontaneous joint or muscle bleed
	• *Immune-mediated reaction resulting in platelet destruction in the circulation.*
	  ○ Idiopathic thrombocytopenic purpura (ITP) is most common (1/25,000 distributed evenly between sexes)
	  ○ Mild ITP symptoms may not be evident; history may reveal non-specific viral infection that preceded sudden onset of bruising/petechiae
	• *Disorders of coagulation or platelet function (acquired or inherited) recognised after an abnormal bleeding episode:*
	  ○ Haemophilia (A and B)
	  ○ von Willebrand's disease (vWD)
	  ○ Glanzmann's disease
	  ○ Acquired drug reaction (aspirin, sulphonamides, chloramphenicol, warfarin)

• Lethargy, pyrexia, malaise, vomiting with purpura/ bruising, and/or lymphadenopathy	• *Systemic disease:*
	  ○ Meningitis/septicaemia
	  ○ Viral infection (coxsackie, echo or enterovirus)
	  ○ Liver disease
	• *Malignancy or bone marrow failure:*
	  ○ Leukaemia
	  ○ Aplastic anaemia

• Unusual episodes of bruising/ bleeding	• *Factitial purpura:*
	  ○ Non-accidental injury (NAI)
	  ○ Self abuse/harm

• Associated abdominal pain +/− purpuric rash, throat infection and haematuria	• *Vascular/autoimmune:*
	  ○ Henoch–Schönlein purpura (HSP)
	  ○ Systemic lupus erythematosus (SLE)

• Associated joint pain or limitation of movement	• Fracture, dislocation or malignancy (see Ch. 13)

Note that bruising confined mostly to legs is associated with Henoch–Schönlein purpura (HSP) and normal activity, whereas petechiae above the nipple line is seen with severe cough, viral infections and Valsalva manoeuvre. Suspect non-accidental injury (NAI) with bruising in different stages, ecchymoses on head, trunk, genitals or lesions with a distinctive pattern (handmarks, belt or paddle marks) that is inconsistent with history.

✚ MANAGEMENT

- **Additional diagnostics:**
  - Full blood count (FBC) with differential white cell count (Diff) is the initial laboratory test that should be performed. Information will be gained regarding the three cell lines in peripheral blood; most blood abnormalities are associated with a derangement of at least one of the lines (red cells, white cells and platelets).
  - Urine and stool should also be checked for blood (urine dipstick and faecal occult blood).
  - Other tests of coagulation function (if history, physical or above tests indicate) include prothrombin time (PT), activated partial thromboplastin time (APTT), thrombin clotting time (TCT), von Willebrand's screen, fibrinogen levels, bleeding time and, in some situations, a bone marrow aspirate (to confirm a diagnosis of ITP or exclude leukaemia).

- **Pharmacotherapeutics:** use of drugs is largely aetiology-specific. In unusually severe cases of bruising or bleeding (attributed to ITP), oral corticosteroids or intravenous immunoglobulins may be given. However, this level of management is unlikely to occur outside the specialist and/or acute care setting where it would be administered in collaboration with medical colleagues. Aspirin (or any NSAID) if being administered to a child with explained bruising/bleeding should be discontinued.

- **Behavioural interventions:** none required for children with normal FBC parameters and no unusual findings with the exception of reassurance and education (see below).

- **Patient education:**
  - Parents and children *with/without* coagulation problems should be given reassurance and routine safety counselling, e.g. head injury and the use of cycle safety helmets.
  - Anticipatory guidance regarding the 'normalcy' of nosebleeds and their relationship to nose-picking, dry nasal membranes, trauma and URTI. Initial management of nosebleeds includes the application of ice and pressure to the nasal dorsum for a few minutes. The head should be held forward to prevent the blood from trickling down the throat. A possible ENT referral may be required if episodes are not easily controlled or self-contained. Nasal cautery may be needed for a recurrent bleeding area within the nostril.
  - If a bleeding disorder is suspected, the child and family should be counselled on the services available from a paediatric haematology team within a comprehensive care centre. These include diagnosis of mild, moderate and severe bleeding disorders; prophylaxis and treatment monitoring; patient education and preventative care; genetic and prenatal counselling; and regular follow-up.

⇨ FOLLOW-UP

- Aetiology-specific.

⇄ MEDICAL CONSULT/ SPECIALIST REFERRAL

- Children with suspected bleeding disorder (irrespective of the aetiology).
- Children with moderate to severe thrombocytopenia (platelets $<30 \times 10^9$/litre).
- An episode of copious bleeding (indicative of haemorrhage) is considered a medical emergency. *Note:* major haemorrhage is rare in patients with bleeding disorders;

bleeding is prolonged rather than profuse.

- A gravely ill or quickly deteriorating child with purpuric rash, malaise, pyrexia, vomiting, irritability (meningococcal septicaemia).
- A seemingly healthy child with vague history of non-specific infection and abnormal clinical findings on examination (hepatosplenomegaly, generalised purpuric lesions), as leukaemia and lymphoma need to be ruled out.

PAEDIATRIC PEARLS

- Abnormal bruising as a presenting problem or an incidental finding must be explored and fully documented, not ignored; when in doubt, check the FBC, urinalysis and faecal occult blood. Be wary of NAI if unexplained bleeding/bruising.
- *Do not* delay referral for any suspicious/unexplained bleeding/bruising while awaiting laboratory results; delays could be costly and leukaemia (while uncommon) does occur.
- Always beware spreading petechiae in an unwell child (meningococcal septicaemia).
- Babies of ethnic or oriental origin commonly have a large, flat, black and blue area found on the buttocks and in the lumbosacral region (mongolian spot). It is a normal finding resulting from pigmented cells in the dermis that fade in early childhood.
- Never pre-judge or make assumptions; routine blood tests can support suspicions.
- Children with bleeding disorders or reduced platelet counts should not be given aspirin, but may have paracetamol. If stronger pain relief is required, families should contact their provider. Even small doses of aspirin can dramatically prolong the bleeding time and cause bleeding in patients with thrombocytopenia or bleeding problems. *Note*: some commonly available teething gels contain salicylates.

- The extent of bruising (with or without petechiae) may not correlate with the presence of internal bleeding and, conversely, a child with ITP may have widespread bruising (with or without petechiae) with a normal haemoglobin (Hgb).
- Despite a markedly reduced platelet count (and varying symptomatology) in acute onset ITP, serious complications are rare. The disease is self-limiting in approximately 90% of patients and requires only observation. External bleeding is usually seen in the form of epistaxis; the risk of severe intracranial or gastrointestinal bleeding is rare.

BIBLIOGRAPHY

Buchanan GR. ITP: How much is enough? Contemp Pediatr 2000; 17(4):112–121.

George J. The clinical importance of acquired abnormalities of platelet function. New Engl J Med 1991; 324:28.

Manno CS. Difficult pediatric diagnoses: bleeding and bruising. Pediatr Clin North Am 1991; 38(3):637–655.

APPENDICES

APPENDIX 1

Overview of Child Development

Katherine Jenner

- The information given in Tables A1.1–A1.6 is for use as a *guide* for the assessment of development. The references in the Further Reading section are sources of additional information.
- It is important to remember that each child is an individual and will have their own rate of growth and development.
- Physical, psychological, sociological and spiritual development are normally interrelated along a continuum.
- Although children have a genetic propensity for development, they need the *opportunity* to maximise their potential—this must be taken into account when assessing milestones.
- The milestone format is adapted from Sheridan's (1997) aspects of developmental progress.

☰ BIBLIOGRAPHY

Bee H. The developing child, 8th edn. New York: Longman; 1997.

Donaldson M. Children's minds. London: Fontana; 1986.

Hall DMB. Health for all children, 3rd edn. Oxford: Oxford University Press; 1996.

http://www.kidsource.com/education/on.track.html, 30/01/01.

Smith PK, Cowie H, Blades M. Understanding children's development, 3rd edn. Oxford: Blackwell Science; 1998.

Taylor JD, Muller DJ, Wattley L, et al. Nursing children: psychology, research and practice, 3rd edn. London: Chapman and Hall; 1999.

Sheridan MD. From birth to 5 years. London: Routledge; 1997.

Wong DL. Whaley and Wong's nursing care of infants and children, 6th edn. St Louis: Mosby, 1999.

Table A1.1 Milestones of Growth and Development: Birth to 6 months (Full-Term Baby). Adapted from Sheridan (1997)

Milestone	Age (months)					
	1	2	3	4	5	6
Physical growth gains	Weight: 180 g/week Height: 2.5 cm/month Head circumference: 2 cm/month → 1 cm/month →					→ Birth weight doubles
Gross motor ability	• Lifts head in prone position	• Lifts head in prone position to 45°	• Kicks vigorously	• Sits (supported) head steady • Rolls to supine	• Control of head and arm movements	• May sit unaided • Stands, hands held
Fine motor movements/manipulative/adaptive skills	• Grasp reflex (fisted hand)	• Control of eye muscles: follows objects with eyes, past the midline • Oral exploration		• Hands open • Brings objects to mouth	• Purposeful grasping	• Palmar grasp of objects
Vision, hearing and other sensory capacities Cognition Communication/speech	• Cries • Facial response to sound • Able to stare at an object if within 20 cm • Other basic responses to smell, taste, touch, temperature and pain	• Colour perception • Visual exploration • Coos (vowel sounds), grunts		• Laughs and squeals • Turns towards voice/other sounds	• Can accommodate to near objects	• Hand–eye coordination developing • Babbles (most vowel sounds and many consonant sounds)
Social/emotional	• Stares at faces • Helpless • Asocial • Generalised tension	• Smiles in response to others • Soothed by rocking (maybe!)		• Smiles spontaneously	• Recognises main carer	• Reaches for toys • Recognises strangers • Smiles discriminatingly • Expects feeding, dressing and washing

Table A1.2 Milestones of Growth and Development: 7–12 months (Full-Term Baby). Adapted from Sheridan (1997)

Milestone	Age (months)					
	7	8	9	10	11	12
Physical growth gains	Weight: 85–140 g/week Height: 1.25 cm/month Head circumference: 1 cm/month --->					Birth weight trebles Birth length increases by approx. 50%
Gross motor ability	• Sits—self-supporting • Control of trunk and hands • Beginning to crawl/shuffle	• Sits unaided • Crawls/shuffles (usually)	• Pulls to stand	• Control of legs and feet	• Cruises (walks whilst holding onto furniture or hands held)	• Stands unaided • Cruises • Walks, one hand held
Fine motor movements/ manipulative/ adaptive skills	• Can transfer objects from one hand to another • Can hold an object in each hand simultaneously	• Crude pincer (thumb and forefinger) grasp		• Can pick up small round objects • Can let go of objects at will	• Neat pincer grasp	• Can help turn pages of book • Tries to build a tower (with bricks—usually fails)
Vision, hearing and other sensory capacities Cognition Communication/speech	• Can fixate on tiny objects • Developing depth perception	• Utters 'mama' and 'dada' arbitrarily • Appears to understand 'no' • Imitates sounds		• Speaks 1 or 2 words • Responds to simple commands • Can ascribe meaning to early words		• Visual acuity 20/40–20/60 • Speaks 2–4 words with meaning • Follows command with gesture (e.g. Where is the cat?) • Points to indicate desires
Social/emotional	• Imitates actions and noises • Reacts to different facial expressions • Sensitive to emotional changes in others	• Feeds self • Waves 'bye bye'		• Fear of strangers • Responds to own name • Plays 'pat-a-cake' • Gives and takes objects	• Shows anger, affection, curiosity and exploration	• Self-feeding—fingers and spoon • Drinks (with spills) from cup • Enjoys attention

Table A1.3 Milestones of Growth and Development: 15–36 months. Adapted from Sheridan (1997)

Milestone	Age			
	15 months	18 months	2 years	36 months
Physical growth gains	Weight: (birth weight triples 14 months) Height: 12 cm in 2nd year	◄------ 2–3 kg/year ------►	(birth weight quadruples)	
Gross motor ability	• Walks unaided • Stoops and recovers (16 months)	• Creeps up stairs • Walks backwards • Climbs • Stiff-legged run	• Can walk up steps—brings 2nd foot to join 1st unaided • Jumps • Runs without falling • Kicks large ball	• Rides tricycle using peddles
Fine motor movements/ manipulative/ adaptive skills	• Scribbles (16 months) holding pencil in fist	• Pushes/pulls objects • Can turns pages of books	• Builds 6–7 cube tower • Aligns and manipulates cubes • Can unravel, undo, untie • Solves single-piece puzzle	• Imitates horizontal and vertical lines • Builds with cubes
Communication Language Cognition	• 4–6 words • Can follow command without associated gesture	• 10–20 words • Names objects • Few phrases: 'lets go', 'stop it' • Can point to approx. four external body parts • Beginning use of symbols • Plays matching games	• Combines 2–3 words • Uses 'I' and 'you' • Verbalises wants • Understands more than says • 50% speech intelligible to strangers	• Can name all external body parts • Language development strongly influenced by environment
Social/emotional	• Drinks from cup • Imitates activities	• Feeds self with spoon • Forms relationships • Solitary play • Hugs dolls/cuddly toys • Temperament apparent • Self-comforting behaviours	• Removes coat • Differentiates self from others • Imitates adult activities (cooking, hammering) • Tolerates some separation from main carer • Temper tantrums • Parallel play	• Pulls up pants • Washes and dries hands

Table A1.4 Milestones of Development: 3–5 years. Adapted from Sheridan (1997)

Milestone	Age				
	3 years	3½ years	4 years	4½ years	5 years
Physical growth gains	Weight: 2–3 kg/year ————————————————→ Slow and steady Height: 6–8 cm/year ——→ birth length doubles ——→ 5–7.5 cm/year ——————→ Slow and steady				
Gross motor ability	• Walks up and down steps—alternating feet • Can tip toe • Jumps from a step	• Stands on one foot for 2–3 s	• Competent walking, running, skipping, jumping • Hops on one foot (?earlier)	• Broad jumps (24 inches)	• Skips—alternating feet
Fine motor movements/ manipulative/ adaptive skills	• Copies circle • Draws a three-part person • Draws a person's head	• Copies a cross	• Eye–hand and muscle coordination evident (throws and catches ball readily) • Drawings demonstrate advancing perception of shape and form	• Copies square • Draws a six-part person	• Prints first name
Communication Language Cognition	• 500 words • 75% of speech intelligible to strangers • Beginning to use complete sentences • Bilingual children may mix languages • Gives full name, age and sex • Knows two colours • Asks 'why' • Thinks symbolically but one dimensionally—no concept of conservation (if shown equal volumes of water which are then poured into glasses of different heights, will think that there is more water in the taller glass)	• Understands cold, tired, hungry	• Counts 4 objects • Identifies some letters and numbers • Understands prepositions (under, on, behind, in front of) • Uses more words to convey a meaning • Asks how and why • No concept of conservation • Follows simple directional demands	• Understands opposites • Bosses and criticises	• Counts 10 objects • Continence day and night should be achieved • Asks meaning of words • Refinement of language skills and linguistic competence—uses longer words, larger vocabulary, more complex sentences, better grammar, grasps subtle grammar exceptions
Social/emotional	• Toilet trained • Puts on shirt • Knows front from back • Some impulse control, self-regulation • More independent but with need for attachment security • Some evidence of turn taking with other children	• Engages in associative play	• Dresses with little assistance • Shoes on correct feet • Play becomes important method of expression/working through of ideas • Feelings of guilt and anxiety • Ability to consider other viewpoints • Developing sense of right and wrong	• Shows off	• Ties shoes

Table A1.5   Milestones of Growth and Development: 6–11 years. Adapted from Sheridan (1997)

Milestone	Age	
	6 years	7–10/11 years
Physical growth	• Slow and steady: weight gain 2–3 kg/year; height gain 5–7.5 cm/year • Face and body begin to elongate, longer limbs • Eruption of permanent teeth begins	• Cranium completed growth by now
Gross motor ability Fine motor skills	• Steadier on feet • Refining of coordination—begin to become more poised	• Gaining in stamina during exercise • Fundamental motor skills locomotion and dexterity fully developed by 7 years (climbing, jumping, hopping, skipping, throwing, catching)
Communication Language	• Continues to refine language skills and linguistic competence—longer words, larger vocabulary, more complex sentences, better grammar, grasps subtle grammar exceptions	• 23,000 words (8 years) • 75% grammar (potentially) correct • Speech becoming less egocentric
Cognition	• Developing concrete thinking; beginning to understand conservation (of amounts); understands rules and logical mathematical operations, e.g. reversibility of + and −; × and ÷ (*Note: needs written/pictorial explanations to achieve this*) • Beginning to understand others—what they are likely to do/think	
Social/emotional	• Gender aware • Can judge comparisons/differences between self and others • Developing close friendships—peer groups, best friend • Developing sense of productivity, worth, achievement, skill mastery and self-assurance	

Table A1.6   Milestones of Growth and Development: 11–18 years.[a] Adapted from Sheridan (1997)

Milestone	Girls	Boys
Physical growth	• Pubertal growth spurt 10–14 years (approx.) • Weight gain 7–25 kg (17 kg = mean) • Height gain 5–25 cm (20.5 cm = mean) • Dentition of 28 teeth complete—second molars erupt (12 years approx.) • Onset of menarche	• Pubertal growth spurt 11–16 years (approx.) • Weight gain 7–30 kg (23.7 kg = mean) • Height gain 10–30 cm (27.5 cm = mean) • Dentition of 28 teeth complete—second molars erupt (12 years approx.) • Capacity for nocturnal emissions
Gross motor ability	• Increasing endurance and strength	
Fine motor skills	• Increased neuronal processing allows for finer control	
Social/emotional	• Need to fit in with peer group • Experimentation • Turbulence • Preoccupied with body image • Can spend hours daydreaming (e.g. re: future) • Can be vain and self-centred	
Communication Language Cognition	• Sophisticated use of language • Developing abstract thinking and formal logical thinking (Piaget)	

[a]For further information on sexual maturation and Tanner's staging of puberty, see Chapter 12.

APPENDIX 2

Age-Appropriate Vital Signs and Blood Pressure

Breidge Boyle

Table A2.1 shows age-appropriate vital signs and blood pressure.

Table A2.1 Age-Appropriate Vital Signs and Blood Pressure. Adapted from the Resuscitation Department, Great Ormond Street Hospital for Children NHS Trust			
Age	Heart rate	Respiratory rate	Blood pressure
1 month	120–160	30–60	60–90/40–60
3 months	120–160	30–60	74–100/50–70
6 months	120–160	30–60	74–100/50–70
9 months	120–160	30–60	74–100/50–70
1 year	90–140	24–40	80–112/50–60
15 months	90–140	24–40	80–112/50–80
18 months	90–140	24–40	80–112/50–80
21 months	90–140	24–40	80–112/50–80
2 years	90–140	24–40	80–112/50–80
30 months	90–140	24–40	80–112/50–80
3 years	80–110	22–34	82–110/50–78
4 years	80–110	22–34	82–110/50–78
5 years	80–110	22–34	82–110/50–78
6 years	75–100	18–30	84–120/54–80
8 years	75–100	18–30	84–120/54–80
10 years	60–90	18–30	84–120/54–80
12 years	60–90	12–16	94–140/62–88
14 years	60–90	12–16	94–140/62–88
16 years	60–90	12–16	84–140/62–88

The author would like to acknowledge the contribution of Sheila Simpson, from the Resuscitation Department, Great Ormond Street Hospital NHS Trust in the preparation of this table.

Growth Charts

Growth charts (Figs A.3.1–A.3.14) are shown on the following pages.

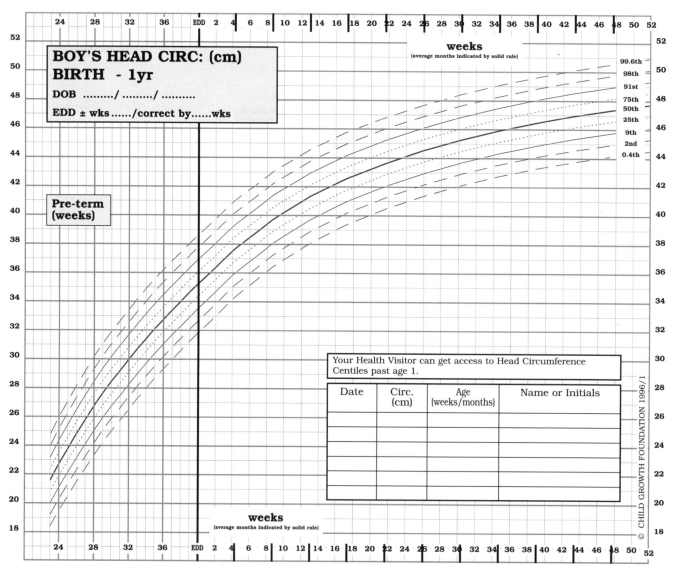

Figure A3.1 Growth chart for boy's head circumference (cm) for birth to 1 year. © Child Growth Foundation. Reproduced with permission. This chart may not be reproduced in any form whatsoever.

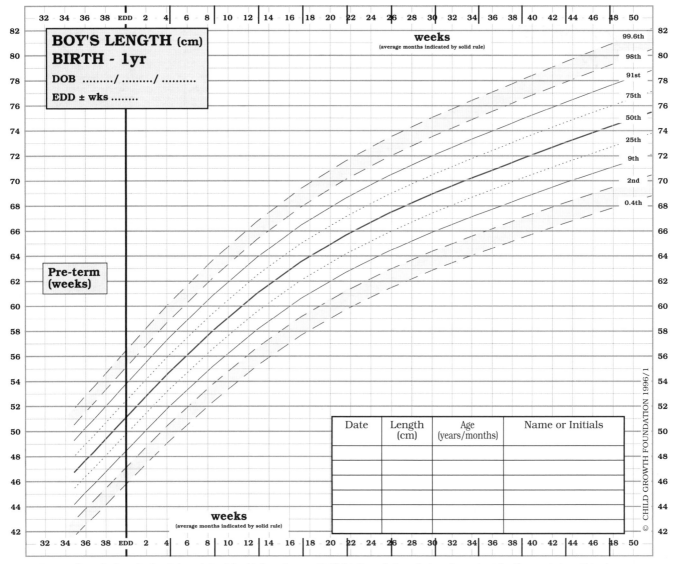

Figure A3.2 Growth chart for boy's length (cm) for birth to 1 year. © Child Growth Foundation. Reproduced with permission. This chart may not be reproduced in any form whatsoever.

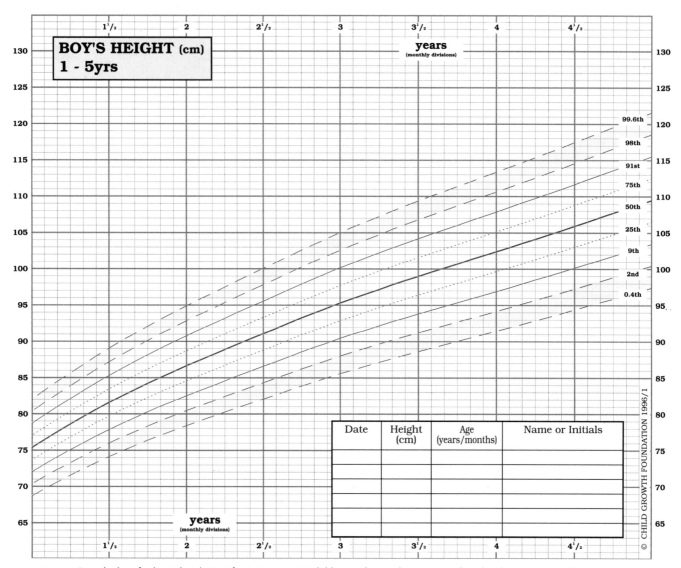

Figure A3.3 Growth chart for boy's height (cm) for 1–5 years. © Child Growth Foundation. Reproduced with permission. This chart may not be reproduced in any form whatsoever.

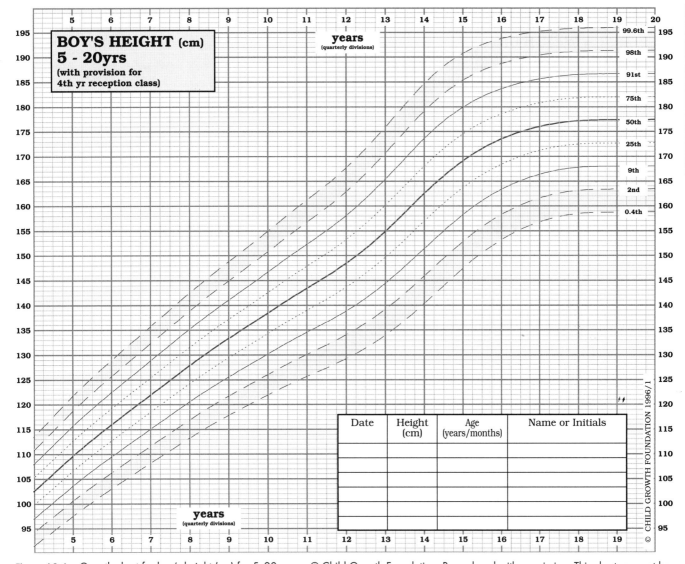

BOY'S HEIGHT (cm)
5 - 20yrs
(with provision for
4th yr reception class)

Date	Height (cm)	Age (years/months)	Name or Initials

© CHILD GROWTH FOUNDATION 1996/1

Figure A3.4 Growth chart for boy's height (cm) for 5–20 years. © Child Growth Foundation. Reproduced with permission. This chart may not be reproduced in any form whatsoever.

APPENDICES

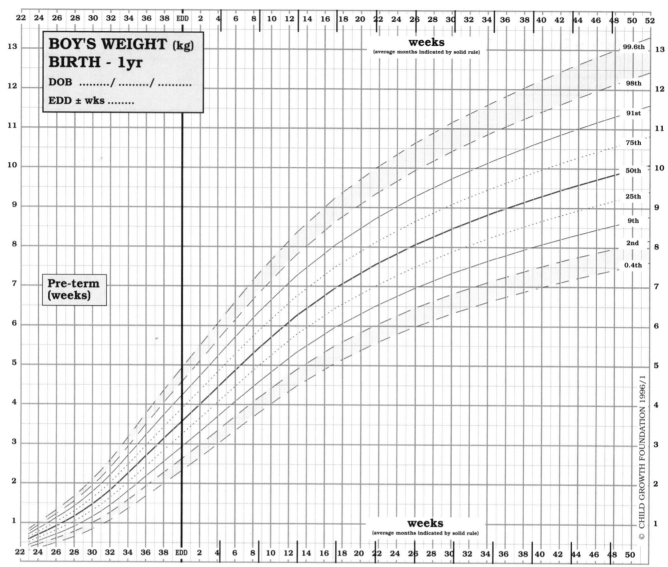

Figure A3.5 Growth chart for boy's weight (kg) for birth to 1 year. © Child Growth Foundation. Reproduced with permission. This chart may not be reproduced in any form whatsoever.

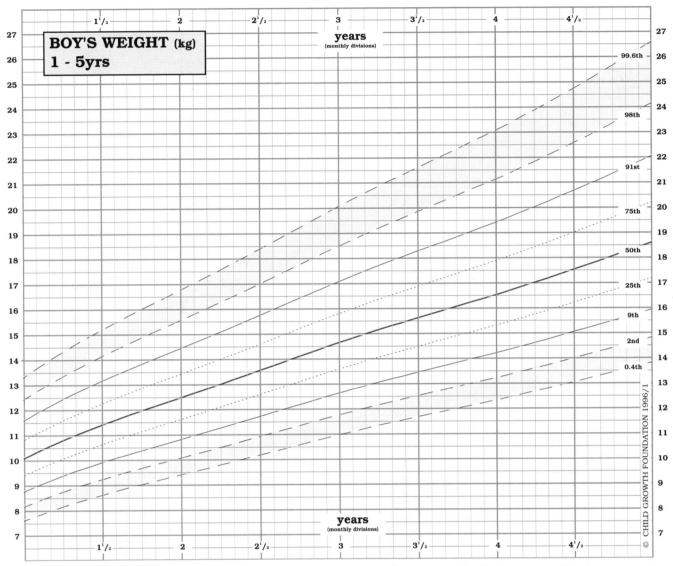

BOY'S WEIGHT (kg) 1 - 5yrs

years (monthly divisions)

99.6th
98th
91st
75th
50th
25th
9th
2nd
0.4th

© CHILD GROWTH FOUNDATION 1996/1

years (monthly divisions)

Figure A3.6 Growth chart for boy's weight (kg) for 1–5 years. © Child Growth Foundation. Reproduced with permission. This chart may not be reproduced in any form whatsoever.

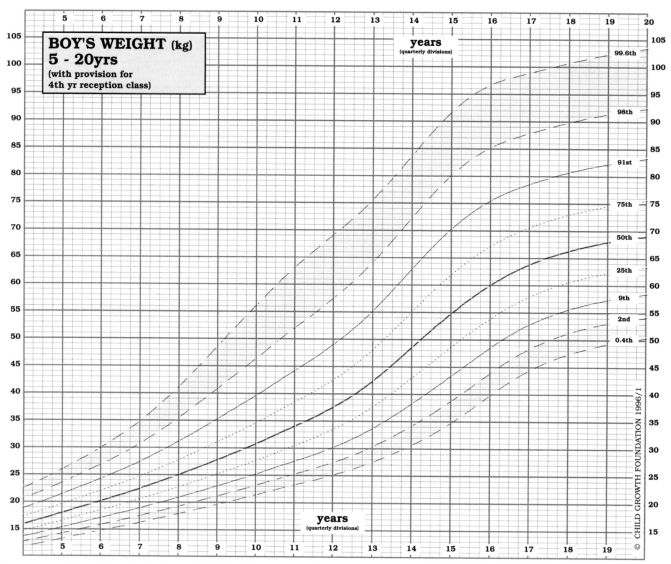

Figure A3.7 Growth chart for boy's weight (kg) for 5–20 years. © Child Growth Foundation. Reproduced with permission. This chart may not be reproduced in any form whatsoever.

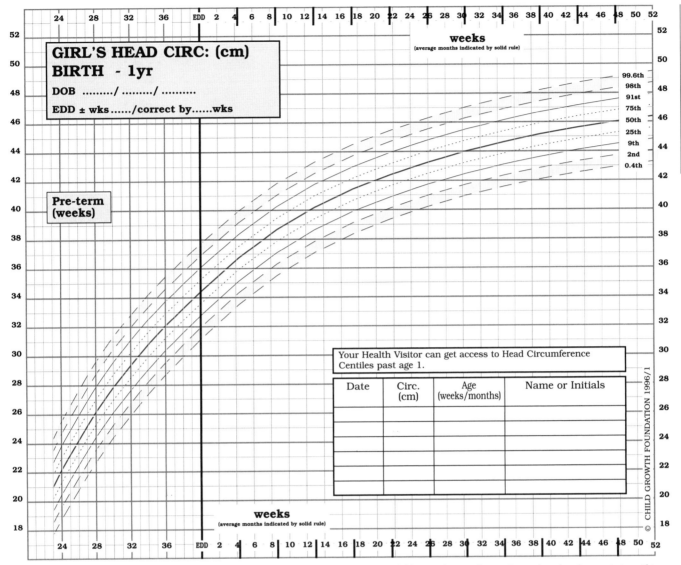

GIRL'S HEAD CIRC: (cm)
BIRTH - 1yr

DOB ..../ ..../ ....

EDD ± wks ....../correct by......wks

Pre-term (weeks)

weeks
(average months indicated by solid rule)

99.6th
98th
91st
75th
50th
25th
9th
2nd
0.4th

weeks
(average months indicated by solid rule)

Your Health Visitor can get access to Head Circumference Centiles past age 1.

Date	Circ. (cm)	Age (weeks/months)	Name or Initials

© CHILD GROWTH FOUNDATION 1996/1

Figure A3.8 Growth chart for girl's head circumference (cm) for birth to 1 year. © Child Growth Foundation. Reproduced with permission. This chart may not be reproduced in any form whatsoever.

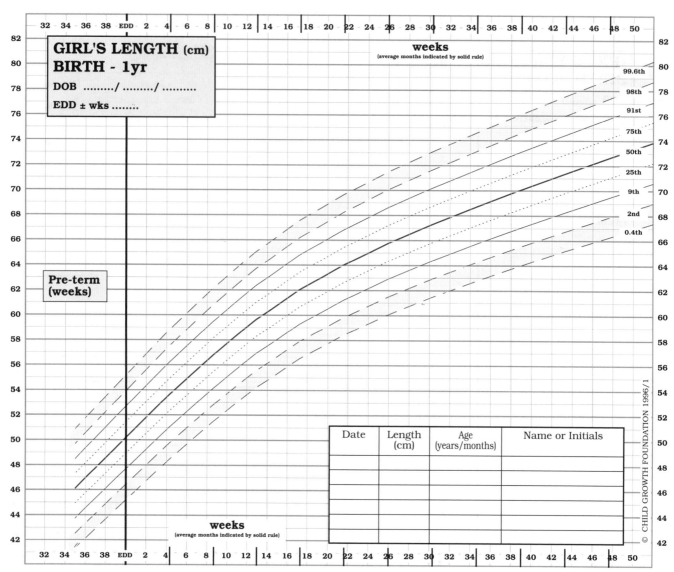

Figure A3.9   Growth chart for girl's length (cm) for birth to 1 year. © Child Growth Foundation. Reproduced with permission. This chart may not be reproduced in any form whatsoever.

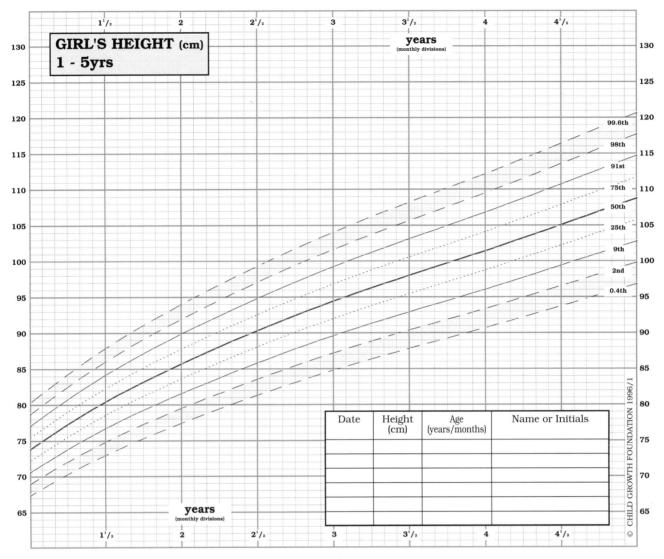

Figure A3.10 Growth chart for girl's height (cm) for 1–5 years. © Child Growth Foundation. Reproduced with permission. This chart may not be reproduced in any form whatsoever.

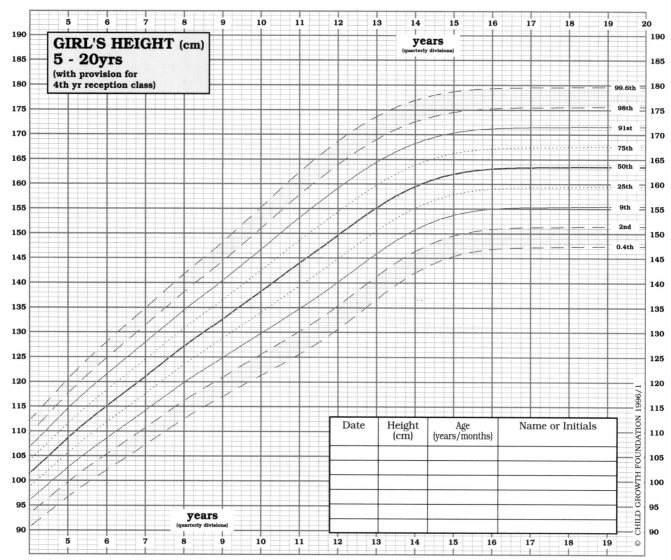

Figure A3.11   Growth chart for girl's height (cm) for 5–20 years. © Child Growth Foundation. Reproduced with permission. This chart may not be reproduced in any form whatsoever.

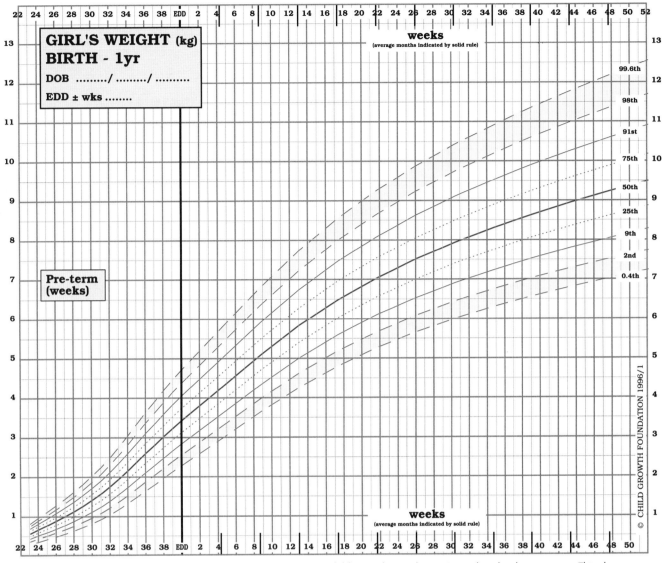

Figure A3.12   Growth chart for girl's weight (kg) for birth to 1 year. © Child Growth Foundation. Reproduced with permission. This chart may not be reproduced in any form whatsoever.

APPENDICES

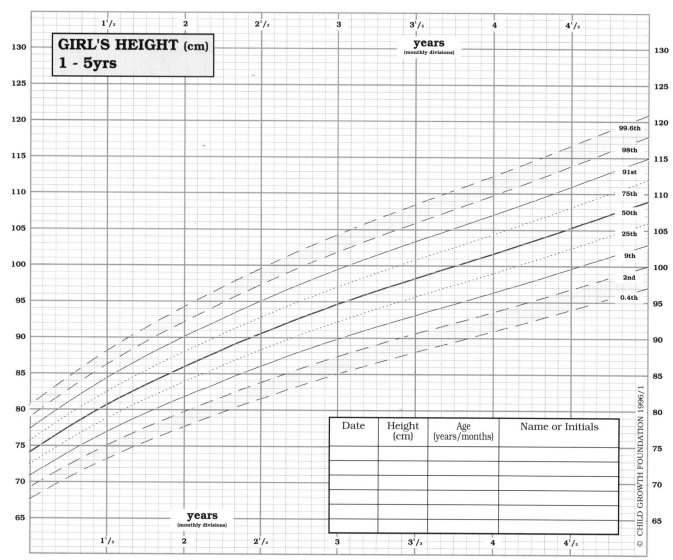

GIRL'S HEIGHT (cm) 1 - 5yrs

Figure A3.13 Growth chart for girl's weight (kg) for 1–5 years. © Child Growth Foundation. Reproduced with permission. This chart may not be reproduced in any form whatsoever.

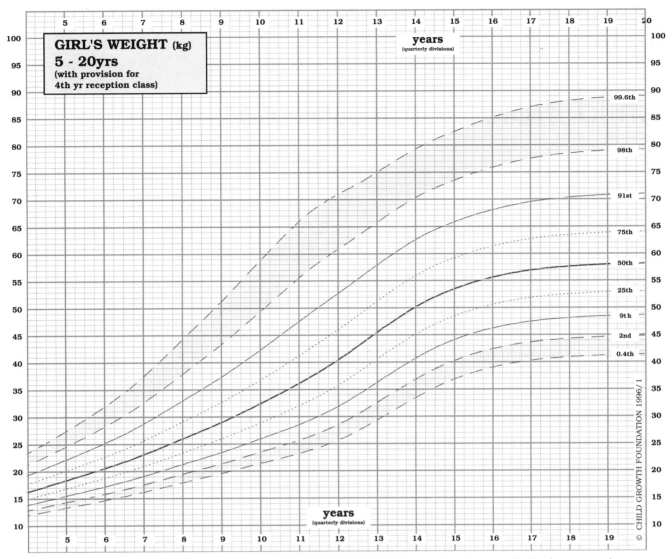

Figure A3.14   Growth chart for girl's weight (kg) for 5–20 years. © Child Growth Foundation. All rights reserved. This chart may not be reproduced in any form whatsoever.

APPENDIX 4

Child Protection Resources

Debbie Laws

An in-depth discussion of child protection issues is outside the scope of this text. However, the nurse practitioner (NP) who cares for children is professionally obligated to be knowledgeable and up-to-date in the area of child protection (i.e. theories, processes and resources in her practice setting). These may include the child protection nurse advisor, the Area Child Protection Committee and/or additional configurations of professionals dedicated to child protection. In addition, each practice setting should have in place a current child protection strategy that outlines specific contacts and procedures to be followed when a child protection concern arises. Lastly, it is important that the NP always maintains an index of suspicion with regard to child protection in order that an issue of child abuse or neglect is never overlooked.

▤ BIBLIOGRAPHY

Alderson P. Young children's rights. Exploring beliefs, principles and practice. London: Save the Children; 2000.

British Medical Association. Domestic violence: a health care issue? London: BMA; 1998.

Cawson P, Wattam C, Brooker S, et al. Child maltreatment in the United Kingdom: a study of the prevalence of child abuse and neglect. London: NSPCC; 2000.

Cleaver H, Freeman P. Parental perspectives in suspected cases of child abuse. London: HMSO; 1995.

Cleaver H, Wattam C, Gordon R. Assessing risk in child protection. London: NSPCC; 1998.

Cloke C, Naish J. Key issues in child protection for health visitors and nurses. London: NSPCC & HVA; 1994.

Corby B. Child abuse: towards a knowledge base. Buckingham: Open University Press; 1993.

Cunningham C. Realising children's rights: policy, practice and Save the Children's work in England. London: Save the Children; 1999.

Department of Health. Child protection: messages from research. London; HMSO; 1995.

Department of Health. Working together to safeguard children: a guide to inter-agency working to safeguard and promote the welfare of children. London: HMSO; 1999.

Farmer E, Owen M. Child protection practice: private risks and public remedies. London: HMSO; 1995.

Health Visitors Association. Protecting the child. London: Health Visitors Association; 1994.

Howitt D. Child abuse errors: when good intentions go wrong. London: Havester Wheatsheaf Press; 1992.

Jones DPH, Ramchandani P. Child sexual abuse. Informing practice from research. Abington: Radcliffe Medical Press; 1999.

Kemshall H. Risk assessment and risk management. London: Jessica Kingsley; 1997.

Marchant R, Page M. Bridging the gap: child protection and children with disabilities: London: NSPCC; 1993.

Meadows R. The ABC of child abuse. London: BMA; 1992.

National Commission of Inquiry. Childhood matters. London: HMSO; 1997.

Newell P. Taking children seriously: a proposal for a children's rights commissioner, revised edn. London: Calouste Gulbenkian Foundation; 2000.

O'Hagan K. Emotional and psychological abuse. Buckingham: Open University Press; 1993.

Parton N. The politics of child abuse. Houndswood: Macmillan; 1991.

Parton N, Wattam C. Child sexual abuse: responding to the experiences of children. Chichester: Wiley; 1999.

Platt D, Shemmings D. Making enquiries into alleged child abuse and neglect: partnership with families. London: Wiley; 1996.

Reder P. Beyond blame: child abuse tragedies revisited. London: Routledge; 1993.

Royal College of Nursing. Domestic violence: guidance for nurses. London: RCN; 2000.

Save the Children Alliance. Children's rights: reality or rhetoric? The UN convention on the rights of the child, the first ten years. London: Save the Children; 2000.

Stevenson O. Neglected children: issues and dilemmas (working together for children, young people and their families series). Oxford: Blackwell Science; 1998.

The Violence Against Children Study Group. Children, child abuse and child protection: placing children centrally. Chichester: Wiley; 1999.

Thorbur J, Lewis A, Shemmings D. Partnership or paternalism? Family involvement in child protection. London: HMSO; 1996.

Thorpe D. Evaluating child protection. Buckingham; Open University Press; 1993.

Wilson K, James A. The child protection handbook. London: BallièreTindall; 1995.

Wolfe D. Preventing physical and emotional abuse of children. New York: Guildford Press; 1991.

Inquiry Reports

The Bridge Child Care Consultancy. Paul: death through neglect. Marlborough: Chapman & Chapman; 1995.

Waterhouse R, Clough M, Fleming M. Lost in care: report of the tribunal of inquiry into child abuse in North Wales (The Waterhouse Report). London: The Stationery Office; 2000.

Williamson E. Domestic violence and health: the response of the medical profession. Bristol: The Policy Press; 2000.

National Contacts/Sources of Information and Advice

Community Practitioner and Health Visitor
Association (CPHVA).
National Society for the Prevention of Cruelty
to Children (NSPCC).
Royal College of Nursing (RCN).

Local Contacts

Area Child Protection Committee
(see website address below).
Constabulary: Child Protection Team.
NSPCC (see website address below).

Nurse Advisor for Hospital/Unit/
Community for Child Protection.

Website Addresses

www.nspcc.org.uk
National Society for the Prevention of Cruelty
to Children.

www.childline.org.uk
National website for Childline: many links to
other useful sites and information.

www.yesican.org
International Child Abuse Network: mission
statement is 'Working world-wide to break
the cycle of child abuse'.

www.doh.gov.uk/acpc
National website for Area Child Protection
Committees: many links to other useful
sites and information.

www.unicef.org/crc/crc
National website for UNICEF—many links
to other useful sites and information,
including the Children's Parliament, which
is one of the emerging forums which gives
children the opportunity to voice their
opinions and concerns.

APPENDICES

Index

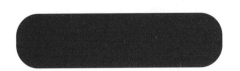